Pass the HESI A2!

A complete Study Guide and Practice Test Questions

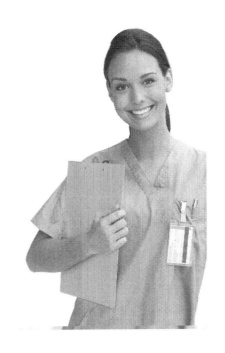

Complete Test Preparation

Test Preparation Publishing
Victoria BC Canada

We strongly recommend that students check with exam providers for up-to-date information regarding test content.

Please note that HESI is a registered trademark of the Health Education Systems Inc., which was not involved in the production of, and does not endorse, this product.

ISBN-13: 978-1478296966
ISBN-10: 1478296968

About Complete Test Preparation

The Complete Test Preparation Team has been publishing high quality study materials since 2005. Millions of students visit our websites every year, and thousands of students, teachers and parents all over the world have purchased our teaching materials, curriculum, study guides and practice tests.

Complete Test Preparation is committed to providing students with the best study materials and practice tests available on the market. Members of our team combine years of teaching experience, with experienced writers and editors, all with advanced degrees.

Team Members for this publication

Editor: Brian Stocker MA
Contributor: Dr. C. Gregory
Contributor: Dr. G. A. Stocker DDS
Contributor: D. A. Stocker M. Ed.
Contributor: Dr. N. Wyatt

Published by
Complete Test Preparation
921 Foul Bay Rd.
Victoria BC Canada V8S 4H9
Visit us on the web at http://www.test-preparation.ca
Printed in the USA

Contact us at feedback@test-preparation.ca

Contents

Getting Started

CONGRATULATIONS! By deciding to take the Health Education Systems (HESI A2) Exam, you have taken the first step toward a great future! Of course, there is no point in taking this important examination unless you intend to do your very best in order to earn the highest grade you possibly can. That means getting yourself organized and discovering the best approaches, methods and strategies to master the material. Yes, that will require real effort and dedication on your part but if you are willing to focus your energy and devote the study time necessary, before you know it you will be opening that letter of acceptance to the school of your dreams.

We know that taking on a new endeavour can be a little scary, and it is easy to feel unsure of where to begin. That's where we come in. This study guide is designed to help you improve your test-taking skills, show you a few tricks of the trade and increase both your competency and confidence.

The Health Education Systems A2 Exam

The HESI A2 exam is composed of modules and not all schools use all of the modules. It is therefore very important that you find out what modules your school will use! That way you won't waste valuable study time learning something that isn't on your exam!

The HESI A2 Modules are: Math, Vocabulary, Reading Comprehension, Biology, Chemistry, Physics, Basic Scientific principals and Anatomy and Physiology.

You don`t have to worry because these sections are included in this study guide. However, to maximize your study time, it is very important to check which modules your university offers before studying everything under the sun!

While we seek to make our guide as comprehensive as possible, it is important to note that like all entrance exams, the HESI A2 Exam might be adjusted at some future point. New material might be added, or content that is no longer relevant or applicable might be removed. It is always a good idea to give the materials you receive when you register to take the HESI a careful review.

How this study guide is organized

This study guide is divided into four sections. The first section, Self-Assessments, which will help you recognize your areas of strength and weaknesses. This will be a boon when it comes to managing your study time most efficiently; there is not much point of focusing on material you have already got firmly under control. Instead, taking the self-assessments will show you where that time could be much better spent. In this area you will begin with a few questions to quickly evaluate your understanding of material that is likely to appear on the HESI. If you do poorly in certain areas, simply work carefully through those sections in the tutorials and then try the self-assessment again.

The second section, Tutorials, offers information in each of the content areas, as well as strategies to help you master that material. The tutorials are not intended to be a complete course, but cover general principals. If you find that you do not understand the tutorials, it is recommended that you seek out additional instruction. Most Universities recommend student take introductory courses in Math, English and Science before taking the HESI.

Third, we offer two sets of practice test questions, similar to those on the HESI A2 Exam. Again, we cover all modules, so make sure to check with your school!

In addition to all these materials, the last three chapters give you important information on how to answer multiple choice questions, how to prepare for a test, and how to take a test.

The HESI Study Plan

Now that you have made the decision to take the HESI, it is time to get started. Before you do another thing, you will need to figure out a plan of attack. The very best study tip is to start early! The longer the time period you devote to regular study practice, the more likely you will be to retain the material and be able to access it quickly. If you thought that 1x20 is the same as 2x10, guess what? It really is not, when it comes to study time. Reviewing material for just an hour per day over the course of 20 days is far better than studying for two hours a day for only 10 days. The more often you revisit a particular piece of information, the better you will know it. Not only will your grasp and understanding be better, but your ability to reach into your brain and quickly and efficiently pull out the tidbit you need, will be greatly enhanced as well.

The great Chinese scholar and philosopher Confucius believed that true knowledge could be defined as knowing both what you know and what you do not know. The first step in preparing for the HESI Exam is to assess your strengths and weaknesses. You may already have an idea of what you know and what you do not know, but evaluating yourself using our Self- Assessment modules for each of the three areas, Math, English and Reading Comprehension, will clarify the details.

Making a Study Schedule

In order to make your study time most productive you will need to develop a study plan. The purpose of the plan is to organize all the bits of pieces of information in such a way that you will not feel overwhelmed. Rome was not built in a day, and learning everything you will need to know in order to pass the HESI Exam is going to take time, too. Arranging the material you need to learn into manageable chunks is the best way to go. Each study session should make you feel as though you have succeeded in accomplishing your goal, and your goal is simply to learn what you planned to learn during that particular session. Try to organize the content in such a way that each study session builds upon previous ones. That way, you will retain the information, be better able to access it, and review the previous bits and pieces at the same time.

Self-assessment

The Best Study Tip! The very best study tip is to start early! The longer you study regularly, the more you will retain and 'learn' the material. Studying for 1 hour per day for 20 days is far better than studying for 2 hours for 10 days.

What don't you know?

The first step is to assess your strengths and weaknesses. You may already have an idea of where your weaknesses are, or you can take our Self-assessment modules for each of the areas, Math, English, Science and Reading Comprehension.

Exam Component	Rate from 1 to 5
Reading Comprehension	
Paragraph & Passage Comprehension	
Drawing inferences & conclusions	
English Grammar	
Vocabulary	
Math	
Fractions	
Decimals	
Percent	
Science	
Anatomy and Physiology	
Biology	
Chemistry	

 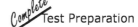

Making a Study Schedule

The key to making a study plan is to divide the material you need to learn into manage-able size and learn it, while at the same time reviewing the material that you already know.

Using the table above, any scores of 3 or below, you need to spend time learning, going over and practicing this subject area. A score of 4 means you need to review the material, but you don't have to spend time re-learning. A score of 5 and you are OK with just an occasional review before the exam.

A score of 0 or 1 means you really need to work on this area and should allocate the most time and the highest priority. Some students prefer a 5-day plan and others a 10-day plan. It also depends on how much time you have until the exam.

Here is an example of a 5-day plan based on an example from the table above:

Fractions: 1 Study 1 hour everyday – review on last day
Biology: 3 Study 1 hour for 2 days then ½ hour a day, then review
Vocabulary: 4 Review every second day
Word Problems: 2 Study 1 hour on the first day – then ½ hour everyday
Reading Comprehension: 5 Review for ½ hour every other day
Algebra: 5 Review for ½ hour every other day
Chemistry: 5 very confident – review a few times.

Using this example, Chemistry and Grammar are good and only need occasional review. Biology is also good and needs 'some' review. Decimals need a bit of work, Word Problems need a lot of work and Fractions are very weak and need the majority of time. Based on this, here is a sample study plan:

Day	Subject	Time
Monday		
Study	Fractions	1 hour
Study	Word Problems	1 hour
½ **hour break**		
Study	Biology	1 hour
Review	Chemistry	½ hour
Tuesday		
Study	Fractions	1 hour
Study	Word Problems	½ hour
½ **hour break**		
Study	Decimals	½ hour
Review	Vocabulary	½ hour
Review	Grammar	½ hour
Wednesday		
Study	Fractions	1 hour
Study	Word Problems	½ hour
½ **hour break**		
Study	Biology	½ hour
Review	Chemistry	½ hour
Thursday		
Study	Fractions	½ hour
Study	Word Problems	½ hour
Review	Biology	½ hour
½ **hour break**		
Review	Grammar	½ hour
Review	Vocabulary	½ hour
Friday		
Review	Fractions	½ hour
Review	Word Problems	½ hour
Review	Biology	½ hour
½ **hour break**		
Review	Vocabulary	½ hour
Review	Grammar	½ hour

Reading Comprehension Self-Assessment

THIS SECTION CONTAINS A SELF-ASSESSMENT AND READING COMPREHENSION TUTORIALS. The Tutorials are designed to familiarize general principals and the Self-Assessment contains general questions similar to the questions likely to be on the HESI exam, but are not intended to be identical to the exam questions. Many Universities recommend that students take an introductory courses before taking the HESI Exam. The tutorials are not designed to be a complete course, and it is assumed that students have some familiarity with reading comprehension. If you do not understand parts of the tutorial, or find the tutorial difficult, it is recommended that you seek out additional instruction.

The purpose of the self-assessment is:

- Identify your strengths and weaknesses.

- Develop your personalized study plan (above)

- Get accustomed to the HESI format

- Extra practice – the self-assessments are almost a full 3rd practice test!

Since this is a Self-assessment, and depending on how confident you are with Reading Comprehension, timing is optional. The HESI has 47 reading comprehension questions, to be answered in 60 minutes. Note that some schools do not have a time limit. The self-assessment has 10 questions, so allow about 13 minutes to complete this assessment.

The questions below are not exactly the same as you will find on the HESI - that would be too easy! And nobody knows what the questions will be and they change all the time. Below are general Reading Comprehension questions that cover the same areas as the HESI. So while the format and exact wording of the questions may differ slightly, and change from year to year, if you can answer the questions below, you will have no problem with the Reading Comprehension section of the HESI.

The self-assessment is designed to give you a baseline score in the different areas covered. Here is a brief outline of how your score on the self-assessment relates to your understanding of the material.

75% - 100%	Excellent – you have mastered the content
50 – 75%	Good. You have a working knowledge. Even though you can just pass this section, you may want to review the Tutorials and do some extra practice to see if you can improve your mark.
25% - 50%	Below Average. You do not understand the reading comprehension problems. Review the tutorials, and retake this quiz again in a few days, before proceeding to the rest of the Practice Test.
Less than 25%	Poor. You have a very limited understanding of the reading comprehension problems. Please review the Tutorials, and retake this quiz again in a few days, before proceeding to the rest of the study guide.

After taking the Self-Assessment, use the table above to assess your understanding. If you scored low, read through the Tutorial, Help with Reading Comprehension, and if you need more practice, see Chapter 8 Multiple Choice Secrets for more practice and strategy answering reading comprehension multiple choice.

 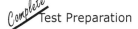

Reading Comprehension Self-Assessment Answer Sheet

1. (A) (B) (C) (D)

2. (A) (B) (C) (D)

3. (A) (B) (C) (D)

4. (A) (B) (C) (D)

5. (A) (B) (C) (D)

6. (A) (B) (C) (D)

7. (A) (B) (C) (D)

8. (A) (B) (C) (D)

9. (A) (B) (C) (D)

10. (A) (B) (C) (D)

Directions: The following questions are based on a number of reading passages. Each passage is followed by a series of questions. Read each passage carefully, and then answer the questions based on it. You may reread the passage as often as you wish. When you have finished answering the questions based on one passage, go right on to the next passage. Choose the best answer based on the information given and implied.

Questions 1 – 4 refer to the following passage.

Passage 1 - The Immune System

An immune system is a system of biological structures and processes that protects against disease by identifying and killing pathogens and other threats. The immune system can detect a wide variety of agents, from viruses to parasitic worms, and distinguish them from the organism's own healthy cells and tissues. Detection is complicated as pathogens evolve rapidly to avoid the immune system defences, and successfully infect their hosts.

The human immune system consists of many types of proteins, cells, organs, and tissues, which interact in an elaborate and dynamic network. As part of this more complex immune response, the human immune system adapts over time to recognize specific pathogens more efficiently. This adaptation process is referred to as "adaptive immunity" or "acquired immunity" and creates immunological memory. Immunological memory created from a primary response to a specific pathogen, provides an enhanced response to future encounters with that same pathogen. This process of acquired immunity is the basis of vaccination. [1]

1. What can we infer from the first paragraph in this passage?

    a. When a person's body fights off the flu, this is the immune system in action

    b. When a person's immune system functions correctly, they avoid all sicknesses and injuries

    c. When a person's immune system is weak, a person will likely get a terminal disease

    d. When a person's body fights off a cold, this is the circulatory system in action

2. The immune system's primary function is to:

    a. Strengthen the bones

    b. Protect against disease

    c. Improve respiration

    d. Improve circulation

 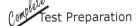

3. Based on the passage, what can we say about evolution's role in the immune system?

    a. Evolution of the immune system is an important factor in the immune system's efficiency

    b. Evolution causes a person to die, thus killing the pathogen

    c. Evolution plays no known role in immunity

    d. The least evolved earth species have better immunity

4. Acquired immunity is another term for what?

    a. White blood cells

    b. AIDS

    c. Adaptive immunity

    d. Disease

Questions 5 – 8 refer to the following passage.

Passage 2 - White Blood Cells

White blood cells (WBCs), or leukocytes (also spelled "leucocytes"), are cells of the immune system that defend the body against both infectious disease and foreign material. Five different and diverse types of leukocytes exist, but they are all produced and derived from a powerful cell in the bone marrow known as a hematopoietic stem cell. Leukocytes are found throughout the body, including the blood and lymphatic system.

The number of WBCs in the blood is often an indicator of disease. There are normally between 4×10^9 and 1.1×10^{10} white blood cells in a liter of blood, making up approximately 1% of blood in a healthy adult. The physical properties of white blood cells, such as volume, conductivity, and granularity, changes due to the presence of immature cells, or malignant cells.

The name white blood cell derives from the fact that after processing a blood sample in a centrifuge, the white cells are typically a thin, white layer of nucleated cells. The scientific term leukocyte directly reflects this description, derived from Greek leukos (white), and kytos (cell). [2]

5. What can we infer from the first paragraph in this selection?

    a. Red blood cells are not as important as white blood cells

    b. White blood cells are the culprits in most infectious diseases

    c. White blood cells are essential to fight off infectious diseases

    d. Red blood cells are essential to fight off infectious diseases

6. What can we say about the number of white blood cells in a liter of blood?

   a. They make up about 1% of a healthy adult's blood

   b. There are 10^{10} WBCs in a healthy adult's blood

   c. The number varies according to age

   d. They are a thin white layer of nucleated cells

7. What is a more scientific term for "white blood cell"?

   a. Red blood cell

   b. Anthrocyte

   c. Leukocyte

   d. Leukemia

8. Can the number of leukocytes indicate cancer?

   a. Yes, the white blood cell count can indicate disease.

   b. No, the white blood cell count is not a reliable indicator.

   c. Yes, disease can indicate a high white cell count.

   d. None of the choices are correct.

Questions 9 - 10 refer to the following passage.

Thunderstorms I

Warm air is less dense than cool air, so warm air rises within cooler air like a hot air balloon or warm water in an ocean current. Clouds form as warm air carrying moisture rises. As the warm air rises, it cools, and the moist water vapor begins to condense. This releases energy that keeps the air warmer than its surroundings, and as a result, continues to rise. If enough instability is present in the atmosphere, this process will continue long enough for cumulonimbus clouds to form, which support lightning and thunder. All thunderstorms, regardless of type, go through three stages: the cumulus stage, the mature stage, and the dissipation stage. Depending on the conditions in the atmosphere, these three stages can take anywhere from 20 minutes to several hours. [3]

9. This passage tells us

   a. Warm air is denser than cool air

   b. All thunderstorms go through three stages

   c. Thunderstorms may occur without clouds present

   d. The stages of a thunderstorm conclude within just a few minutes

10. When warm air rises through colder air, it results in

    a. Evaporation

    b. Humidity

    c. Clear skies

    d. Condensation

Reading Comprehension Self-Assessment Answer Key

1. A

The passage does not mention the flu specifically, however we know the flu is a pathogen (A bacterium, virus, or other microorganism that can cause disease). Therefore, we can infer, when a person's body fights off the flu, this is the immune system in action.

2. B

The immune system's primary function is to protect against disease.

3. A

The passage refers to evolution of the immune system being important for efficiency. In paragraph three, there is a discussion of adaptive and acquired immunity, where the immune system "remembers" pathogens.
We can conclude, evolution of the immune system is an important factor in the immune system's efficiency.

4. C

This is taken directly from the passage. Acquired immunity is another term for adaptive immunity.

5. C

We can infer white blood cells are essential to fight off infectious diseases, from the passage, "cells of the immune system that defend the body against both infectious disease and foreign material."

6. A

We can say the number of white blood cells in a liter of blood make up about 1% of a healthy adult's blood. This is a fact-based question that is easy and fast to answer. The question asks about a percentage. You can quickly and easily scan to passage for the percent sign, or the word percent and find the answer.

7. C

A more scientific term for "white blood cell" is leukocyte, from the first paragraph, first sentence of the passage.

8. A

The white blood cell count can indicate disease (cancer). We know this from the last sentence of paragraph two, "The physical properties of white blood cells, such as volume, conductivity, and granularity, changes due to the presence of immature cells, or malignant cells."

9. B

All thunderstorms will go through three stages. This is taken directly from the text, "All thunderstorms, regardless of type, go through three stages: the cumulus stage, the mature stage, and the dissipation stage."

10. D

Condensation. From the passage, "As the warm air rises, it cools, and the moist water vapor begins to condense."

Help with Reading Comprehension

At first sight, reading comprehension tests look challenging especially if you are given long essays to answer only two to three questions. While reading, you might notice your attention waning, or feeling sleepy. Do not be discouraged because there are various tactics and long range strategies that make comprehending even long, boring essays easier.

Your friends before your foes. It is always best to tackle essays or passages with familiar subjects rather than those with unfamiliar ones. This approach applies the same logic as tackling easy questions before hard ones. Skip passages that do not interest you and leave them for later when there is more time left.

Don't use 'special' reading techniques. This is not the time for speed-reading or anything like that – just plain ordinary reading – not too slow and not too fast.

Read through the entire passage and the questions before you do anything. Many students try reading the questions first and then looking for answers in the passage thinking this approach is more efficient. What these students do not realize is that it is often hard to navigate in unfamiliar roads. If you do not familiarize yourself with the passage first, looking for answers become not only time-consuming but also dangerous because you might miss the context of the answer you are looking for. If you read the questions first you will only confuse yourself and lose valuable time.

Familiarize yourself with reading comprehension questions. If you are familiar with the common types of reading comprehension questions, you are able to take note of important parts of the passage, saving time. There are six major kinds of reading comprehension questions.

- **Main Idea**- Questions that ask for the central thought or significance of the passage.

- **Specific Details** - Questions that asks for explicitly stated ideas.

- **Drawing Inferences** - Questions that ask for a statement's intended meaning.

- **Tone or Attitude** - Questions that test your ability to sense the emotional state of the author.

- **Context Meaning** – Questions that ask for the meaning of a word depending on the context.

- **Technique** – Questions that ask for the method of organization or the writing style of the author.

Read. Read. Read. The best preparation for reading comprehension tests is always to read, read and read. If you are not used to reading lengthy passages, you will probably lose concentration. Increase your attention span by making a habit out of reading.

Reading Comprehension tests become less daunting when you have trained yourself to read and understand fast. Always remember that it is easier to understand passages you are interested in. Do not read through passages hastily. Make mental notes of ideas that you think might be asked.

Reading Comprehension Strategy

When facing the reading comprehension section of a standardized test, you need a strategy to be successful. You want to keep several steps in mind:

• First, make a note of the time and the number of sections. Time your work accordingly. Typically, four to five minutes per section is sufficient. Second, read the directions for each selection thoroughly before beginning (and listen well to any additional verbal instructions, as they will often clarify obscure or confusing written guidelines). You must know exactly how to do what you're about to do!

• Now you're ready to begin reading the selection. Read the passage carefully, noting significant characters or events on a scratch sheet of paper or underlining on the test sheet. Many students find making a basic list in the margins helpful. Quickly jot down or underline one-word summaries of characters, notable happenings, numbers, or key ideas. This will help you better retain information and focus wandering thoughts. Remember, however, that your main goal in doing this is to find the information that answers the questions. Even if you find the passage interesting, remember your goal and work fast but stay on track.

• Now read the question and all of the choices. Now you have read the passage, have a general idea of the main ideas, and have marked the important points. Read the question and all of the choices. Never choose an answer without reading them all! Questions are often designed to confuse – stay focussed and clear. Usually the answer choices will focus on one or two facts or inferences from the passage. Keep these clear in your mind.

• Search for the answer. With a very general idea of what the different choices are, go back to the passage and scan for the relevant information. Watch for big words, unusual or unique words. These make your job easier as you can scan the text for the particular word.

• Mark the Answer. Now you have the key information the question is looking for. Go back to the question, quickly scan the choices and mark the correct one.

Understand and practice the different types of standardized reading comprehension

 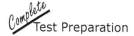

tests. See the list above for the different types. Typically, there will be several questions dealing with facts from the selection, a couple more inference questions dealing with logical consequences of those facts, and periodically an application-oriented question surfaces to force you to make connections with what you already know. Some students prefer to answer the questions as listed, and feel classifying the question and then ordering is wasting precious time. Other students prefer to answer the different types of questions in order of how easy or difficult they are. The choice is yours and do whatever works for you. If you want to try answering in order of difficulty, here is a recommended order, answer fact questions first; they're easily found within the passage. Tackle inference problems next, after re-reading the question(s) as many times as you need to. Application or 'best guess' questions usually take the longest, so save them for last.

Use the practice tests to try out both ways of answering and see what works for you.

For more help with reading comprehension, see Multiple Choice Secrets.

Mathematics Self-Assessment and Tutorials

THIS SECTION CONTAINS A SELF-ASSESSMENT AND MATH TUTORIALS. The Tutorials are designed to familiarize general principals and the Self-Assessment contains general questions similar to the math questions likely to be on the HESI exam, but are not intended to be identical to the exam questions. Many Universities recommend that students take an introductory math course before taking the HESI Exam. The tutorials are not designed to be a complete math course, and it is assumed that students have some familiarity with math. If you do not understand parts of the tutorial, or find the tutorial difficult, it is recommended that you seek out additional instruction.

Mathematics Self-assessment

Below is a Mathematics Self-assessment. The purpose of the self-assessment is:

- Identify your strengths and weaknesses.

- Develop your personalized study plan (above)

- Get accustomed to the HESI format

- Extra practice – the self-assessments are almost a full 3rd practice test!

Since this is a Self-assessment, and depending on how confident you are with Math, timing yourself is optional. The HESI includes a comprehensive Math Exam that covers decimals, whole numbers, fractions, number system conversions, percentages and basic algebra. There is generally a section where you are asked to solve medical related word problems, such as calculating dosages. There are a total of 50 questions, which must be answered in 50 minutes. The self-assessment has 50 questions, so allow 50 minutes to complete this assessment.

The questions below are not exactly the same as you will find on the HESI - that would be too easy! And nobody knows what the questions will be and they change all the time. Below are general Math questions that cover the same areas as the HESI. So while the format and exact wording of the questions may differ slightly, and change from year to year, if you can answer the questions below, you will have no problem with the Math section of the HESI.

The self-assessment is designed to give you a baseline score in the different areas covered. Here is a brief outline of how your score on the self-assessment relates to your understanding of the material.

75% - 100%	Excellent – you have mastered the content
50 – 75%	Good. You have a working knowledge. Even though you can just pass this section, you may want to review the tutorials and do some extra practice to see if you can improve your mark.
25% - 50%	Below Average. You do not understand the content. Review the tutorials, and retake this quiz again in a few days, before proceeding to the rest of the Practice Test Course.
Less than 25%	Poor. You have a very limited understanding. Please review the Tutorials, and retake this quiz again in a few days, before proceeding to the rest of the course.

Math Self-Assessment Answer Sheet

1. (A) (B) (C) (D)
2. (A) (B) (C) (D)
3. (A) (B) (C) (D)
4. (A) (B) (C) (D)
5. (A) (B) (C) (D)
6. (A) (B) (C) (D)
7. (A) (B) (C) (D)
8. (A) (B) (C) (D)
9. (A) (B) (C) (D)
10. (A) (B) (C) (D)
11. (A) (B) (C) (D)
12. (A) (B) (C) (D)
13. (A) (B) (C) (D)
14. (A) (B) (C) (D)
15. (A) (B) (C) (D)
16. (A) (B) (C) (D)
17. (A) (B) (C) (D)

18. (A) (B) (C) (D)
19. (A) (B) (C) (D)
20. (A) (B) (C) (D)
21. (A) (B) (C) (D)
22. (A) (B) (C) (D)
23. (A) (B) (C) (D)
24. (A) (B) (C) (D)
25. (A) (B) (C) (D)
26. (A) (B) (C) (D)
27. (A) (B) (C) (D)
28. (A) (B) (C) (D)
29. (A) (B) (C) (D)
30. (A) (B) (C) (D)
31. (A) (B) (C) (D)
32. (A) (B) (C) (D)
33. (A) (B) (C) (D)
34. (A) (B) (C) (D)

35. (A) (B) (C) (D)
36. (A) (B) (C) (D)
37. (A) (B) (C) (D)
38. (A) (B) (C) (D)
39. (A) (B) (C) (D)
40. (A) (B) (C) (D)
41. (A) (B) (C) (D)
42. (A) (B) (C) (D)
43. (A) (B) (C) (D)
44. (A) (B) (C) (D)
45. (A) (B) (C) (D)
46. (A) (B) (C) (D)
47. (A) (B) (C) (D)
48. (A) (B) (C) (D)
49. (A) (B) (C) (D)
50. (A) (B) (C) (D)

Complete Test Preparation

Basic Math

1. 389 + 454 =

    a. 853

    b. 833

    c. 843

    d. 863

2. 9,177 + 7,204 =

    a. 16,4712

    b. 16,371

    c. 16,381

    d. 15,412

3. 2,199 + 5,832 =

    a. 8,331

    b. 8,041

    c. 8,141

    d. 8,031

4. 8,390 - 5,239 =

    a. 3,261

    b. 3,151

    c. 3,161

    d. 3,101

5. 643 - 587 =

    a. 56

    b. 66

    c. 46

    d. 55

6. 3,406 - 2,767 =

    a. 629

    b. 720

    c. 639

    d. 649

7. 149 × 7 =

    a. 1032

    b. 1043

    c. 1059

    d. 1063

8. 467 × 41 =

    a. 19,147

    b. 21,227

    c. 23,107

    d. 18,177

9. 309 × 17 =

    a. 5,303

    b. 4,913

    c. 4,773

    d. 5,253

10. 491 ÷ 9 =

    a. 54 r5

    b. 56 r6

    c. 57 r5

    d. 51 r

Decimals, Fractions and Percent

11. 15 is what percent of 200?

     a. 7.5%

     b. 15%

     c. 20%

     d. 17.50%

12. A boy has 5 red balls, 3 white balls and 2 yellow balls. What percent of the balls are yellow?

     a. 2%

     b. 8%

     c. 20%

     d. 12%

13. Add 10% of 300 to 50% of 20

     a. 50%

     b. 40%

     c. 60%

     d. 45%

14. Convert 75% to a fraction.

     a. 2/100

     b. 75/100

     c. 3/4

     d. 4/7

15. Convert 90% to a fraction

     a. 1/10

     b. 9/9

     c. 10/100

     d. 9/10

16. Multiply 3 by 25% of 40

    a. 75

    b. 30

    c. 68

    d. 35

17. What is 10% of 30 multiplied by 75% of 200?

    a. 450

    b. 750

    c. 20

    d. 45

18. Convert 0.28 to a fraction.

    a. 7/25

    b. 3.25

    c. 8/25

    d. 5/28

19. Convert 0.45 to a fraction

    a. 7/20

    b. 7/45

    c. 9/20

    d. 3/20

20. Convert 1/5 to percent.

    a. 10%

    b. 5%

    c. 20%

    d. 25%

21. Convert 4/20 to percent

    a. 25%

    b. 20%

    c. 40%

    d. 30%

22. Convert 0.55 to percent

    a. 45%

    b. 15%

    c. 75%

    d. 55%

23. Convert 0.33 to percent

    a. 77%

    b. 67%

    c. 33%

    d. 57%

24. A man buys an item for $420 and has a balance of $3000.00. How much did he have before?

    a. $2,580

    b. $3,420

    c. $2,420

    d. $342

25. Divide 9.60 by 3.2

    a. 2.50

    b. 3

    c. 2.3

    d. 6.4

26. What is the best approximate solution for 1.135 - 113.5?

    a. -110

    b. 100

    c. -90

    d. 110

Medical Dosage Problems

27. The physician orders 40 mg Depo-Medrol; 80 mg/ml is on hand. How many milliliters will you give?

    a. 0.5 ml

    b. 0.80 ml

    c. 0.25 ml

    d. 0.40 ml

28. The physician orders 750 mg Tagamet liquid; 1500 mg/tsp is on hand. How many teaspoons will you give?

    a. 0.75 tsp

    b. 0.5 tsp

    c. 1 tsp

    d. 0.55 tsp

29. The physician ordered 75 mg of Seconal; 50 mg/mL is on hand. How many mL will you give?

    a. 1.25 ml

    b. 1.75 ml

    c. 1 ml

    d. 1.5 ml

30. The physician ordered 1,500 mg Duricef; 1g/tablet is on hand. How many tablets will you give?

    a. .5 tablets

    b. .75 tablets

    c. 1 tablet

    d. 1.5 tablets

31. The physician orders 150 mg morphine sulphate; 1 g/ml is on hand. How many ml will you give?

    a. 0.15 ml

    b. 1.5 ml

    c. 0.25 ml

    d. 0.015

32. The physician ordered 10 units of regular insulin; 100 U/mL is on hand. How many milliliters will you give?

    a. 1.01ml

    b. 1 ml

    c. 0.01 ml

    d. 0.1 ml

Metric Conversion

33. Convert 10 kg. to grams.

    a. 10,000 grams

    b. 1,000 grams

    c. 100 grams

    d. 10.11 grams

34. Convert 0.55 metric tons to kilograms.

    a. 55 kg.

    b. 5500 kg.

    c. 550 kg.

    d. 505 kg.

35. Convert 2.5 liters to milliliters.

    a. 1050 ml.

    b. 2,500 ml.

    c. 2050 ml.

    d. 1500 ml.

36. Convert 210 mg. to grams.

    a. 0.21 mg.

    b. 2.1 g.

    c. 0.21 g.

    d. 2.12 g.

37. Convert 10 pounds to kilograms.

    a. 4.54 kg.

    b. 11.25 kg.

    c. 15 kg.

    d. 10.25 kg.

38. Convert 450 cm. to decameter.

    a. 4500 dm.

    b. 450 dm.

    c. 45 dm.

    d. 0.45 dm.

39. Convert 850 ml. to deciliters.

    a. 8.5 dl.

    b. 85 dl.

    c. 8.5 ml.

    d. 850 dl.

40. Convert 0.539 grams to milligrams.

    a. 539 g.

    b. 539 mg.

    c. 53.9 mg.

    d. 0.53 g.

Word Problems

41. Two trains leave a station at the same time in opposite directions. One has an average speed of 72km/hr. and the other 52km/hr. How far apart are they in 20 minutes?

    a. 6.67 km.

    b. 17.33 km.

    c. 24.3 km.

    d. 41.33 km.

42. The average weight of 13 students in a class of 15 (two were absent that day) is 42 kg. When the remaining two are weighed, the average became 42.7kg. If one of the remaining students weighs 48, how much does the other weigh?

    a. 44.7 kg.

    b. 45.6 kg.

    c. 46.5 kg.

    d. 47.4 kg.

43. The total expense of building a fence around a square-shaped field is $2000 at a rate of $5 per meter. What is the length of one side?

    a. 40 meters.

    b. 80 meters.

    c. 100 meters.

    d. 320 meters.

44. There were some oranges in a basket. By adding 8/5 of the total to the basket, the new total is 130. How many oranges were in the basket?

    a. 60

    b. 50

    c. 40

    d. 35

45. Two trains started at the same time from points 200 km. apart. The first train travels at 40 km/hr and the second train travels at 65 km/hr. How many minutes will it take them to cross?

    a. 92 minutes.

    b. 106 minutes.

    c. 114 minutes.

    d. 118 minutes.

46. A person earns $25,000 per month and pays $9,000 income tax per year. The Government increased income tax by 0.5% per month and his monthly earning was increased $11,000. How much more income tax will he pay per month?

    a. $1260

    b. $1050

    c. $750

    d. $510

47. A company gives a 12% discount to customers on the retail price, and on total purchases over $10,000, they give an additional 3% discount. A customer's total came to $13,500 (discounted price). How much did he save?

    a. $2315

    b. $1850

    c. $2025

    d. $2225

48. Brian jogged 7 times around a circular track 75 meters in diameter. How much linear distance did he cover?

    a. 1250 meters

    b. 1450 meters

    c. 1650 meters

    d. 1725 meters

49. A mother is 7 times older than her child is. In 25 years, her age will be double that of her child. How old is the mother now?

    a. 25

    b. 30

    c. 33

    d. 35

50. John purchased a jacket at a 7% discount. He had a membership that gave him an additional 2% discount. If he paid $425, what is the retail price of the jacket?

    a. $448

    b. $460

    c. $466

    d. $472

Math Self-assessment Answer Key

Basic Math

1. C
389 + 454 = 843

2. C
9,177 + 7,204 = 16,381

3. D
2,199 + 5,832 = 8,031

4. B
8,390 - 5,239 = 3,151

5. A
643 - 587 = 56

6. C
3,406 - 2,767 = 639

7. B
149 × 7 = 1043

8. A
467 × 41 = 19,147

9. D
309 × 17 = 52,53

10. A
491 ÷ 9 = 54 r5

Decimals, Percent and Fractions

11. A
15% = 15/100 X 200 = 7.5%
Notice that the questions asks, What 15 is what percent of 200? The question does not ask, what is 15% of 200! The answers are very different.

12. C
Total no. of balls = 10, no. of yellow balls = 2, ans. = 2/10 X 100 = 20%

13. B

Study >> Practice >> Succeed!

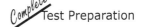
Complete Test Preparation

10% of 300 = 30 and 50% of 20 = 10 so 30 + 1- = 40.

14. C
75%= 75/100 = ¾

15. D
90% = 90/100 = 9/10

16. B
25% of 40 = 10 and 10 x 3 = 30

17. A
10% of 30 = 3 and 75% of 200 = 150, 3 X 150 = 450

18. A
0.28 = 28/100 = 7/25

19. C
0.45 = 45/100 = 9/20

20. C
1/5 X 100 = 20%

21. B
4/20 X 100 = 1/5 X 100 = 20%

22. D
0.55 X 100 = 55%

23. C
0.33 X 100 = 33%

24. B
(Amount Spent) $420 + $3000 (Balance) = $3420

25. B
9.60/3.2 = 3

26. A
1.135 -113.5 = -113.5 + 1-135 = -112.37. Best approximate = -110

Medical Dosage Problems

27. A
Set up the formula -
Dose ordered/Dose on hand X Quantity/1 = Dosage

40 mg/80 mg X 1 ML/1 = 40/80 = 0.5 mL

28. B
Set up the formula -
Dose ordered/Dose on hand X Quantity/1 = Dosage
750 mg/1500 mg X 1 tsp/1 = 750/1500 = 0.5 tsp

29. D
75 mg/50mg X 1 mL/1 = 75/50 = 1.5 mL

30. D
1500 mg/1000 mg X 1 tab/1 = 1500/1000 = 1.5 tablets
(Convert 1 g = 1000 mg)

31. A
150 mg/1000 mg X 1ml/1 = 150/1000 =   0.15 mL (Convert 1 g = 1000 mg)

32. D
10 units/100 units X 1 ML/1 = 10/100 = 0.1 mL

Metric Conversion

33. A
1kg = 1,000 g and 10 kg = 10 x 1,000 = 10,000 g

34. C
1,000 kilograms = 1 ton, 0.55 ton = 1,000 x 0.55 = 550 kilograms

35. B
1 liter = 1,000 milliliters, 2.5 liters = 2.5 x 1,000 = 2,500 milliliters

36. C
1,000 mg = 1 g, 210 mg = 210/1,000 = 0.21 g

37. A
1 pound = 0.45 kg, 10 pounds = 4.53592 or, 4.54 kg

38. D
1000 cm=1 dm, 450 cm = 1,000/450 = 0.45 dm

39. A
5.8 dl   100 ml = 1 dl., 850 ml = 850/100 = 8.5 dl.

40. B 1 g = 1,000 mg. 0.539 g = 0.539 x 1000 = 539 mg.

Word Problems

41. A
Distance traveled by 1st train in 20 minutes = (72 km/hr × 20 minutes) /60 minutes = 24 km. Distance traveled by 2nd train in 20 minutes = (52 km/hr × 20 minutes)/60 minutes = 17.33 km. Difference in distance=24 - 17.33 = 6.67 km

42. C
Total weight of 13 students with average 42 will be = 42 × 13 = 546 kg.
Total weight of 15 students with average 42.7 will be = 42.7 × 15 = 640.5 kg. So total weight of the remaining 2 will be = 640.5 - 546 = 94.5 kg. Weight of the other will be = 94.5 – 48 = 46.5 kg

43. C
Total length of the fence will be = 2000/5 = 400 meters. This will equal to the perimeter of the square field, so the length of one side will be = 400/4 = 100 meters.

44. B
Let the number of oranges in the basket before additions = x
Then: X + 8x/5 = 130
5x + 8x = 650
X = 50

45. C
Let the time to cross be x hours. The equation will be
40x + 65x = 200
X = 1.9047 hours
X = 1.9047 X 60 = 114.28 minutes

46. D
With the new tax rate, income tax is 3.5% so the per month income tax = $9000/12 = $750. Per month income tax rate = $750 X 100/$25,000 = 3%. Income per month = $25,000 + $11,000 = $36,000. Monthly tax amount = $36,000 X 0.035 = $1260

Amount of addition tax = $1260 - $750 = $510

47. A
To calculate the balance before the 3% was taken solve the equation: 13500 = 0.97x, x = 13917.53 Then use this number to solve what the total was before the 12% discount, with the equation: 13917.53 = 0.88x, x = 15,815.37. Then subtract 13500 from this to get a savings of $2315

48. C
In one round trip he covers the distance equal to the circumference of the circular path.
Circumference/Diameter = π = 3.14159
75/X = 3.14159
75 X 3.14159 = X
Circumference of the path = X = 235.65 meters.

Distance covered 7 times around = 235.65 × 7=1650 meters.

49. D

Suppose the mother's age is x years and that of child's is y. Then according to first condition y = 7x

After 25 years the equation will be

y + 25 = 2(x + 25)

Solving it y + 25 = 2x + 50

Putting the value of y = 7x in the below equation

7x + 25 = 2x + 50

x = 5 years

So the child is 5 years old and mother is 35.

50. C

Let the original price be x, then at the rate of 7% the discounted price will be=0.93x

2% discounted amount then will be=0.02×0.93x=0.0186x

Remaining price = 0.93x -0.0186x = 0.9114x

This is the amount which John has paid so 0.9114x = 425

X = 425/0.9114

X = 466.31

The retail price will be $466

Metric Conversion – A Quick Tutorial

Conversion between metric and standard units can be tricky since the units of distance, volume, area and temperature can seem rather arbitrary when compared to one another. Although the metric system (using SI units) is the standard system of measure in most parts of the world many countries still use at least some of their traditional units of measure. In North America those units come from the old British system.

When measuring distance the relation between metric and standard units looks like this:

0.039 in	1 millimeter		1 inch	25.4 mm
3.28 ft	1 meter		1 foot	.305 m
0.621 mi	1 kilometer		1 mile	1.61 km

Here, you can see that 1 millimeter is equal to .039 inches and 1 inch equals 25.4 millimeters.

When measuring **area** the relation between metric and standard looks like this:

.0016 in2	1 square millimeter		1 square inch	645.2 mm2
10.764 ft2	1 square meter		1 square foot	.093 m2
.386 mi2	1 square kilometer		1 square mile	2.59 km2
2.47 ac	hectare		1 acre	.405 ha

Similarly, when measuring **volume** the relation between metric and standard units looks like this:

3034 fl oz	1 milliliter		1 fluid ounce	29.57 ml
.0264 gal	1 liter		1 gallon	3.785 L
35.314 ft3	1 cubic meter		1 cubic foot	.028 m3

When measuring **weight** and **mass** the relation between metric and standard units looks like this:

.035 oz	1 gram		1 ounce	28.35 g
2.202 lbs	1 kilogram		1 pound	.454 kg
1.103 T	1 metric ton		1 ton	.907 t

Complete Test Preparation

It is important to note that in science, the metric units of grams and kilograms are always used to denote the mass of an object rather than its weight.

In predominantly metric countries the standard unit of temperature is degrees Celsius while in countries with only limited use of the metric system, such as the United States, degrees Fahrenheit is used. This chart shows the difference between Fahrenheit and Celsius:

0° Celsius	32° Fahrenheit
10° Celsius	50° Fahrenheit
20° Celsius	68° Fahrenheit
30° Celsius	86° Fahrenheit
40° Celsius	104° Fahrenheit
50° Celsius	122° Fahrenheit
60° Celsius	140° Fahrenheit
70° Celsius	158° Fahrenheit
80° Celsius	176° Fahrenheit
90° Celsius	194° Fahrenheit
100° Celsius	212° Fahrenheit

As you can see 0° C is freezing while 32° F is freezing. Similarity 100° C is boiling while the Fahrenheit system takes until 212° F. To convert from Celsius to Fahrenheit you need to multiply the temperature in Celsius by 1.8 and then add 32 to it. (x° F = (y° C*1.8) + 32) To convert from Fahrenheit to Celsius you do the opposite. First subtract 32 from the temperature then divide by 1.8. (x° C = (y° -32) / 1.8)

Fraction Tips, Tricks and Shortcuts

When you are writing an exam, time is precious, and anything you can do to answer questions faster, is a real advantage. Here are some ideas, shortcuts, tips and tricks that can speed up answering fraction problems.

Remember that a fraction is just a number which names a portion of something. For instance, instead of having a whole pie, a fraction says you have a part of a pie--such as a half of one or a fourth of one.

Two digits make up a fraction. The digit on top is known as the numerator. The digit on the bottom is known as the denominator. To remember which is which, just remember that "denominator" and "down" both start with a "d." And the "downstairs" number is the denominator. So for instance, in ½, the numerator is the 1 and the denominator (or "downstairs") number is the 2.

- It's easy to add two fractions if they have the same denominator. Just add the digits on top and leave the bottom one the same: 1/10 + 6/10 = 7/10.

- It's the same with subtracting fractions with the same denominator: 7/10 - 6/10 = 1/10.

- Adding and subtracting fractions with different denominators is a little more complicated. First, you have to get the problem so that they do have the same denominators. One of the easiest ways to do this is to multiply the denominators: For 2/5 + 1/2 multiply 5 by 2. Now you have a denominator of 10. But now you have to change the top numbers too. Since you multiplied the 5 in 2/5 by 2, you also multiply the 2 by 2, to get 4. So the first number is now 4/10. Since you multiplied the second number times 5, you also multiply its top number by 5, to get a final fraction of 5/10. Now you can add 5 and 4 together to get a final sum of 9/10.

- Sometimes you'll be asked to reduce a fraction to its simplest form. This means getting it to where the only common factor of the numerator and denominator is 1. Think of it this way: Numerators and denominators are brothers that must be treated the same. If you do something to one, you must do it to the other, or it's just not fair. For instance, if you divide your numerator by 2, then you should also divide the denominator by the same. Let's take an example: The fraction 2/10 . This is not reduced to its simplest terms because there is a number that will divide evenly into both: the number 2. We want to make it so that the only number that will divide evenly into both is 1. What can we divide into 2 to get 1? The number 2, of course! Now to be "fair," we have to do the same thing to the denominator: Divide 2 into 10 and you get 5. So our new, reduced fraction is 1/5.

- In some ways, multiplying fractions is the easiest of all: Just multiply the two top numbers and then multiply the two bottom numbers. For instance, with this problem:
  2/5 X 2/3 you multiply 2 by 2 and get a top number of 4; then multiply 5 by 3 and get a bottom number of 15. Your answer is 4/15.

- Dividing fractions is a bit more involved, but still not too hard. You once again multiply, but only AFTER you have turned the second fraction upside-down. To divide ⅞ by ½, turn the ½ into 2/1, then multiply the top numbers and multiply the bottom numbers: ⅞ X 2/1 gives us 14 on top and 8 on the bottom.

Converting Fractions to Decimals

There are a couple of ways to become good at converting fractions to decimals. One -- the one that will make you the fastest in basic math skills -- is to learn some basic fraction facts. It's a good idea, if you're good at memory, to memorize the following:

1/100 is "one hundredth," expressed as a decimal, it's .01.

1/50 is "two hundredths," expressed as a decimal, it's .02.

1/25 is "one twenty-fifths" or "four hundredths," expressed as a decimal, it's .04.

1/20 is "one twentieth" or ""five hundredths," expressed as a decimal, it's .05.

1/10 is "one tenth," expressed as a decimal, it's .1.

1/8 is "one eighth," or "one hundred twenty-five thousandths," expressed as a decimal, it's .125.

1/5 is "one fifth," or "two tenths," expressed as a decimal, it's .2.

1/4 is "one fourth" or "twenty-five hundredths," expressed as a decimal, it's .25.

1/3 is "one third" or "thirty-three hundredths," expressed as a decimal, it's .33.

1/2 is "one half" or "five tenths," expressed as a decimal, it's .5.

3/4 is "three fourths," or "seventy-five hundredths," expressed as a decimal, it's .75.

Of course, if you're no good at memorization, another good technique for converting a fraction to a decimal is to manipulate it so that the fraction's denominator is 10, 10, 1000, or some other power of 10. Here's an example: We'll start with ¾. What is the first number in the 4 "times table" that you can multiply and get a multiple of 10? Can you multiply 4 by something to get 10? No. Can you multiply it by something to get 100? Yes! 4 X 25 is 100. So let's take that 25 and multiply it by the numerator in our fraction ¾. The numerator is 3, and 3 X 25 is 75. We'll move the decimal in 75 all the way to the left, and we find that ¾ is .75.

We'll do another one: 1/5. Again, we want to find a power of 10 that 5 goes into evenly. Will 5 go into 10? Yes! It goes 2 times. So we'll take that 2 and multiply it by our numerator, 1, and we get 2. We move the decimal in 2 all the way to the left and find that 1/5 is equal to .2.

Converting Fractions to Percent

Working with either fractions or percents can be intimidating enough. But converting from one to the other? That's a genuine nightmare for those who are not math wizards. But really, it doesn't have to be that way. Here are two ways to make it easier and faster to convert a fraction to a percent.

☐ First, you might remember that a fraction is nothing more than a division problem: you're dividing the bottom number into the top number. So for instance, if we start with a fraction 1/10, we are making a division problem with the 10 on the outside of the bracket and the 1 on the inside. As you remember from your lessons on dividing by decimals, since 10 won't go into 1, you add a decimal and make it 10 into 1.0. 10 into 10 goes 1 time, and since it's behind the decimal, it's .1. And how do we say .1? We say "one tenth," which is exactly what we started with: 1/10. So we have a number we can work with now: .1. When we're dealing with percents, though, we're dealing strictly with hundredths (not tenths). You remember from studying decimals that adding a zero to the right of the number on the right side of the decimal does not change the value. Therefore, we can change .1 into .10 and have the same number--except now it's expressed as hundredths. We have 10 hundredths. That's ten out of 100--which is just another way of saying ten percent (ten per hundred or ten out of 100). In other words .1 = .10 = 10 percent. Remember, if you're changing from a decimal to a percent, get rid of the decimal on the left and replace it with a percent mark on the right: 10%. Let's review those steps again: Divide 10 into 1. Since 10 doesn't go into 1, turn 1 into 1.0. Now divide 10 into 1.0. Since 10 goes into 10 1 time, put it there and add your decimal to make it .1. Since a percent is always "hundredths," let's change .1 into .10. Then remove the decimal on the left and replace with a percent sign on the right. The answer is 10%.

If you're doing these conversions on a multiple-choice test, here's an idea that might be even easier and faster. Let's say you have a fraction of 1/8 and you're asked what the percent is. Since we know that "percent" means hundredths, ask yourself what number we can multiply 8 by to get 100. Since there is no number, ask what number gets us close to 100. That number is 12: 8 X 12 = 96. So it gets us a little less than 100. Now, whatever you do to the denominator, you have to do to the numerator. Let's multiply 1 X 12 and we get 12. However, since 96 is a little less than 100, we know that our answer will be a percent a little MORE than 12%. So if your possible answers on the multiple-choice test are these:

a) 8.5%   b) 19%   c) 12.5%   d) 25%

then we know the answer is c) 12.5%, because it's a little MORE than the 12 we got in our math problem above.

Another way to look at this, using multiple choice strategy is you know the answer will be "about" 12. Looking at the other choices, they are all either too large or too small and can be eliminated right away.

This was an easy example to demonstrate, so don't be fooled! You probably won't get such an easy question on your exam, but the principle holds just the same. By estimating your answer quickly, you can eliminate choices immediately and save precious exam time.

Decimal Tips, Tricks and Shortcuts

Converting Decimals to Fractions

One of the most important tricks for correctly converting a decimal to a fraction doesn't involve math at all. It's simply to learn to say the decimal correctly. If you say "point one" or "point 25" for .1 and .25, you'll have more trouble getting the conversion correct.

But if you know that it's called "one tenth" and "twenty-five hundredths," you're on the way to a correct conversion. That's because, if you know your fractions, you know that "one tenth" looks like this: 1/10. And "twenty-five hundredths" looks like this: 25/100.

Even if you have digits before the decimal, such as 3.4, learning how to say the word will help you with the conversion into a fraction. It's not "three point four," it's "three and four tenths." Knowing this, you know that the fraction which looks like "three and four tenths" is 3 4/10.

Of course, your conversion is not complete until you reduce the fraction to its lowest terms: It's not 25/100, but 1/4.

Converting Decimals to Percent

Changing a decimal to a percent is easy if you remember one math formula: multiply by 100. For instance, if you start with .45, you change it to a percent by simply multiplying it by 100. You then wind up with 45. Add the % sign to the end and you get 45%.

That seems easy enough, right? In this case think of it this way: You just take out the decimal and stick in a percent sign on the opposite sign. In other words, the decimal on the left is replaced by the % on the right.

It doesn't work quite that easily if the decimal is in the middle of the number. Let's use 3.7 as an example. In this case, take out the decimal in the middle and replace it with a 0 % at the end. So 3.7 converted to decimal is 370%.

Percent Tips, Tricks and Shortcuts

Percent problems are not nearly as scary as they appear, if you remember this neat trick:

Draw a cross as in:

Portion	Percent
Whole	100

In the upper left, write PORTION. In the bottom left write WHOLE. In the top right, write PERCENT and in the bottom right, write 100. Whatever your problem is, you will leave blank the unknown, and fill in the other four parts. For example, let's suppose your problem is: Find 10% of 50. Since we know the 10% part, we put 10 in the percent corner. Since the whole number in our problem is 50, we put that in the corner marked whole. You always put 100 underneath the percent, so we leave it as is, which leaves only the top left corner blank. This is where we'll put our answer. Now simply multiply the two corner numbers that are NOT 100. In this case, it's 10 X 50. That gives us 500. Now multiply this by the remaining corner, or 100, to get a final answer of 5. 5 is the number that goes in the upper-left corner, and is your final solution.

Another hint to remember: Percents are the same thing as hundredths in decimals. So .45 is the same as 45 hundredths or 45 percent.

Converting Percents to Decimals

Percents are simply a specific type of decimals, so it should be no surprise that converting between the two is actually fairly simple. Here are a few tricks and shortcuts to keep in mind:

- Remember that percent literally means "per 100" or "for every 100." So when you speak of 30% you're saying 30 for every 100 or the fraction 30/100. In basic math, you learned that fractions that have 10 or 100 as the denominator can easily be turned into a decimal. 30/100 is thirty hundredths, or expressed as a decimal, .30.
- Another way to look at it: To convert a percent to a decimal, simply divide the number by 100. So for instance, if the percent is 47%, divide 47 by 100. The result will be .47. Get rid of the % mark and you're done.
- Remember that the easiest way of dividing by 100 is by moving your decimal two spots to the left.

Converting Percents to Fractions

Converting percents to fractions is easy. After all, a percent is nothing except a type of fraction; it tells you what part of 100 that you're talking about. Here are some simple ideas for making the conversion from a percent to a fraction:

- If the percent is a whole number -- say 34% -- then simply write a fraction with 100 as the denominator (the bottom number). Then put the percentage itself on top. So 34% becomes 34/100.
- Now reduce as you would reduce any percent. In this case, by dividing 2 into 34 and 2 into 100, you get 17/50.
- If your percent is not a whole number -- say 3.4% --then convert it to a decimal expressed as hundredths. 3.4 is the same as 3.40 (or 3 and forty hundredths). Now ask yourself how you would express "three and forty hundredths" as a fraction. It would, of course, be 3 40/100. Reduce this and it becomes 3 2/5.

How to Answer Basic Math Multiple Choice

Math is the one section where you need to make sure that you understand the processes before you ever tackle it. That's because the time allowed on the math portion is typically so short that there's not much room for error. You have to be fast and accurate. It's imperative that before the test day arrives, you've learned all of the main formulas that will be used, and then to create your own problems (and solve them).

On the actual test day, use the "Plug-Check-Check" strategy. Here's how it goes.

Read the problem, but not the answers. You'll want to work the problem first and come up with your own answers. If you did the work right, you should find your answer among the options given.

If you need help with the problem, plug actual numbers into the variables given. You'll find it easier to work with numbers than it is to work with letters. For instance, if the question asks, "If Y-4 is 2 more than Z, then Y+5 is how much more than Z?" try selecting a value for Y. Let's take 6. Your question now becomes, "If 6-4 is 2 more than Z, then 6 plus 5 is how much more than Z?" Now your answer should be easier to work with.

Check the answer options to see if your answer matches one of those. If so, select it.

If no answer matches the one you got, re-check your math, but this time, use a different method. In math, it's common for there to be more than one way to solve a problem. As a simple example, if you multiplied 12 X 13 and did not get an answer that matches one of the answer options, you might try adding 13 together 12 different times and see if you get a good answer.

Math Multiple Choice Strategy

The two strategies for working with basic math multiple choice are Estimation and Elimination.

Math Strategy 1 - Estimation.

Just like it sounds, try to estimate an approximate answer first. Then look at the choices.

Math Strategy 2 - Elimination.

For every question, no matter what type, eliminating obviously incorrect answers narrows the possible choices. Elimination is probably the most powerful strategy for answering multiple choice.

Here are a few basic math examples of how this works.

Solve 2/3 + 5/12

    a. 9/17

    b. 3/11

    c. 7/12

    d. 1 1/12

First estimate the answer. 2/3 is more than half and 5/12 is about half, so the answer is going to be very close to 1.

Next, Eliminate. Choice A is about 1/2 and can be eliminated, Choice B is very small, less than 1/2 and can be eliminated. Choice C is close to 1/2 and can be eliminated. Leaving only Choice D, which is just over 1.

Work through the solution, a common denominator is needed, a number which both 3 and 12 will divide into.
2/3 = 8/12. So, 8+5/12 = 13/12 = 1 1/12

Choice D is correct.

Solve 4/5 – 2/3

    a. 2/2

    b. 2/13

    c. 1

    d. 2/15

You can eliminate Choice A, because it is 1 and since both of the numbers are close to one, the difference is going to be very small. You can eliminate Choice C for the same reason.

Next, look at the denominators. Since 5 and 3 don't go in to 13, you can eliminate Choice B as well.

That leaves Choice D.

Checking the answer, the common denominator will be 15. So 12-10/15 = 2/15. Choice D is correct.

Fractions shortcut - Cancelling out.

In any operation with fractions, if the numerator of one fractions has a common multiple with the denominator of the other, you can cancel out. This saves time and simplifies the problem quickly, making it easier to manage.

Solve 2/15 ÷ 4/5

     a. 6/65

     b. 6/75

     c. 5/12

     d. 1/6

To divide fractions, we multiply the first fraction with the inverse of the second fraction. Therefore we have

2/15 x 5/4. The numerator of the first fraction, 2, shares a multiple with the denominator of the second fraction, 4, which is 2. These cancel out, which gives, 1/3 x 1/2 = 1/6

Cancelling Out solved the questions very quickly, but we can still use multiple choice strategies to answer.

Choice B can be eliminated because 75 is too large a denominator. Choice C can be eliminated because 5 and 15 don't go in to 12.

Choice D is correct.

Decimal Multiple Choice strategy and Shortcuts.

Multiplying decimals gives a very quick way to estimate and eliminate choices. Anytime that you multiply decimals, it is going to give a answer with the same number of decimal places as the combined operands.

So for example,

2.38 X 1.2 will produce a number with three places of decimal, which is 2.856.

Here are a few examples with step-by-step explanation:

Solve 2.06 x 1.2

     a. 24.82

     b. 2.482

     c. 24.72

     d. 2.472

This is a simple question, but even before you start calculating, you can eliminate several choices. When multiplying decimals, there will always be as many numbers behind the decimal place in the answer as the sum of the ones in the initial problem, so Choice A and C can be eliminate.

The correct answer is D: 2.06 x 1.2 = 2.472

Solve 20.0 ÷ 2.5

    a. 12.05

    b. 9.25

    c. 8.3

    d. 8

First estimate the answer to be around 10, and eliminate Choice A. And since it'd also be an even number, you can eliminate Choice B and C., leaving only choice D.

The correct Answer is D: 20.0 ÷ 2.5 = 8

How to Solve Word Problems

Most students find math word problems difficult. Tackling word problems is much easier if you have a systematic approach which we outline below.

Here is the biggest tip for studying word problems.

Practice regularly and systematically. Sounds simple and easy right? Yes it is, and yes it really does work.

Word problems are a way of thinking and require you to translate a real word problem into mathematical terms.

Some math instructors go so far as to say that learning how to think mathematically is the main reason for teaching word problems.

So what do we mean by Practice regularly and systematically? Studying word problems and math in general requires a logical and mathematical frame of mind. The only way you can get this is by practicing regularly, which means everyday.

It is critical that you practice word problems everyday for the 5 days before the exam as a bare minimum.

If you practice and miss a day, you have lost the mathematical frame of mind and the benefit of your previous practice is pretty much gone. Anyone who has done any amount of math will agree – you have to practice everyday.

Everything is important. The other critical point about word problems is that all of the information given in the problem has some purpose. There is no unnecessary information! Word problems are typically around 50 words in 1 to 3 sentences. If the sometimes complicated relationships are to be explained in that short an explanation, every word has to count. Make sure that you use every piece of information.

Here are 9 simple steps to help you resolve word problems.

Step 1 – Read through the problem at least three times. The first reading should be a quick scan, and the next two readings should be done slowly with a view to finding answers to these important questions:

What does the problem ask? (Usually located towards the end of the problem)

What does the problem imply? (This is usually a point you were asked to remember).

Mark all information, and underline all important words or phrases.

Step 2 – Try to make a pictorial representation of the problem such as a circle and an arrow to indicate travel. This makes the problem a bit more real and sensible to you.

A favorite word problem is something like, 1 train leaves Station A travelling at 100 km/hr and another train leaves Station B travelling at 60 km/hr. ...

Draw a line, the two stations, and the two trains at either end. This will help solidify the situation in your mind.

Step 3 – Use the information you have to make a table with a blank portion to indicate information you do not know.

Step 4 – Assign a single letter to represent each unknown data in your table. You can write down the unknown that each letter represents so that you do not make the error of assigning answers to the wrong unknown, because a word problem may have multiple unknowns and you will need to create equations for each unknown.

Step 5 – Translate the English terms in the word problem into a mathematical algebraic equation. Remember that the main problem with word problems is that they are not expressed in regular math equations. You ability to correctly identify the variables and translate the word problem into an equation determines your ability to solve the problem.

Step 6 – Check the equation to see if it looks like regular equations that you are used to seeing and whether it looks sensible. Does the equation appear to represent the information in the question? Take note that you may need to rewrite some formulas needed to solve the word problem equation. For example, word distance problems may need you rewriting the distance formula, which is Distance = Time x Rate. If the word problem requires that you solve for time you will need to use Distance/Rate and Distance/Time to solve for Rate. If you understand the distance word problem you should be able to identify the variable you need to solve for.

Step 7 – Use algebra rules to solve the derived equation. Take note that the laws of equation demands that what is done on this side of the equation has to also be done on the other side. You have to solve the equation so that the unknown ends up alone on one side. Where there are multiple unknowns you will need to use elimination or substitution methods to resolve all the equations.

Step 8 – Check your final answers to see if they make sense with the information given in the problem. For example if the word problem involves a discount, the final price should be less or if a product was taxed then the final answer has to cost more.

Step 9 – Cross check your answers by placing the answer or answers in the first equation to replace the unknown or unknowns. If your answer is correct then both side of the equation must equate or equal. If your answer is not correct then you may have derived a wrong equation or solved the equation wrongly. Repeat the necessary steps to correct.

Types of Word Problems

Word problems can be classified into 12 types. Below are examples of each type with a complete solution. Some types of word problems can be solved quickly using multiple choice strategies and some can not. Always look for ways to estimate the answer and then eliminate choices.

1. Age

A girl is 10 years older than her brother. By next year, she will be twice the age of her brother. What are their ages now?

    a. 25, 15
    b. 19, 9
    c. 21, 11
    d. 29, 19

Solution: B

We will assume that the girl's age is "a" and her brother's is "b". This means that based on the information in the first sentence,
$a = 10 + b$

Next year, she will be twice her brother's age, which gives
$a + 1 = 2(b+1)$

We need to solve for one unknown factor and then use the answer to solve for the other. To do this we substitute the value of "a" from the first equation into the second equation. This gives

$10+b + 1 = 2b + 2$
$11 + b = 2b + 2$
$11 - 2 = 2b - b$
$b= 9$

$9 = b$ this means that her brother is 9 years old. Solving for the girl's age in the first equation gives $a = 10 + 9$. $a = 19$ the girl is aged 19. So, the girl is aged 19 and the boy

Complete Test Preparation

is 9

2. Distance or speed

Two boats travel down a river towards the same destination, starting at the same time. One of the boats is traveling at 52 km/hr, and the other boat at 43 km/hr. How far apart will they be after 40 minutes?

    a. 46.67 km

    b. 19.23 km

    c. 6.4 km

    d. 14.39 km

Solution: C

After 40 minutes, the first boat will have traveled = 52 km/hr x 40 minutes/60 minutes = 34.7 km

After 40 minutes, the second boat will have traveled = 43 km/hr x 40/60 minutes = 28.66 km

Difference between the two boats will be 34.7 km – 28.66 km = 6.04 km.

Multiple Choice Strategy

First estimate the answer. The first boat is travelling 9 km. faster than the second, for 40 minutes, which is 2/3 of an hour. 2/3 of 9 = 6, as a rough guess of the distance apart.

Choices A, B and D can be eliminated right away.

3. Ratio

The instructions in a cookbook states that 700 grams of flour must be mixed in 100 ml of water, and 0.90 grams of salt added. A cook however has just 325 grams of flour. What is the quantity of water and salt that he should use?

    a. 0.41 grams and 46.4 ml

    b. 0.45 grams and 49.3 ml

    c. 0.39 grams and 39.8 ml

    d. 0.25 grams and 40.1 ml

Solution: A

The Cookbook states 700 grams of flour, but the cook only has 325. The first step is to determine the percentage of flour he has 325/700 x 100 = 46.4%

That means that 46.4% of all other items must also be used.

46.4% of 100 = 46.4 ml of water

46.4% of 0.90 = 0.41 grams of salt.

Multiple Choice Strategy

The recipe calls for 700 grams of flour but the cook only has 325, which is just less than half, the amount of water and salt are going to be approximately half.

Choices C and D can be eliminated right away.   Choice B is very close so be careful. Looking closely at Choice B, it is exactly half, and since 325 is slightly less than half of 700, it can't be correct.

Choice A is correct.

4. Percent

An agent received $6,685 as his commission for selling a property. If his commission was 13% of the selling price, how much was the property?

> a. $68,825
> b. $121,850
> c. $49,025
> d. $51,423

Solution: D

Let's assume that the property price is x
That means from the information given, 13% of x = 6,685
Solve for x,
x = 6685 x 100/13 = $51,423

Multiple Choice Strategy

The commission,13%, is just over 10%, which is easier to work with. Round up $6685 to $6700, and multiple by 10 for an approximate answer. 10 X 6700 = $67,000. You can do this in your head. Choice B is much too big and can be eliminated. Choice C is too small and can be eliminated. Choices A and D are left and good possibilities.

Do the calculations to make the final choice.

5. Sales & Profit

A store owner buys merchandise for $21,045. He transports them for $3,905 and pays his staff $1,450 to stock the merchandise on his shelves. If he does not incur further costs, how much does he need to sell the items to make $5,000 profit?

    a. $32,500

    b. $29,350

    c. $32,400

    d. $31,400

Solution: D

Total cost of the items is $21,045 + $3,905 + $1,450 = $26,400
Total cost is now $26,400 + $5000 profit = $31,400

Multiple Choice Strategy

Round off and add the numbers up in your head quickly.
21,000 + 4,000 + 1500 = 26500. Add in 5000 profit for a total of 31500.

Choice B is too small and can be eliminated. Choice C and Choice A are too large and can be eliminated.

6. Tax/Income

A woman earns $42,000 per month and pays 5% tax on her monthly income. If the Government increases her monthly taxes by $1,500, what is her income after tax?

    a. $38,400

    b. $36,050

    c. $40,500

    d. $39, 500

Solution: A

Initial tax on income was 5/100 x 42,000 = $2,100
$1,500 was added to the tax to give $2,100 + 1,500 = $3,600
Income after tax left is $42,000 - $3,600 = $38,400

7. Interest

A man invests $3000 in a 2-year term deposit that pays 3% interest per year. How much will he have at the end of the 2-year term?

    a. $5,200
    b. $3,020
    c. $3,182.7
    d. $3,000

Solution: C

This is a compound interest problem. The funds are invested for 2 years and interest is paid yearly, so in the second year, he will earn interest on the interest paid in the first year.

3% interest in the first year = 3/100 x 3,000 = $90
At end of first year, total amount = 3,000 + 90 = $3,090
Second year = 3/100 x 3,090 = 92.7.
At end of second year, total amount = $3090 + $92.7 = $3,182.7

8. Averaging

The average weight of 10 books is 54 grams. 2 more books were added and the average weight became 55.4. If one of the 2 new books added weighed 62.8 g, what is the weight of the other?

    a. 44.7 g
    b. 67.4 g
    c. 62 g
    d. 52 g

Solution: C
Total weight of 10 books with average 54 grams will be=10×54=540 g
Total weight of 12 books with average 55.4 will be=55.4×12=664.8 g
So total weight of the remaining 2 will be= 664.8 – 540 = 124.8 g
If one weighs 62.8, the weight of the other will be= 124.8 g – 62.8 g = 62 g

Multiple Choice Strategy

Averaging problems can be estimated by looking at which direction the average goes. If additional items are added and the average goes up, the new items much be greater than the average. If the average goes down after new items are added, the new items must be less than the average.

In this case, the average is 54 grams and 2 books are added which increases the average to 55.4, so the new books must weight more than 54 grams.

Choices A and D can be eliminated right away.

9. Probability

A bag contains 15 marbles of various colors. If 3 marbles are white, 5 are red and the rest are black, what is the probability of randomly picking out a black marble from the bag?

    a. 7/15
    b. 3/15
    c. 1/5
    d. 4/15

Solution: A

Total marbles = 15
Number of black marbles = 15 – (3 + 5) = 7
Probability of picking out a black marble = 7/15

10. Two Variables

A company paid a total of $2850 to book for 6 single rooms and 4 double rooms in a hotel for one night. Another company paid $3185 to book for 13 single rooms for one night in the same hotel. What is the cost for single and double rooms in that hotel?

    a. single= $250 and double = $345
    b. single= $254 and double = $350
    c. single = $245 and double = $305
    d. single = $245 and double = $345

Solution: D

We can determine the price of single rooms from the information given of the second company. 13 single rooms = 3185.
One single room = 3185 / 13 = 245
The first company paid for 6 single rooms at $245. 245 x 6 = $1470
Total amount paid for 4 double rooms by first company = $2850 - $1470 = $1380
Cost per double room = 1380 / 4 = $345

 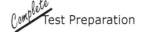

11. Geometry

The length of a rectangle is 5 in. more than its width. The perimeter of the rectangle is 26 in. What is the width and length of the rectangle?

    a. width = 6 inches, Length = 9 inches

    b. width = 4 inches, Length = 9 inches

    c. width =4 inches, Length = 5 inches

    d. width = 6 inches, Length = 11 inches

Solution: B

Formula for perimeter of a rectangle is 2(L + W)
p=26, so 2(L+W) = p
The length is 5 inches more than the width, so
2(w+5) + 2w = 26
2w + 10 + 2w = 26
2w + 2w = 26 - 10
4w = 18

W = 16/4 = 4 inches

L is 5 inches more than w, so L = 5 + 4 = 9 inches.

12. Totals and fractions

A basket contains 125 oranges, mangos and apples. If 3/5 of the fruits in the basket are mangos and only 2/5 of the mangos are ripe, how many ripe mangos are there in the basket?

    a. 30

    b. 68

    c. 55

    d. 47

Solution: A
Number of mangos in the basket is 3/5 x 125 = 75
Number of ripe mangos = 2/5 x 75 = 30

Algebraic Equations – A Quick Tutorial

Algebra is a basic form of mathematics designed to define unknown quantities called **variables**. Variables in algebra are represented by letters, often **x**, **y** and **z** or **a**, **b** and **c**, and they are placed in equations alongside known quantities. An algebraic equation can be as simple as **2x=6** where simple division can tell us that **x=6/2** or **x=3**. Equations can also have variables on both sides such as **2x+3=8x**. For this equation, we need to take more steps. First, subtracting **2x** from both sides we get the equation **3=6x**. From there it is again a simple matter of division to show that **x=.5**. The point of an equation is that it demonstrates that two distinct pieces of information have the same value. (It *equates* them.) Even though we do not know what **2x+3** is or what **8x** is, we at least know that they are the same.

There are three types of equalities in algebra. There are reflexive equalities that say **x=x**. There are symmetric equalities that say that if **x=y** then **y=x** as well. And there are transitive equalities that say that if **x=y** and **y=z** then **x=z**.

The definite number next to the variable in each equation is called its **coefficient**. A variable can always be thought of as having a coefficient; if there is no number next to it, the coefficient equals 1, and if it has a negative sign in front of it, the coefficient equals -1.

Often, algebra is presented in the form of word problems and it is up to you to figure out the equation. For instance, a question might describe a hockey team that has 6 wins, 3 losses in regulation time and 1 loss in overtime over their last 10 games. It will then tell you that the team has 13 points (awarded for wins and overtime losses in order to organize the league's standings) in their last 10 games and ask, given that a regulation loss earns a team 0 points: How many points is a win worth? How many is an overtime loss worth?

This question will give you the variables **x = a win, y = a regulation loss** and **z = an overtime loss**, from which you can derive the equation **6x+3y+1z=13**. Since you already know that **y=0 points**, you can rewrite the equation as **6x+z=13**. Now we have a two variable or **polynomial** equation to solve. First, we need to find a way to rewrite it so that there is only one variable in the equation. If we solve for **x** we get the equation **6x=13-1z** which can be simplified to **x=2z**. We can then plug that into the original equation and get **6(2z)+z=13** or **13z=13** or **z=1**. Now we know two variables that we can use to solve for **x** and we can write the equation **6x+1=13** or **x=2**. Thus, we can tell that in hockey teams get 2 points for each regulation win (**x=2**) and 1 point for each overtime win (**z=1**).

This is a highly simplified example of algebra, but the same process works with any basic mathematical function provided you follow the **order of operations**. The order of operations is the order in which you have to perform each mathematical function in order to get the correct answer. Following the order of operations is important because while some operations can be done in any order:

(1+2)+3 = 3+3 = 6 is the same as **(2+3)+1 = 5+1 = 6**

others cannot:

(10-2)/4 = 8/4 = 2 is not the same as **(10/4)-2 = 2.5-2 = .5**

Doing the operations in any order you want can give you very incorrect results.

The order of operations goes: **parentheses, exponents, multiplication, division, addition, subtraction**. It can be remembered through the acronym **P**lease **E**xcuse **M**y **D**ear **A**unt **S**ally.

English Self-Assessment and Tutorials

THIS SECTION CONTAINS A SELF-ASSESSMENT AND ENGLISH TUTORIALS. The Tutorials are designed to familiarize general principals and the Self-Assessment contains general questions similar to the English questions likely to be on the HESI exam, but are not intended to be identical to the exam questions. Many Universities recommend that students take an introductory English course before taking the HESI Exam. The tutorials are *not* designed to be a complete English course, and it is assumed that students have some familiarity with English. If you do not understand parts of the tutorial, or find the tutorial difficult, it is recommended that you seek out additional instruction.

The purpose of the self-assessment is:

- Identify your strengths and weaknesses.

- Develop your personalized study plan (above)

- Get accustomed to the HESI format

- Extra practice – the self-assessment is a 3rd test!

Since this is a self-assessment, and depending on how confident you are with English Grammar, timing yourself is optional. There are a total of 50 questions which must be answered in 50 minutes. The self-assessment has 20 questions, so allow 20 minutes to complete this assessment.

The questions below are not exactly the same as you will find on the HESI - that would be too easy! And nobody knows what the questions will be and they change all the time. Below are general English questions that cover the same areas as the HESI. So while the format and exact wording of the questions may differ slightly, and change from year to year, if you can answer the questions below, you will have no problem with the English section of the HESI.

NOTE: The English section is an optional module and not all schools include in their HESI. We strongly suggest that you check with your school for the HESI A2 exam details. It is always a good idea to give the materials you receive when you register to take the HESI a careful review.

75% - 100%	Excellent – you have mastered the content
50 – 75%	Good. You have a working knowledge. Even though you can just pass this section, you may want to review the Tutorials and do some extra practice to see if you can improve your mark.
25% - 50%	Below Average. You do not understand the content.

Review the tutorials, and retake this quiz again in a few days, before proceeding to the rest of the Practice Test Course. |
| Less than 25% | Poor. You have a very limited understanding.

Please review the Tutorials, and retake this quiz again in a few days, before proceeding to the rest of the course. |

English Self-Assessment Answer Sheet

1. Ⓐ Ⓑ Ⓒ Ⓓ 11. Ⓐ Ⓑ Ⓒ Ⓓ 21. Ⓐ Ⓑ Ⓒ Ⓓ

2. Ⓐ Ⓑ Ⓒ Ⓓ 12. Ⓐ Ⓑ Ⓒ Ⓓ 22. Ⓐ Ⓑ Ⓒ Ⓓ

3. Ⓐ Ⓑ Ⓒ Ⓓ 13. Ⓐ Ⓑ Ⓒ Ⓓ 23. Ⓐ Ⓑ Ⓒ Ⓓ

4. Ⓐ Ⓑ Ⓒ Ⓓ 14. Ⓐ Ⓑ Ⓒ Ⓓ 24. Ⓐ Ⓑ Ⓒ Ⓓ

5. Ⓐ Ⓑ Ⓒ Ⓓ 15. Ⓐ Ⓑ Ⓒ Ⓓ 25. Ⓐ Ⓑ Ⓒ Ⓓ

6. Ⓐ Ⓑ Ⓒ Ⓓ 16. Ⓐ Ⓑ Ⓒ Ⓓ 26. Ⓐ Ⓑ Ⓒ Ⓓ

7. Ⓐ Ⓑ Ⓒ Ⓓ 17. Ⓐ Ⓑ Ⓒ Ⓓ 27. Ⓐ Ⓑ Ⓒ Ⓓ

8. Ⓐ Ⓑ Ⓒ Ⓓ 18. Ⓐ Ⓑ Ⓒ Ⓓ 28. Ⓐ Ⓑ Ⓒ Ⓓ

9. Ⓐ Ⓑ Ⓒ Ⓓ 19. Ⓐ Ⓑ Ⓒ Ⓓ 29. Ⓐ Ⓑ Ⓒ Ⓓ

10. Ⓐ Ⓑ Ⓒ Ⓓ 20. Ⓐ Ⓑ Ⓒ Ⓓ 30. Ⓐ Ⓑ Ⓒ Ⓓ

Part 1 – English Grammar

1. Choose the sentence with the correct grammar.

a. He would have postponed the camping trip, if he would have known about the forecast.

b. If he would have known about the forecast, he would have postponed the camping trip.

c. If he have known about the forecast, he would have postponed the camping trip.

d. If he had known about the forecast, he would have postponed the camping trip.

2. Choose the sentence with the correct grammar.

a. If Joe had told me the truth, I wouldn't have been so angry.

b. If Joe would have told me the truth, I wouldn't have been so angry.

c. I wouldn't have been so angry if Joe would have told the truth.

d. If Joe would have telled me the truth, I wouldn't have been so angry.

3. Choose the sentence with the correct grammar.

a. He doesn't have any money to buy clothes, and neither do I.

b. He doesn't have any money to buy clothes, and neither does I.

c. He don't have any money to buy clothes, and neither do I.

d. He don't have any money to buy clothes, and neither does I.

4. Choose the sentence with the correct grammar.

a. Because it really don't matter, I don't care if I go there.

b. Because it really doesn't matter, I doesn't care if I go there.

c. Because it really doesn't matter, I don't care if I go there.

d. Because it really don't matter, I don't care if I go there.

5. Choose the sentence with the correct grammar.

a. The dog took the stuffed toy to his master's empty chair.

b. The dog brang the stuffed toy to his master's empty chair.

c. The dog brought the stuffed toy to his master's empty chair.

d. The dog taken the stuffed toy to his master's empty chair.

6. Choose the sentence with the correct grammar.

a. Until you take the overdue books to the library, you can't take any new ones home.

b. Until you take the overdue books to the library, you can't bring any new ones home.

c. Until you bring the overdue books to the library, you can't take any new ones home.

d. Until you take the overdue books to the library, you can't take any new ones home.

7. Choose the sentence with the correct grammar.

a. Newer cars use fewer gasoline and produce fewer emissions.

b. Newer cars use less gasoline and produce less emissions.

c. Newer cars use less gasoline and produce fewer emissions.

d. Newer cars fewer less gasoline and produce less emissions.

8. Choose the sentence with the correct grammar.

a. His doctor suggested that he eat less snacks and do fewer lounging on the couch.

b. His doctor suggested that he eat fewer snacks and do less lounging on the couch.

c. His doctor suggested that he eat less snacks and do less lounging on the couch.

d. His doctor suggested that he eat fewer snacks and do fewer lounging on the couch.

9. Choose the sentence with the correct grammar.

a. However, I believe that he didn't really try that hard.

b. However I believe that he didn't really try that hard.

c. However; I believe that he didn't really try that hard.

d. However: I believe that he didn't really try that hard.

10. Choose the sentence with the correct grammar.

a. There was however, very little difference between the two.

b. There was, however very little difference between the two.

c. There was; however, very little difference between the two.

d. There was, however, very little difference between the two.

Part II – Vocabulary

Choose the word that best suits the given definition.

11. ADJECTIVE Corrupted, Impure.

 e. Adulterate

 f. Harbor

 g. Infuriate

 h. Inculcate

12. NOUN Eagerness and enthusiasm.

 a. Alacrity

 b. Happiness

 c. Donator

 d. Marital

13. VERB To make less severe.

 a. Suspense

 b. Alleviate

 c. Ingrate

 d. Action

14. VERB To make blissful or happy.

 a. Brand

 b. Negate

 c. Beatify

 d. Train

15. NOUN One who gives a gift or who gives money to a charity organization.

 a. Captain

 b. Benefactor

 c. Source

 d. Teacher

Complete Test Preparation

16. ADJECTIVE Hidden, secret, disguised.

    a. Accustomed

    b. Covert

    c. Hide

    d. Carriage

17. VERB Straightforward, open and sincere.

    a. Lawful

    b. Candid

    c. True

    d. Lawful

18. VERB Fearless or invulnerable to intimidation and fear.

    a. Feeble

    b. Strongest

    c. Dauntless

    d. Super

19. VERB To remove a leader or high official from position.

    a. Sack

    b. Suspend

    c. Depose

    d. Dropped

20. VERB To build up or strengthen in relation to morals or religion.

    a. Sanctify

    b. Amplify

    c. Edify

    d. Wry

Choose the best definition of the given word.

21. Choose the best definition for virago.

    a. Loud and domineering woman

    b. A quiet woman

    c. A load domineering Man

    d. A quiet man

22. Choose the best definition of deprecate.

    a. Approve

    b. Indifference

    c. Disapprove

    d. None of the above

23. Choose the best definition for succor.

    a. To suck on

    b. To hate

    c. To like

    d. Give help of assistance

24. Choose the best definition of specious.

    a. Logical

    b. Illogical

    c. Emotional

    d. 2 species

25. Choose the best definition of proscribe.

    a. Welcome

    b. Write a prescription

    c. Banish

    d. Give a diagnosis

26. Choose the best definition of pernicious.

    a. Deadly

    b. Infectious

    c. Common

    d. Rare

27. Choose the best definition of pedestrian.

    a. Rare

    b. Often

    c. Walking or Running

    d. Commonplace

28. Choose the best definition of petulant.

    a. Patient

    b. Childish

    c. Impatient

    d. Mature

29. Choose the best definition of stint.

    a. Thrifty

    b. Annoyed

    c. Dislike

    d. Insult

30. Choose the best definition of precipitate.

    a. To rain

    b. To throw down

    c. To throw up

    d. To snow

Answer Key

1. D

The third conditional is used for talking about an unreal situation (a situation that did not happen) in the past. For example, "If I had studied harder, [if clause] I would have passed the exam [main clause]. This has the same meaning as, "I failed the exam because I didn't study hard enough."

2. A

The third conditional is used for talking about an unreal situation (a situation that did not happen) in the past. For example, "If I had studied harder, [if clause] I would have passed the exam [main clause]. This has the same meaning as, "I failed the exam because I didn't study hard enough."

3. A

Shows agreement with a negative statement by using "neither."

4. C

Doesn't, does not, or does is used with the third person singular--the pronouns he, she, and it. Don't, do not, or do is used with first, second, and third person plural.

5. A

Whether to use "bring" or "take" depends on location. Something coming toward the subject's location is brought. Something going away from the subject's location is taken.

6. C

Whether to use "bring" or "take" depends on location. Something coming toward the subject's location is brought. Something going away from the subject's location is taken.

7. C

"Fewer" is used with countable nouns and "less" is used with uncountable nouns.

8. B

"Fewer" is used with countable nouns and "less" is used with uncountable nouns.

9. A

"However" is bracketed with a comma after it at the beginning of a sentence.

10. D

"However" is bracketed with a comma before and after it within a sentence.

Part II – Vocabulary

11. A
Adulterate VERB corrupted; impure; adulterated.

12. A
Alacrity NOUN eagerness; liveliness; enthusiasm.

13. B
Alleviate VERB to make less severe, as a pain or difficulty.

14. C
Beatify VERB to make blissful.

15. B
Benefactor NOUN somebody who gives one a gift. Usually refers to someone who gives money to a charity or another form of organization.

16. B
Covert ADJECTIVE Partially hidden, disguised, secret, surreptitious.

17. B
Candid ADJECTIVE straightforward, open and sincere.

18. C
Dauntless ADJECTIVE invulnerable to fear or intimidation.

19. C
Depose VERB to remove (a leader) from (high) office, without killing the incumbent.

20. C
Edify VERB to instruct or improve morally or intellectually.

21. A
Virago NOUN given to undue belligerence or ill manner at the slightest provocation; a shrew.

22. C
Deprecate VERB to belittle or express disapproval of.

23. D
Succor NOUN aid, assistance or relief given to one in distress; ministration.

24. B
Specious ADJECTIVE seemingly well-reasoned or factual, but actually fallacious or insincere; strongly held but false.

25. C
Proscribe ADJECTIVE seemingly well-reasoned or factual, but actually fallacious or insincere; strongly held but false.

26. A
Pernicious ADJECTIVE causing much harm in a subtle way.

Complete Test Preparation

27. D
Pedestrian ADJECTIVE ordinary, dull; everyday; unexceptional.

28. C
Petulant ADJECTIVE childishly irritable, impatient.

29. A
Stint VERB to be sparing, thrifty.

30. A
Precipitate VERB to have water in the air fall to the ground, for example as rain, snow, sleet. [17]

English Tutorials

How to Answer English Grammar Multiple Choice - Verb Tense

This tutorial is designed to help you answer English Grammar multiple choice questions as well as a very quick refresher on verb tenses. It is assumed that you have some familiarity with the verb tenses covered here. If you find these questions difficulty or do not understand the tense construction, we recommend you seek out additional instruction.

Tenses Covered

1. Past Progressive
2. Present Perfect
3. Present Perfect Progressive
4. Present Progressive
5. Simple Future
6. Simple Future – "Going to" Form
7. Past Perfect Progressive
8. Future Perfect Progressive
9. Future Perfect
10. Future Progressive
11. Past Perfect

1. The Past Progressive Tense

How to Recognize This Tense

He *was running* very fast when he fell.

They *were drinking* coffee when he arrived.

About the Past Progressive Tense

This tense is used to speak of an action that was in progress in the past when another event occurred.

The action was unfolding at a point in the past.

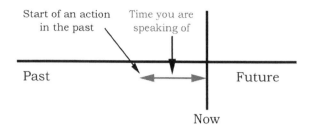

Past Progressive Tense Construction

This tense is formed by using the past tense of the verb "to be" plus the present participle of the main verb.

Sample Question

Bill _____ lunch when we arrived.

    a. will eat

    b. is eating

    c. eats

    d. was eating

How to Answer This Type of Question

1. First examine the question for clues about the time frame.

The sentence ends with "when we arrived," so we know the time frame is a point ("when") in the past (arrived).

The correct answer will refer to an ongoing action at a point of time in the past.

2. Examine the choices and eliminate any obviously incorrect answers.

Choice A is the future tense so we can eliminate.

Choice B is the present continuous so we can eliminate.

Choice C is present tense so we can eliminate.

Choice D refers to an action that takes place at a point of time in the past ("was eating").

2. The Present Perfect Tense

How to Recognize This Tense

I *have had* enough to eat.

We *have been* to Paris many times.

I *have known* him for five years.

I *have been* coming here since I was a child.

About the Present Perfect Tense

This tense expresses the idea that something happened (or didn't happen) at an unspecific time in the past up until the present. The action happened at an unspecified time in the past. (If there is a specific time mentioned, the simple past tense is used.) It can be used for repeated action, accomplishments, changes over time and uncompleted action.

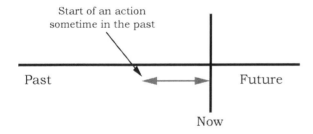

Present Perfect Tense Construction

It is also used with "for" and "since".

This tense is formed by using the present tense of the verb "to have" plus the past participle of the main verb.

Sample Question

I _____ these birds many times.

  a. am seeing

  b. will saw

  c. have seen

  d. have saw

How to Answer This Type of Question

1. First examine the question for clues about the time frame.

"Many times" tells us that the action is repeated and in the past.

2. Examine the choices and eliminate any obviously incorrect answers.

Choice A, "am seeing" is incorrect because it is a continuing action, i.e. in the present; it also doesn't use a form of 'have'.

Choice B is grammatically incorrect.

Choice C is tells of something that has happened in the past and is now over. Best choice so far.

Choice D is grammatically incorrect.

3. The Present Perfect Progressive Tense

How to Recognize This Tense

We *have been seeing* a lot of rainy days.

I *have been reading* some very good books.

About the Present Perfect Progressive Tense

This tense expresses the idea that something happened (or didn't happen) in the relatively recent past, but <u>the action is not finished.</u> It is used to express the duration of the action.

NOTE: The present perfect speaks of an action that happened sometime in the past, but this action is finished. In the present perfect progressive tense, the action that started in the past is still going on.

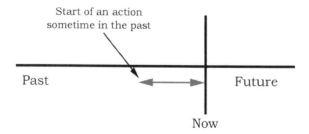

Present Perfect Progressive Tense Construction

This tense is formed by using the present tense of the verb "to have," plus "been," plus the present participle of the main verb.

Sample Question

Bill _____ there for two hours.

    a. sits

    b. sitting

    c. has been sitting

    d. will sat

How to Answer This Type of Question

1. First examine the question for clues about the time frame.

"For two hours" tells us that the action, "sits," is continuous up to now, and may continue into the future.

Note this sentence could also be the simple past tense,

Bill sat there for two hours.

Or the future tense,

Bill will sit there for two hours.

However, these are not among the options.

2. Examine the choices and eliminate any obviously incorrect answers.

Choice A is incorrect because it is the present tense.
Choice B is incorrect because it is the present continuous. Choice C is correct. "Has been sitting" expresses a continuous action in the past that isn't finished.
Choice D is grammatically incorrect.

4. The Present Progressive Tense

How to Recognize This Tense

We *are having* a delicious lunch.

They *are driving* much too fast.

About the Present Progressive Tense

This tense is used to express what the action is <u>right now</u>. The action started in the recent past, and is continuing into the future.

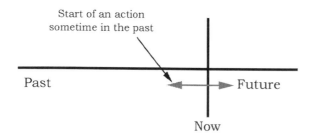

Start of an action
sometime in the past

Past

Future

Now

Present Perfect Tense Construction

The Present Progressive Tense is formed by using the present tense of "to be" plus the present participle of the main verb.

Sample Question

She _____ very hard these days.

 a. works

 b. is working

 c. will work

 d. worked

How to Answer This Type of Question

1. First examine the question for clues about the time frame.

The end of the sentence includes "these days" which tell us the action started in the past, continues into the present, and may continue into the future.

2. Examine the choices and eliminate any obviously incorrect answers.

Choice A, the simple present is incorrect.
Choice B, "is working" is correct.
Check the other two choices just to be sure. Choice C is future tense, and Choice D is past tense, so they can be eliminated.

The correct answer is Choice B.

5. The Simple Future Tense

How to Recognize This Tense

I *will see* you tomorrow.
We *will drive* the car.

About the Simple Future Tense

This tense shows that the action will happen some time in the future.

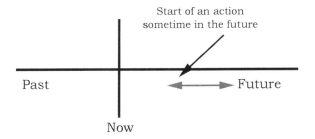

Simple Future Tense Construction

The tense is formed by using "will" plus the root form of the verb. (The root form of the verb is the infinitive without "to." Examples: read, swim.)

Sample Question

We _____ to Paris next year.

    a. went

    b. had been

    c. will go

    d. go

How to Answer This Type of Question

1. First examine the question for clues about the time frame.

The last two words of the sentence, "next year," clearly identify this sentence as referring to the future.

2. Examine the choices and eliminate any obviously incorrect answers.

Choice A is the past tense and can be eliminated.

Choice B is the past perfect tense and can be eliminated.

Choice D is the simple present and can be eliminated.

Choice C is the only one left and is the correct simple future tense.

6. The Simple Future Tense – The "Going to" Form

How to Recognize This Tense

I *am going to* see you tomorrow.

We *are going to* drive the car.

About the Simple Future Tense

This form of the future tense is used to show the intention of doing something in the future. (This is the strict grammatical meaning, but in daily speech, it is often used interchangeably with the simple future tense, the "will" form.)

The tense is formed by using the present conditional tense of "to go," plus the infinitive of the verb.

Sample Question

I _____ shopping in an hour.

    a. go

    b. have gone

    c. am going to go

    d. went

How to Answer This Type of Question

1. First examine the question for clues about the time frame.

"In an hour" clearly identifies the action as taking place in the future.

2. Examine the choices and eliminate any obviously incorrect answers.

Choice A is the simple present tense and can also be eliminated.

Choice B is the past perfect and can be eliminated.

Choice C is the correct answer.

Choice D is the past tense and can be eliminated.

7. The Past Perfect Progressive Tense

How to Recognize This Tense

I *had been sleeping* for an hour when you phoned.

We *had been eating* our dinner when they all came into the dining room.

About the Past Perfect Progressive Tense

This tense is used to show that the action had been going on for a period of time in the past when another action, also in the past, occurred.

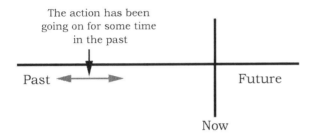

Past Perfect Tense Construction

The tense is formed by using the past perfect tense of the verb "to be" plus the present participle of the main verb.

Sample Question

How long _____ you _____ when I saw you?

    a. are _____ running

    b. had _____ running

    c. had _____ been running

    d. was _____ running

How to Answer This Type of Question

1. First examine the question for clues about the time frame.

"When I saw" tells us the sentence happened at a point of time ("when") in the past ("saw").

2. Examine the choices and eliminate any obviously incorrect answers.

Choice A, "are running" is incorrect and can be eliminated.

Choice B, "Had ___ running" is grammatically incorrect and can be eliminated.

Choice C is correct.

Choice D is grammatically incorrect so the answer is Choice C.

8. Future Perfect Progressive Tense

How to Recognize This Tense

I *will have been working* here for two years in March.

I *will have been driving* for four hours when I get there, so I will be tired.

About the Future Perfect Progressive Tense

This tense is used to show that the action continues up to a point of time in the future.

Future Prefect Progressive Tense Construction

This tense is formed by using the future perfect tense of "to be" plus the present participle of the main verb.

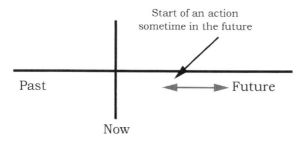

Sample Question

_____ you _____ all the time I am gone?

    a. have _____ been working

    b. will _____ have been working

    c. are _____ worked

    d. will _____ worked

How to Answer This Type of Question

1. First examine the question for clues about the time frame.

"All the time I am gone" refers to an action in the future ("time I am gone") and the action is progressive ("all the time"). The progressive action means the correct choice will be a verb tense that ends in "ing."

2. Examine the choices and eliminate any obviously incorrect answers.

Choice A, the past perfect, refers to a past continuous event and is also grammatically incorrect in the sentence, so Choice A can be eliminated.

Choice B looks correct because it refers to an action will be going on for a period of time in the future.

Examine Choices C and D just to be sure. Both choices are grammatically incorrect and can be eliminated.
Choice B is the correct answer.

9. The Future Perfect Tense

How to Recognize This Tense

By next November, I *will have received* my promotion.

By the time he gets home, she is going *to have cleaned* the entire house.

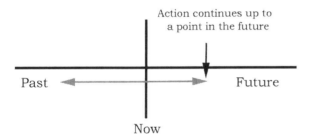

About the Future Perfect Tense

The future perfect tense expresses action in the future before another action in the future. This is the past in the future. For example:

He *will have prepared* dinner when she arrives.

Future Perfect Tense Construction

This tense is formed by "will + have + past participle."

Sample Question

They _____ their seats before the game begins.

    a. will have find

    b. will find

    c. will have found

    d. found

How to Answer This Type of Question

1. First examine the question for clues about the time frame.

This question could be several different tenses. The only clue about the time frame is "before the game begins," which refers to a specific point of time.

We know it isn't in the past, because "begins" is incorrect for the past tense. Similarly with the present. So the question is about something that happens in the future, before another event in the future.

2. Examine the choices and eliminate any obviously incorrect answers.

Choice A can be eliminated as incorrect.
Choice B looks good, so mark it and check the others before making a final decision.
Choice C is the past perfect and can be eliminated because the time frame is incorrect.
Choice D is the simple past tense and can be eliminated for the same reason.

10. Future Progressive Tense

How to Recognize This Tense

The teams *will be playing* soccer when we arrive.

At 3:45 the soccer fans *will be waiting* for the game to start at 4:00 o'clock

At 3:45 the soccer players *will be preparing* to play at 4:00 o'clock

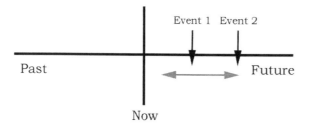

About the Future Progressive Tense

The future progressive tense talks about a continuing action in the future.

Future Progressive Tense Construction

will+ be + (root form) + ing = will be playing

Sample Question

Many excited fans _____ a bus to see the game at 4:00.

     a. catch

     b. catching

     c. have been catching

     d. will be catching

How to Answer This Type of Question

1. First examine the question for clues about the time frame.

"At 4:00," tells us the sentence is either in the past OR in the future.

2. Examine the choices and eliminate any obviously incorrect answers.

From the time frame of the sentence, the answer will be past or future tense.

Choice A is the present tense and can be eliminated.
Choice B is the present continuous tense and can be eliminated.
Choice C is the past perfect continuous and can be eliminated.
Choice D is the only one left. Quickly examining the tense, it is future progressive and is correct in the sentence.

11. The Past Perfect Tense

How to Recognize This Tense

The party *had* just *started* when the coach arrived.

We *had waited* for twenty minutes when the bus finally came.

About the Past Perfect

The past perfect tense talks about two events that happened in the past and establishes which event happened first.

Complete Test Preparation

Another example is, "We had eaten when he arrived."

The two events are "eat" and "he arrived." From the sentence above the past perfect tense tells us the first event, "eat" happened before the second event, "he arrived."

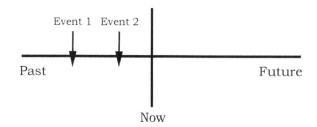

I had already eaten when my friends arrived.

Past Perfect Tense Construction

The past perfect is formed by "have" plus the past participle.

Sample Question

It was time to go home after they _____ the game.

     a. will win

     b. win

     c. had won

     d. wins

How to Answer This Type of Question

1. First examine the question for clues about the time frame.

"Was" tells us the sentence happened in the past. Also notice there are two events, "go home" and "after the game."

2. Examine the choices and eliminate any obviously incorrect answers.

Choice A is the future tense and can be eliminated. Choice B is the simple present and can be eliminated. Choice C is the past perfect and orders the two events in the past. Choice D is the present tense and incorrect and can be eliminated, so Choice C is the correct answer.

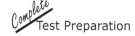

Common English Usage Mistakes - A Quick Review

Like some parts of English grammar, usage is definitely going to be on the exam and there isn't any tricky strategies or shortcuts to help you get through this section. Here is a quick review of common usage mistakes.

1. May and Might

'May' can act as a principal verb, which can express permission or possibility.

Examples:

Lets wait, the meeting may have started.
May I begin now?

'May' can act as an auxiliary verb, which an expresses a purpose or wish

Examples:

May you find favour in the sight of your employer.

May your wishes come true.
People go to school so that they may be educated.

The past tense of may is might.

Examples:

I asked if I might begin

'Might' can be used to signify a weak or slim possibility or polite suggestion.

Examples:

You might find him in his office, but I doubt it.
You might offer to help if you want to.

2. Lie and Lay

The verb lay should always take an object. The three forms of the verb lay are: laid, lay and laid.

The verb lie (recline) should not take any object. The three forms of the verb lie are: lay, lie and lain.

Complete Test Preparation

Examples:

Lay on the bed.
The tables were laid by the students.
Let the little kid lie.
The patient lay on the table.

The dog has lain there for 30 minutes.

Note: The verb lie can also mean "to tell a falsehood". This verb can appear in three forms: lied, lie, and lied. This is different from the verb lie (recline) mentioned above.

Examples:

The accused is fond of telling lies.
Did she lie?

3. Would and should

The past tense of shall is 'should', and so "should" generally follows the same principles as "shall."

The past tense of will is "would," and so "would" generally follows the same principles as "will."

The two verbs 'would and should' can be correctly used interchangeably to signify obligation. The two verbs also have some unique uses too. Should is used in three persons to signify obligation.

Examples:

I should go after work.
People should do exercises everyday.
You should be generous.

"Would" is specially used in any of the three persons, to signify willingness, determination and habitual action.

Examples:

They would go for a test run every Saturday.
They would not ignore their duties.
She would try to be punctual.

 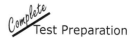

4. Principle and Auxiliary Verbs

Two principal verbs can be used along with one auxiliary verb as long as the auxiliary verb form suits the two principal verbs.

Examples:

A number of people have been employed and some promoted.

A new tree has been planted and the old has been cut down.

Again note the difference in the verb form.

5. Can and Could

A. Can is used to express capacity or ability.

Examples:

I can complete the assignment today
He can meet up with his target.
B. Can is also used to express permission.

Examples:

Yes, you can begin

In the sentence below, "can" was used to mean the same thing as "may." However, the difference is that the word "can" is used for negative or interrogative sentences, while "may" is used in affirmative sentences to express possibility.

Examples:

They may be correct.   Positive sentence - use may.
Can this statement be correct? A question using "can."
It cannot be correct. Negative sentence using "can."

The past tense of can is could. It can serve as a principal verb when it is used to express its own meaning.

Examples:

In spite of the difficulty of the test, he could still perform well.
"Could" here is used to express ability.

 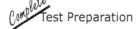

6. Ought

The verb ought should normally be followed by the word to.

Examples:

I *ought to* close shop now.

The verb 'ought' can be used to express:

A. Desirability

You ought to wash your hands before eating.   It is desirable to wash your hands.

B. Probability

She ought to be on her way back by now.   She is probably on her way.

C. Moral obligation or duty

The government ought to protect the oppressed.   It is the government's duty to protect the oppressed.

7. Raise and Rise

Rise
The verb rise means to go up, or to ascend.
The verb rise can appear in three forms, rose, rise, and risen. The verb should not take an object.

Examples:

The bird rose very slowly.
The trees rise above the house.
My aunt has risen in her career.

Raise
The verb raise means to increase, to lift up.
The verb raise can appear in three forms, raised, raise and raised.

Examples:

Complete Test Preparation

He raised his hand.
The workers requested a raise.
Do not raise that subject.

8. Past Tense and Past Participle

Pay attention to the proper use these verbs: sing, show, ring, awake, fly, flow, begin, hang and sink.

Mistakes usually occur when using the past participle and past tense of these verbs as they are often mixed up.

Each of these verbs can appear in three forms:

Sing, Sang, Sung.
Show, Showed, Showed/Shown.
Ring, Rang, Rung.
Awake, awoke, awaken
Fly, Flew, Flown.
Flow, Flowed, Flowed.
Begin, Began, Begun.
Hang, Hanged, Hanged (a criminal)
Hang, Hung, Hung (a picture)
Sink, Sank, Sunk.

Examples:

The stranger rang the door bell. (simple past tense)
I have rung the door bell already. (past participle - an action completed in the past)

The stone sank in the river. (simple past tense)
The stone had already sunk. (past participle - an action completed in the past)

The meeting began at 4:00.
The meeting has begun.

9. Shall and Will

When speaking informally, the two can be used interchangeably. In formal writing, they must be used correctly.

"Will" is used in the second or third person, while "shall" is used in the first person. Both verbs are used to express a time or even in the future.

 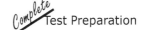

Examples:
I shall, We shall (First Person)
You will (Second Person)
They will (Third Person)

This principle however reverses when the verbs are to be used to express threats, determination, command, willingness, promise or compulsion. In these instances, will is now used in first person and shall in the second and third person.

Examples:

I will be there next week, no matter what.
This is a promise, so the first person "I" takes "will."

You shall ensure that the work is completed.
This is a command, so the second person "you" takes "shall."

I will try to make payments as promised.
This is a promise, so the first person "I" takes "will."

They shall have arrived by the end of the day.
This is a determination, so the third person "they" takes shall.

Note
A. The two verbs, shall and will should not occur twice in the same sentence when the same future is being referred to

Example:

I shall arrive early if my driver is here on time.

B. Will should not be used in the first person when questions are being asked

Examples:

Shall I go ?
Shall we go?

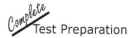

Subject Verb Agreement

Verbs in any sentence must agree with the subject of the sentence both in person and number. Problems usually occur when the verb doesn't correspond with the right subject or the verb fails to match the noun close to it.

Unfortunately, there is no easy way around these principals - no tricky strategy or easy rule. You just have to memorize them.

Here is a quick review:

The verb to be, present (past)

Person	Singular	Plural
First	I am (was)	we are (were)
Second	you are (were)	you are (were)
Third	he, she, it is (was)	they are (were)

The verb to have, present (past)

Person	Singular	Plural
First	I have (had)	we have (had)
Second	you have (had)	you have (had)
Third	he, she, it has (had)	they have (had)

Regular verbs, e.g. to walk, present (past)

Person	Singular	Plural
First	I walk (walked)	we walk (walked)
Second	you walk (walked)	you walk (walked)
Third	he, she, it walks (walked)	they work (walked)

1. Every and Each

When nouns are qualified by "every" or "each," they take a singular verb even if they are joined by 'and'

Examples:

Each mother and daughter *was* a given separate test.
Every teacher and student *was* properly welcomed.

2. Plural Nouns

Nouns like measles, tongs, trousers, riches, scissors etc. are all plural.

Examples:

The trousers *are* dirty.
My scissors *have* gone missing.
The tongs *are* on the table.

3. With and As Well

Two subjects linked with "with" or "as well" should have a verb that matches the first subject.

Examples:

The pencil, with the papers and equipment, *is* on the desk.
David as well as Louis is coming.

4. Plural Nouns

The following nouns take a singular verb:

> politics, mathematics, innings, news, advice, summons, furniture, information, poetry, machinery, vacation, scenery

Examples:

The machinery *is* difficult to assemble
The furniture *has* been delivered
The scenery *was* beautiful

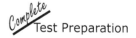

5. Single Entities

A proper noun in plural form that refers to a single entity requires a singular verb. This is a complicated way of saying; some things appear to be plural, but are really singular, or some nouns refer to a collection of things but the collection is really singular.

Examples:

The United Nations Organization *is* the decision maker in the matter.

Here the "United Nations Organization" is really only one "thing" or noun, but is made up of many "nations."

The book, "The Seven Virgins" *was* not available in the library.

Here there is only one book, although the title of the book is plural.

6. Specific Amounts are always singular

A plural noun that refers to a specific amount or quantity that is considered as a whole (dozen, hundred, score etc) requires a singular verb.

Examples:

60 minutes *is* quite a long time.
Here "60 minutes" is considered a whole, and therefore one item (singular noun).

The first million is the most difficult.

7. Either, Neither and Each are always singular

The verb is always singular when used with: either, each, neither, every one and many.

Examples:

Either of the boys *is* lying.
Each of the employees *has* been well compensated
Many a police officer *has* been found to be courageous
Every one of the teachers *is* responsible

 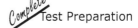

8. Linking with Either, Or, and Neither match the second subject

Two subjects linked by "either," "or,""nor" or "neither" should have a verb that matches the second subject.

Examples:

Neither David nor Paul *will* be coming.
Either Mary or Tina *is* paying.

Note
If one of the subjects linked by "either," "or,""nor" or "neither" is in plural form, then the verb should also be in plural, and the verb should be close to the plural subject.

Examples:
Neither the mother *nor* her kids *have* eaten.
Either Mary *or* her *friends are* paying.

9. Collective Nouns are Plural

Some collective nouns such as poultry, gentry, cattle, vermin etc. are considered plural and require a plural verb.

Examples:

The *poultry are* sick.
The *cattle are* well fed.

Note
Collective nouns involving people can work with both plural and singular verbs.

Examples:

Nigerians are known to be hard working
Europeans live in Africa

10. Nouns that are Singular and Plural

Nouns like deer, sheep, swine, salmon etc. can be singular or plural and require the same verb form.

 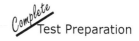

Examples:

The swine is feeding. (singular)
The swine are feeding. (plural)

The salmon is on the table. (singular)
The salmon are running upstream. (plural)

11. Collective Nouns are Singular

Collective nouns such as Army, Jury, Assembly, Committee, Team etc should carry a singular verb when they subscribe to one idea. If the ideas or views are more than one, then the verb used should be plural.

Examples:

The committee is in agreement in their decision.

The committee were in disagreement in their decision.
The jury has agreed on a verdict.
The jury were unable to agree on a verdict.

12. Subjects links by "and" are plural.

Two subjects linked by "and" always require a plural verb

Examples:

David and John are students.

Note
If the subjects linked by "and" are used as one phrase, or constitute one idea, then the verb must be singular

The color of his socks and shoe is black.
Here "socks and shoe" are two nouns, however the subject is "color" which is singular.

 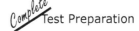

Help with Building your Vocabulary

Vocabulary tests can be daunting when you think of the enormous number of words that might come up in the exam. As the exam date draws near, your anxiety will grow because you know that no matter how many words you memorize, chances are, you will still remember so few. Here are some tips which you can use to hurdle the big words that may come up in your exam without having to open the dictionary and memorize all the words known to humankind.

Build up and tear apart the big words. Big words, like many other things, are composed of small parts. Some words are made up of many other words. A man who lifts weights for example, is a weight lifter. Words are also made up of word parts called prefixes, suffixes and roots. Often times, we can see the relationship of different words through these parts. A person who is skilled with both hands is ambidextrous. A word with double meaning is ambiguous. A person with two conflicting emotions is ambivalent. Two words with synonymous meanings often have the same root. Bio, a root word derived from Latin is used in words like biography meaning to write about a person's life, and biology meaning the study of living organisms.

- **Words with double meanings.** Did you know that the word husband not only means a man married to a woman, but also thrift or frugality? Sometimes, words have double meanings. The dictionary meaning, or the denotation of a word is sometimes different from the way we use it or its connotation.

- **Read widely, read deeply and read daily.** The best way to expand your vocabulary is to familiarize yourself with as many words as possible through reading. By reading, you are able to remember words in a proper context and thus, remember its meaning or at the very least, its use. Reading widely would help you get acquainted with words you may never use every day. This is the best strategy without doubt. However, if you are studying for an exam next week, or even tomorrow, it isn't much help! Below you will find a range of different ways to learn new words quickly and efficiently.

- **Remember.** Always remember that big words are easy to understand when divided into smaller parts, and the smaller words will often have several other meanings aside from the one you already know. Below is an extensive list of root or stem words, followed by one hundred questions to help you learn word stems.

Here are suggested effective ways to help you improve your vocabulary.

Be Committed To Learning New Words. To improve your vocabulary you need to make a commitment to learn new words. Commit to learning at least a word or two a day. You can also get new words by reading books, poems, stories, plays and magazines. Expose yourself to more language to increase the number of new words that you learn.

- **Learn Practical Vocabulary**. As much as possible, learn vocabulary that is associated with what you do and that you can use regularly. For example learn words related to your profession or hobby. Learn as much vocabulary as you can in your favorite subjects.

 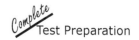

- **Use New Words Frequently**. As soon as you learn a new word start using it and do so frequently. Repeat it when you are alone and try to use the word as often as you can with people you talk to. You can also use flashcards to practice new words that you learn.

- **Learn the Proper Usage.** If you do not understand the proper usage, look it up and make sure you have it right.

- **Use a Dictionary**. When reading textbooks, novels or assigned readings, keep the dictionary nearby. Also learn how to use online dictionaries and WORD dictionary. As soon as you come across a new word, check for its meaning. If you cannot do so immediately, then you should right it down and check it as soon as possible. This will help you understand what the word means and exactly how best to use it.

- **Learn Word Roots, Prefixes and Suffixes.** English words are usually derived from suffixes, prefixes and roots, which come from Latin, French or Greek. Learning the root or origin of a word helps you easily understand the meaning of the word and other words that are derived from the root. Generally, if you learn the meaning of one root word, you will understand two or three words. See our List of Stem Words below. This is a great two-for-one strategy. Most prefixes, suffixes, roots and stems are used in two, three or more words, so if you know the root, prefix or suffix, you can guess the meaning of many words.

- **Synonyms and Antonyms**. Most words in the English language have two or three (at least) synonyms and antonyms. For example, "big," in the most common usage, has about seventy-five synonyms and an equal number of antonyms. Understanding the relationships between these words and how they all fit together gives your brain a framework, which makes them easier to learn, remember and recall.

- **Use Flash Cards**. Flash cards are one of the best ways to memorize things. They can be used anywhere and anytime, so you can make use of odd free moments waiting for the bus or waiting in line. Make your own or buy commercially prepared flash cards, and keep them with you all the time.

- **Make word lists.** Learning vocabulary, like learning many things, requires repetition. Keep a new words journal in a separate section or separate notebook. Add any words that you look up in the dictionary, as well as from word lists. Review your word lists regularly.

Photocopying or printing off word lists from the Internet or handouts is not the same. Actually writing out the word and a few notes on the definition is an important process for imprinting the word in your brain. Writing out the word and definition in your New Word Journal, forces you to concentrate and focus on the new word. Hitting PRINT or pushing the button on the photocopier does not do the same thing.

Notice the verbs in bold in the examples above. They are encircling the subjects of each sentence rather than following them. This is inverse word order.

 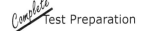

Science Self-Assessment and Tutorials

T HIS SECTION CONTAINS A SELF-ASSESSMENT AND GENERAL SCIENCE TUTORIALS. The Tutorials are designed to familiarize general principals and the Self-Assessment contains general questions similar to the Science questions likely to be on the HESI exam, but are not intended to be identical to the exam questions. Many Universities recommend that students take an introductory science course before taking the HESI Exam. The tutorials are not designed to be a complete science course, and it is assumed that students have some familiarity with science. If you do not understand parts of the tutorial, or find the tutorial difficult, it is recommended that you seek out additional instruction.

The Science Self-Assessment covers basic physics, biology, chemistry, physiology and anatomy. The purpose of the self-assessment is:

- Identify your strengths and weaknesses.

- Develop your personalized study plan (above)

- Get accustomed to the HESI format

- Extra practice – the self-assessment is a 3rd test!

Since this is a self-assessment, and depending on how confident you are with basic science, timing yourself is optional. There are a total of 75 questions (25 biology, 25 chemistry and 25 Anatomy and Physiology) which must be answered in 75 minutes. The self-assessment has 25 questions, so allow 25 minutes to complete this assessment.

The questions below are not exactly the same as you will find on the HESI - that would be too easy! And nobody knows what the questions will be and they change all the time. Below are general Science questions that cover the same areas as the HESI. So while the format and exact wording of the questions may differ slightly, and change from year to year, if you can answer the questions below, you will have no problem with the Science section of the HESI.

NOTE: The Science section is an optional module that not all schools include. We strongly suggest that you check with your school for the HESI A2 exam details. It is always a good idea to give the materials you receive when you register to take the HESI a careful review.

The self-assessment is designed to give you a baseline score in the different areas covered. Here is a brief outline of how your score on the self-assessment relates to your understanding of the material.

75% - 100%	Excellent – you have mastered the content
50 – 75%	Good. You have a working knowledge. Even though you can just pass this section, you may want to review the Tutorials and do some extra practice to see if you can improve your mark.
25% - 50%	Below Average. You do not understand the content. Review the tutorials, and retake this quiz again in a few days, before proceeding to the rest of the Practice Test Course.
Less than 25%	Poor. You have a very limited understanding. Please review the Tutorials, and retake this quiz again in a few days, before proceeding to the rest of the course.

 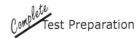

Science Self Assessment Answer Sheet

1. (A) (B) (C) (D)   11. (A) (B) (C) (D)   21. (A) (B) (C) (D)

2. (A) (B) (C) (D)   12. (A) (B) (C) (D)   22. (A) (B) (C) (D)

3. (A) (B) (C) (D)   13. (A) (B) (C) (D)   23. (A) (B) (C) (D)

4. (A) (B) (C) (D)   14. (A) (B) (C) (D)   24. (A) (B) (C) (D)

5. (A) (B) (C) (D)   15. (A) (B) (C) (D)   25. (A) (B) (C) (D)

6. (A) (B) (C) (D)   16. (A) (B) (C) (D)

7. (A) (B) (C) (D)   17. (A) (B) (C) (D)

8. (A) (B) (C) (D)   18. (A) (B) (C) (D)

9. (A) (B) (C) (D)   19. (A) (B) (C) (D)

10. (A) (B) (C) (D)   20. (A) (B) (C) (D)

Physics

1. Which of the following is not true of atomic theory?

a. Originated in the early 19th century with the work of John Dalton.

b. Is the field of physics that describes the characteristics and properties of atoms that make up matter.

c. Explains temperature as the momentum of atoms.

d. Explains macroscopic phenomenon through the behavior of microscopic atoms.

2. Which of these statements about atoms is/are incorrect?

a. Are the largest unit of matter that can take part in a chemical reaction.

b. Can be chemically broken down into much simpler forms.

c. Are composed of protons and neutrons in a central nucleus surrounded by electrons.

d. Do not differ in terms of atomic number or atomic mass.

3. Protons, neutrons, and electrons differ in that:

a. Protons and neutrons form the nucleus of an atom, while electrons are found in fixed energy levels around the nucleus of the atom.

b. Protons and neutrons are charged particles and electrons are neutral.

c. Protons and neutrons form fixed energy levels around the nucleus of the atom and electrons are located near the surface of the atom.

d. Protons, neutrons and electrons are charged particles.

4. Which of the statements about quantum theory is/are false?

a. Quantum theory is concerned with the emission and absorption of energy by matter and with the motion of material particles.

b. Quantum mechanics, a system based on quantum theory, has superseded Newtonian mechanics in the interpretation of physical phenomena on the atomic scale.

c. In quantum theory, energy is treated solely as a continuous phenomenon, while matter is assumed to occupy a very specific region of space and to move in a continuous manner.

d. Quantum theory states that energy is held to be emitted and absorbed in tiny, discrete amounts called quantum.

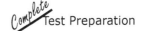

5. Newton's laws of motion consist of three physical laws that form the basis for classical mechanics. Which of the following is/are not included in these laws?

a. Unless acted upon by a force, a body at rest stays at rest.

b. Unless acted upon by a force, a body in motion will change direction and gradually slow until it eventually stops.

c. To every action, there is an equal and opposite reaction.

d. A body acted upon by a force will accelerate in the same direction as the force at a magnitude that is directly proportional to the force.

Biology

6. A _____ _____ is the sequence of developmental stages through which members of a given species must pass.

a. Life cycle

b. Life expectancy

c. Life sequence

d. None of the above

7. Life _____ are the _____ and _____ activities that all _____ systems must be able to carry out in order to maintain life.

a. Life sequences are the chemical and biological activities that all living systems must be able to carry out in order to maintain life.

b. Life expectancies are the biochemical and biophysical activities that all sentient systems must be able to carry out in order to maintain life.

c. Life cycles are the organic and inorganic activities that all living systems must be able to carry out in order to maintain life.

d. Life functions are the biochemical and biophysical activities that all living systems must be able to carry out in order to maintain life.

8. Nutrition is the sum total of activities through which a living organism obtains food; what are the three processes included in nutrition?

a. Ingestion, digestion, and adsorption

b. Ingestion, diffusion, and assimilation

c. Ingestion, digestion, and assimilation

d. Incorporation, digestion, and assimilation

9. _____ is the taking in of food, _____ refers to the chemical changes that take place in the body, and _____ involves the changing of certain nutrients into the protoplasm of cells.

a. Assimilation is the taking in of food, digestion refers to the chemical changes that take place in the body, and ingestion involves the changing of certain nutrients into the protoplasm of cells.

b. Ingestion is the taking in of food, digestion refers to the chemical changes that take place in the body, and assimilation involves the changing of certain nutrients into the protoplasm of cells.

c. Digestion is the taking in of food, ingestion refers to the chemical changes that take place in the body, and assimilation involves the changing of certain nutrients into the protoplasm of cells.

d. Ingestion is the taking in of food, digestion refers to the chemical changes that take place in the body, and diffusion involves the changing of certain nutrients into the protoplasm of cells.

10. The movement of molecules other than water from an area of ____ concentration to an area of _____ concentration is _____.

a. The movement of molecules other than water from an area of high concentration to an area of less concentration is diffusion.

b. The movement of molecules other than water from an area of less concentration to an area of high concentration is diffusion.

c. The movement of molecules other than water from an area of high concentration to an area of less concentration is osmosis.

d. The movement of molecules other than water from an area of lesser concentration to an area of less concentration is dispersal.

11. During _____, a solvent moves through a/an _____ membrane from an area with a_____ concentration of solvents to areas of _____ concentration.

a. During diffusion, a solvent moves through a semipermeable membrane from an area with a lesser concentration of solvents to areas of greater concentration.

b. During osmosis, a solvent moves through an impermeable membrane from an area with a lesser concentration of solvents to areas of greater concentration.

c. During osmosis, a solvent moves through a semipermeable membrane from an area with a greater concentration of solvents to areas of lesser concentration.

d. During osmosis, a solvent moves through a semipermeable membrane from an area with a lesser concentration of solvents to areas of greater concentration.

12. _____ and _____ are forms of _____ transport by which materials pass through plasma membranes.

    a. Diffusion and osmosis are forms of active transport by which materials pass through plasma membranes.

    b. Diffusion and osmosis are forms of passive transport by which materials pass through plasma membranes.

    c. Dispersal and osmosis are forms of passive transport by which materials pass through plasma membranes.

    d. Diffusion and synthesis are forms of active transport by which materials pass through plasma membranes.

13. The scientific discipline that studies the physiological aspects, structures, life cycles and division of cells is called _____.

    a. The scientific discipline that studies the physiological aspects, structures, life cycles and division of cells is called physiology.

    b. The scientific discipline that studies the physiological aspects, structures, life cycles and division of cells is called cell science.

    c. The scientific discipline that studies the physiological aspects, structures, life cycles and division of cells is called biochemistry.

    d. The scientific discipline that studies the physiological aspects, structures, life cycles and division of cells is called cell biology.

14. Which, if any, of the following statements about mitosis are correct?

    a. Mitosis is the process of cell division by which identical daughter cells are produced.

    b. Following mitosis, new cells contain less DNA than did the original cells.

    c. During mitosis, the chromosome number is doubled.

    d. A and C are correct.

15. Which, if any, of the following statements about meiosis are correct?

    a. During meiosis, the number of chromosomes in the cell is halved.

    b. Meiosis only occurs in eukaryotic cells.

    c. Meiosis is the part of the life cycle that involves sexual reproduction.

    d. All of these statements are correct.

Chemistry

16. What are the differences, if any, between mixtures and compounds?

a. A mixture is homogeneous, and the properties of its components are retained, while a compound is heterogeneous and its properties are distinct from those of the elements combined in its formation.

b. A mixture is heterogeneous, and the properties of its components are retained, while a compound is homogeneous and its properties are distinct from those of the elements combined in its formation.

c. A mixture is heterogeneous, and the properties of its components are changed, while a compound is homogeneous and its properties are similar to those of the elements combined in its formation.

d. A compound is heterogeneous, and the properties of its components are retained, while a mixture is homogeneous and its properties are distinct from those of the elements combined in its formation.

17. What are the differences, if any, between chemical changes and physical changes?

a. During a physical change, some aspect of the physical properties of matter is altered, but the identity of the substance remains constant. Chemical changes involve the alteration of both a substance's composition and structure.

b. During a chemical change, some aspect of the physical properties of matter is altered, but the identity of the substance remains constant. Physical changes involve the alteration of both a substance's composition and structure.

c. During a physical change, no aspects of the physical properties of matter are altered, but the identity of the substance remains constant. Chemical changes involve the alteration of both a substance's composition and structure.

d. There is no substantive difference between chemical and physical changes.

18. $\Delta H = H_{products} - H_{reactants}$ is the formula used to determine a _____.

a. Change in hydration

b. Change in haploid bond

c. Change in heat content

d. Change in hypothesis

 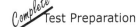

19. In an _____ reaction, the heat content of the products is _____ than the heat content of the reactants, while in an _____ reaction, the heat content of the products is _____ than the heat content of the reactants.

    a. Exothermic, greater, endothermic, less

    b. Endothermic, less, exothermic, greater

    c. Exothermic, greater, exothermic, less

    d. Endothermic, greater, exothermic, less

20. The equation $E = mc^2$ is based on the _____, and states that _____ equals _____ times the _____^{2}.

    a. The equation $E = mc^2$ is based on the 2nd Law of Thermodynamics, and states that Mass equals Energy times (the Velocity of light)^2.

    b. The equation $E = mc^2$ is based on the Law of Conservation of Mass and Energy, and states that Energy equals Mass times (the Velocity of light)^2.

    c. The equation $E = mc^2$ is based on the 1st Law of Thermodynamics, and states that Mass equals Energy times (the Velocity of sound)^2.

    d. The equation $E = mc^2$ is based on the Law of Conservation of Mass and Energy, and states that the Velocity of light equals Energy times (the Mass)^2.

21. When a measurement is recorded, it includes the _____ _____, which are all the digits that are certain plus one uncertain digit.

    a. Major figures

    b. Significant figures

    c. Relative figures

    d. Relevant figures

22. The _____ _____ is based on the lowest theoretical temperature, called _____ _____.

    a. Kelvin scale, absolute zero

    b. Celsius scale, absolute zero

    c. Kelvin scale, boiling point of water

    d. Centigrade scale, freezing point of water

23. Through experiments and calculations, _____ _____ has been verified to be _____° on the _____ scale.

a. Through experiments and calculations, absolute zero has been verified to be −273.15° on the Celsius scale.

b. Through experiments and calculations, unconditional zero has been verified to be 0° on the Kelvin scale.

c. Through experiments and calculations, absolute null has been verified to be -100° on the Celsius scale.

d. Through experiments and calculations, absolute zero has been verified to be −273.15° on the Kelvin scale.

24. When using the scientific notation system to express large numbers, move the _____ _____ until _____ digit(s) remain(s) to the left, then indicate the number of moves of the decimal point as the _____ _ ___.

a. When using the scientific notation system to express large numbers, move the decimal point until only two digits remain to the left, then indicate the number of moves of the decimal point as the exponent of 10.

b. When using the scientific notation system to express large numbers, move the decimal until only one digit remains to the left, then indicate the number of moves of the decimal point as the exponent of 2.

c. When using the scientific notation system to express large numbers, move the decimal until only three digits remain to the left, then indicate the number of moves of the decimal point as the exponent of 10.

d. When using the scientific notation system to express large numbers, move the decimal until only one digit remains to the left, then indicate the number of moves of the decimal point as the exponent of 10.

25. In science, _____ indicates the _____ or _____ of a measurement, while _____ indicates the _____ of a measurement to its known or accepted value.

a. In science, accuracy indicates the reliability or reproducibility of a measurement, while precision indicates the proximity of a measurement to its known or accepted value.

b. In science, exactitude indicates the reliability or reproducibility of a measurement, while contiguity indicates the remoteness of a measurement to its known or accepted value.

c. In science, precision indicates the reliability or reproducibility of a measurement, while accuracy indicates the proximity of a measurement to its known or accepted value.

d. In science, uncertainty indicates the realism or possibility of a measurement, while precision indicates the distance of a measurement to its known or accepted value.

Science Self-Assessment Answer Key

1. C
Answer c is incorrect because atomic theory explains temperature as the motion of atoms (faster = hotter), not the momentum. The momentum of atoms explains the outward pressure that they exert.[4]

2. D
The atoms of different elements differ in atomic number, relative atomic mass, and chemical behavior

3. A
Protons and neutrons form the nucleus of an atom, while electrons are found in fixed energy levels around the nucleus of the atom.

4. C
In quantum theory, energy is treated solely as a continuous phenomenon, while matter is assumed to occupy a very specific region of space and to move in a continuous manner.

5. B
Unless acted upon by a force, a body in motion will change direction and gradually slow until it eventually stops.
This answer is related to Newton's 1st law of motion that states that, unless acted upon by a force, a body at rest stays at rest, and a moving body continues moving at the same speed in a straight line.[4]

Biology

6. A
A **life cycle** is the sequence of developmental stages through which members of a given species must pass.

7. D
Life functions are the biochemical and biophysical activities that all living systems must be able to carry out in order to maintain life.

8. C
The three processes included in nutrition are, **ingestion, digestion, and assimilation.**

9. C
Ingestion is the taking in of food, **digestion** refers to the chemical changes that take place in the body, and **assimilation** involves the changing of certain nutrients into the protoplasm of cells.

 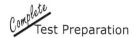

10. A
The movement of molecules other than water from an area of **high** concentration to an area of **less** concentration is **diffusion**.

11. D
During osmosis, a solvent moves through a/an semi permeable membrane from an area with a lesser concentration of solvents to areas of greater concentration.

12. B
Diffusion and **osmosis** are forms of passive transport by which materials pass through plasma membranes.

13. D
The scientific discipline that studies the physiological aspects, structures, life cycles and   division of cells is called **cell biology**.

14. A and C are correct.

   a. Mitosis is the process of cell division by which a cell produces identical daughter cells.

   c. During mitosis, the chromosome number is doubled.

15. D
All of these statements are correct.

Chemistry

16. B
A mixture is heterogeneous, and the properties of its components are retained, while a compound is homogeneous and its properties are distinct from those of the elements combined in its formation.

17. A
During a physical change, some aspects of the physical properties of matter are altered, but the identity of the substance remains constant. Chemical changes involve the alteration of both a substance's composition and structure.
Note: Examples of physical changes include breaking glass, cutting wood and melting ice. Sometimes, the process can be easily reversed. Restoration of the original form is not possible following a chemical change.

18. C
ΔH = Hproducts - Hreactants is the formula used to determine a **change in heat content**.

19. D
In an **Endothermic** reaction, the heat content of the products is **greater** than the heat content of the reactants, while in an **exothermic** reaction, the heat content of the prod-

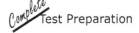

ucts is **less** than the heat content of the reactants.

Because it is virtually impossible to measure the total energy of molecules, the experimental data typically used with reactions is the change in heat content known as enthalpy.

20. B

The equation $E = mc^2$ is based on the **Law of Conservation of Mass and Energy**, and states that **Energy** equals **Mass** times **the Velocity of light**.

21. B

When a measurement is recorded, it includes the **significant figures**, which are all the digits that are certain plus one uncertain digit.

22. A

The Kelvin scale is based on the lowest theoretical temperature, called absolute zero.

23. A

Through experiments and calculations, **absolute zero** has been verified to be **– 273.15°** on the **Celsius** scale.

24. A

When using the scientific notation system to express large numbers, move the **decimal point** until **only two** digits remain to the left, then indicate the number of moves of the decimal point as the **exponent of 10**.

25. C

In science, **precision** indicates the **reliability** or **reproducibility** of a measurement, while **accuracy** indicates the **proximity** of a measurement to its known or accepted value.

Note: Regardless of the precision or accuracy of a measurement, all measurements include a degree of uncertainty, dependent on limitations of the measuring instrument and the skill with which the measurement is completed.

Science Tutorials

Scientific Method

Were it not for the scientific method, people would have no valid method for drawing quantifiable and accurate information about the world. The scientific method is a set of steps that allow people who ask "how" and "why" questions about the world to go about finding valid answers that accurately reflect reality. There are four primary steps to the scientific method: analyzing an aspect of reality and asking "how" or "why" it works or exists, forming a hypothesis that explains "how" or "why," making a prediction about the sort of things that would happen if the hypothesis were true, and performing an experiment to test your prediction.

These steps vary somewhat depending on the field of science you happen to be studying. (In astronomy, for instance, experiments are generally eschewed in favor of observational evidence confirming that predictions are true.) But for the most part this is the model scientists follow.

Observation and Analysis

The first step in the scientific method requires you to determine what it is about reality that you want to explore. You might notice that your friends who eat regular servings of fruits and vegetables are healthier and more athletic than your friends who live off red meat and meals covered in cheese and gravy. This is an observation and, noting it, you are likely to ask yourself "why" it seems to be true. At this stage of the scientific method, scientists will often do research to see if anyone else has explored similar observations and analyze what other people's findings have been. This is an important step not only because it can show you what others have found to be true about their observation, but because it can show what others have found to be false, which can be equally as valuable.

Hypothesis

After making your observation and doing some research, you can form your hypothesis. A hypothesis is an idea you formulate based on the evidence you have already gathered about "how" your observation relates to reality. Using the example of your friends' diets, you may have found research discussing vitamin levels in fruits and vegetables and how certain vitamins will affect a person's health and athleticism. This research may lead you to hypothesize that the foods your healthy friends are eating contain specific types of vitamins, and it is the vitamins making them healthy. Just as importantly, however, is applying research that shows hypotheses that were later proven wrong. Scientists need to know this information, too, as it can help keep them from making errors in their thinking. For instance, you could come across a research paper in which someone hypothesized that the sugars in fruits and vegetables gave people more energy, which then helped them be more athletic. If the paper were to go on to explain that no such link was found, and that the protein and carbohydrates in meat and gravy

 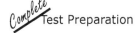

contained far more energy than the sugar, you would know that this hypothesis was wrong and that there was no need for you to waste time exploring it.

Prediction

The third step in the scientific method is making a prediction based on your hypothesis. Forming predictions is vital to the scientific method because if your prediction turns out to be correct, it will demonstrate that your hypothesis can accurately explain some aspect of the world. This is important because one aspect of the scientific method is its ability to prove objectively that your way of understanding the world is valid. We can take the simple example of a car that will not start. If you notice the fuel gauge is pointing towards empty, you can announce your prediction to the other passengers that a careful test of the gas tank will show the car has no fuel. While this seems obvious, it is still important to note since a prediction like this is the only way to really prove to your friends that you understand how a fuel gauge works and what it means.

In the same way a prediction made by a hypothesis is the only way to really show that it represents reality. For instance, based on your vitamin hypothesis you may predict people can be healthy and athletic while eating whatever they want as long as they take vitamin supplements. If this prediction ends up being true, it will show that it is in fact the vitamins, and only the vitamins, in fruits and vegetables that make people healthy and athletic. It will prove that your hypothesis shows how vitamins work.

Experiment

The final step is to perform an experiment that tests your prediction. You may decide to separate your healthy friends into three groups, give one group vitamin supplements and prohibit them from eating vegetables, give another fake supplements and prohibit them from eating vegetables and have the third act normally as the control group. It is always important to have a control group so you have someone acting "normally" to compare your results against. If this experiment shows the real supplement group and the control group maintaining the same level of health and athleticism while the fake supplement group grows weak and sickly, you will know your hypothesis is true. If, on the other hand, you get unexpected results, you will need to go back to step one, analyze your results, make new observations and try again with a different hypothesis.

Any hypothesis that cannot be confirmed with experiment (or in the case of fields such as astronomy, with observation) cannot be considered true and must be altered or abandoned. It is in this stage where scientists—being humans, with human beliefs and prejudices—are most likely to abandon the scientific method. If an experiment or observation gives a scientist results that he or she does not like, the scientist may be inclined to ignore the results rather than reexamine the hypothesis. This was the case for nearly a thousand years in astronomy with astronomers attempting to form accurate models of the solar system based on circular orbits of the planets and on Earth being in the center. For philosophical reasons it was believed that circles were "perfect" and that the Earth was "important," so no model that had the correct elliptical orbits or the sun properly in the center was accepted until the 16th century, even though those models more accurately described all astronomers' observations.

Biology

Biology is a natural science concerned with the study of life and living organisms, including their structure, function, growth, origin, evolution, distribution, and taxonomy. Biology is a vast subject containing many subdivisions, topics, and disciplines. Among the most important topics are five unifying principles that can be said to be the fundamental axioms of modern biology:

- Cells are the basic unit of life

- New species and inherited traits are the product of evolution

- Genes are the basic unit of heredity

- An organism regulates its internal environment to maintain a stable and constant condition

- Living organisms consume and transform energy.

Sub-disciplines of biology are recognized on the basis of the scale at which organisms are studied and the methods used to study them: biochemistry examines the rudimentary chemistry of life; molecular biology studies the complex interactions of systems of biological molecules; cellular biology examines the basic building block of all life, the cell; physiology examines the physical and chemical functions of the tissues, organs, and organ systems of an organism; and ecology examines how various organisms interact and associate with their environment.[6]

Cell Biology

Cell biology (formerly cytology, from the Greek kytos, "contain") is a scientific discipline that studies cells – their physiological properties, their structure, the organelles they contain, interactions with their environment, their life cycle, division and death. This is done both on a microscopic and molecular level. Cell biology research encompasses both the great diversity of single-celled organisms like bacteria and protozoa, as well as the many specialized cells in multi-cellular organisms such as humans.

Knowing the components of cells and how cells work is fundamental to all biological sciences. Appreciating the similarities and differences between cell types is particularly important to the fields of cell and molecular biology as well as to biomedical fields such as cancer research and developmental biology. These fundamental similarities and differences provide a unifying theme, sometimes allowing the principles learned from

 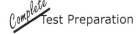

studying one cell type to be extrapolated and generalized to other cell types. Therefore, research in cell biology is closely related to genetics, biochemistry, molecular biology, immunology, and developmental biology.

Each type of protein is usually sent to a particular part of the cell. An important part of cell biology is the investigation of molecular mechanisms by which proteins are moved to different places inside cells or secreted from cells.

Processes – Movement of Proteins

Most proteins are synthesized by ribosomes in the rough endoplasmic reticulum. Ribosomes contain the nucleic acid RNA, which assembles and joins amino acids to make proteins. They can be found alone or in groups within the cytoplasm as well as on the RER. This process is known as protein biosynthesis. Biosynthesis (also called biogenesis) is an enzyme-catalyzed process in cells of living organisms by which substrates are converted to more complex products (also simply known as protein translation). Some proteins, such as those to be incorporated in membranes (known as membrane proteins), are transported into the "rough" endoplasmic reticulum (ER) during synthesis. This process can be followed by transportation and processing in the Golgi apparatus. The Golgi apparatus is a large organelle that processes proteins and prepares them for use both inside and outside the cell. The Golgi apparatus is somewhat like a post office. It receives items (proteins from the ER), packages and labels them, and then sends them on to their destinations (to different parts of the cell or to the cell membrane for transport out of the cell). From the Golgi, membrane proteins can move to the plasma membrane, to other sub-cellular compartments, or they can be secreted from the cell. The ER and Golgi can be thought of as the "membrane protein synthesis compartment" and the "membrane protein processing compartment", respectively. There is a semi-constant flux of proteins through these compartments. ER and Golgi-resident proteins associate with other proteins but remain in their respective compartments. Other proteins "flow" through the ER and Golgi to the plasma membrane. Motor proteins transport membrane protein-containing vesicles along cytoskeletal tracks to distant parts of cells such as axon terminals.

Some proteins that are made in the cytoplasm contain structural features that target them for transport into mitochondria or the nucleus. Some mitochondrial proteins are made inside mitochondria and are coded for by mitochondrial DNA. In plants, chloroplasts also make some cell proteins.

Extracellular and cell surface proteins destined to be degraded can move back into intracellular compartments upon being incorporated into endocytosed vesicles some of which fuse with lysosomes where the proteins are broken down to their individual amino acids. The degradation of some membrane proteins begins while still at the cell surface when they are separated by secretases. Proteins that function in the cytoplasm are often degraded by proteasomes.

Other cellular processes

Active transport and Passive transport - Movement of molecules into and out of cells.

Autophagy - The process whereby cells "eat" their own internal components or microbial invaders.

Adhesion - Holding together cells and tissues.

Reproduction - Made possible by the combination of sperm made in the testiculi (contained in some male cells' nuclei) and the egg made in the ovary (contained in the nucleus of a female cell). When the sperm breaks through the hard outer shell of the egg a new cell embryo is formed, which, in humans, grows to full size in 9 months.

Cell movement - Chemotaxis, Contraction, cilia and flagella.

Cell signaling - Regulation of cell behavior by signals from outside.

DNA repair and Cell death

Metabolism: Glycolysis, respiration, Photosynthesis

Transcription and RNA splicing - gene expression.

Internal cellular structures

Chloroplast - key organelle for photosynthesis (only found in plant cells)

Cilia - motile microtubule-containing structures of eukaryotes

Cytoplasm - contents of the main fluid-filled space inside cells

Cytoskeleton - protein filaments inside cells

Endoplasmic reticulum - major site of membrane protein synthesis

Flagella - motile structures of bacteria, archaea and eukaryotes

Golgi apparatus - site of protein glycosylation in the endomembrane system

Lipid bilayer - fundamental organizational structure of cell membranes

Lysosome - break down cellular waste products and debris into simple compounds (only found in animal cells)

Mitochondrion - major energy-producing organelle by releasing it in the form of ATP

Nucleus - holds most of the DNA of eukaryotic cells and controls all cellular activities

Organelle - term used for major subcellular structures

Ribosome - RNA and protein complex required for protein synthesis in cells

Vesicle - small membrane-bounded spheres inside cells

Heredity: Genes and Mutation

All of the genetic material that tells our cells what jobs they hold is stored in our DNA (deoxyribonucleic acid). When complex creatures such as humans reproduce, our DNA is copied and combined with our mate's DNA to create a new genetic sequence for our offspring. This information is stored in our genes and encoded in DNA base pairs through different combinations of the chemical groupings adenine and thymine (represented by A and T) and guanine and cytosine (represented by G and C). Each gene covers a small portion of our DNA and is responsible for creating the protein that section of DNA holds instructions for.

Genes contain two alleles, one from each of our parents. When we reproduce we will transfer one, and only one, of each allele to our children. Alleles can be either dominant or recessive, and by combining the pairs of alleles we get from our parents, we can determine what our genes say we should be like. This genetic description of ourselves is known as our genotype. Genotype is our exact genetic makeup, and it determines our physical characteristics such as basic hair, eye and skin color. Related to the genotype is our phenotype, which describes the characteristics we display when our genes interact with the environment. For example, skin color is determined by a person's genotype, but the effect the sun has on skin—does the person tan, freckle, bun or even come away without any noticeable effect at all?—is an expression of phenotype.

Under normal circumstances people's genes will transfer directly from their parents following Mendel's Laws of Inheritance. DNA reproduction, however, is not necessarily a flawless process. Errors can develop either at random or due to outside influences such as radiation or chemicals in the environment. These errors, when related to heredity are called de novo mutations; they occur during embryonic development. Some mutations have no effect at all on the person's genetic makeup, but others can alter the way genes express themselves. Whether this is a good thing or not depends entirely on what genes are altered in what ways. Some mutations can cause children to be born sick or to have a higher susceptibility to disease by changing the types of proteins that their genes produce, or even by stopping certain proteins from being produced all together. Others, though, can be an improvement to the child's genetic structure. It is important to remember that the entire process of evolution is based on how random mutations throughout history have affected an individual's ability to interact with the environment.

Several notable examples of beneficial mutations stemming from natural selection can be seen in bubonic plague resistant European populations and malaria resistant African populations. Both groups have genes built from specific alleles that create disease blocking proteins. (The CCR5 protein in people of European descent blocks the plague—and HIV in some cases—and the sickle cell protein in people of African descent blocks malaria.) These genes are widespread throughout their respective populations as a result of natural selection, which killed those who lived in these groups' ancestral regions but who did not possess the mutation. Had these diseases never existed, the mutations would have been considered neutral, providing no benefit yet causing no harm.

There are several ways that errors in DNA reproduction can cause mutations. Chemicals can be inserted into or deleted from base pairs, causing the chemical composition of the pairs to change and, thus, changing the alleles of the gene represented by those pairs.

 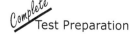

A portion of the DNA strand may also duplicate itself, or it may shift itself, causing the half of the base pair on one side of the DNA strand to link to the wrong half on the other side.

Heredity: Mendelian Inheritance and Punnett Squares

The father of genetics was a 19th century Austrian monk named Gregor Johann Mendel who became famous for his work crossbreeding peas in the garden of his monastery. Aside from his life as a monk, Mendel was a highly educated physicist, studying first at the University of Olomouc (in the modern day Czech Republic) and later at the University of Vienna.

Mendel's work with peas revolutionized the scientific understanding of heredity and yielded two important laws: the Law of Segregation and the Law of Independent Assortment. To better understand these laws, however, we first need to look at the work of another geneticist, Reginald Punnett.

In 1900 while Punnett was doing his graduate work at the University of Cambridge in England, Gregor Mendel's work on genetics, which did not receive much attention during his lifetime, was being rediscovered. Punnett became an early follower of Mendelian genetics and developed the Punnett square as a means to organize the assortment of inherited alleles as Mendel described them. A Punnett square is simply a box with several squares drawn inside of it and with the allele for a particular gene from each parent listed on either the top or the side. Each square shows a possible genotype (or set of alleles that define the gene) that can be inherited by the offspring of those parents. We will see Punnett squares as we explain Mendel's laws.

Law of Segregation

Mendel's Law of Segregation says that only half of the alleles of each parent's genes are transferred to their offspring, with the other half coming from the other parent. Each gene contains two alleles. For instance a gene for trait 'A' could contain the alleles AA, Aa or aa, with the 'A' being the dominant form of the allele and 'a' being the recessive form. (Offspring with one or more dominant alleles exhibit the trait; offspring with only recessive forms do not.) The Law of Segregation says that one allele will come from one parent, and one will come from the other, and it is the parent's combined genetic make-up (rather than one parents particular genotype) that will determine the genes of their offspring.

Mendel also showed that the probability a certain trait would spread from parents to children was 3:1, provided that both parents had one dominant and one recessive form of the gene, also known has having heterozygous alleles. (Having two of the same alleles—AA or aa—is homozygous.) To get a better understanding of this, we can use a Punnett square to demonstrate the process.

 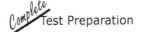

The Punnett square below represents the possible children born to two parents with Aa alleles expressing the 'A' gene.

	A	a
A	**AA**	**Aa**
a	**Aa**	aa

The three genes in bold, with at least one capital letter (AA, Aa and the other Aa), represent cases in which the presence of at least one dominant allele will cause the trait to manifest in the offspring. The remaining one (aa) represents the one case where the child does not manifest the trait even though both his or her parents do. (This could be the one brunette in a family of redheads, for instance.) Provided both parents have one dominant and one recessive allele, the distribution will always be 3:1.

Law of Independent Assortment

Mendel's second law, the Law of Independent Assortment, shows that the alleles of multiple genes will mix independently of one another. When two separate genotypes are tracked, the genes will produce 16 separate possible combinations spread out in a 9:3:3:1 ratio. This is also known as a dihybrid cross, while dealing with a single set of alleles is a monohybrid cross.

We can demonstrate this by assuming that we have a male and a female each with heterozygous alleles making them blond and tall. We can represent this with the genotypes BbTt in each. We should also assume that a 'bb' genotype would give someone brown hair and 'tt' would make them short. Since the Law of Independent Assortment says that each allele will mix independently, we end up with four combinations of genotype that each parent can pass on: BT, Bt, bT and bt. These can then be mapped in a slightly larger Punnett square that looks like this:

	BT	Bt	bT	bt
BT	**BBTT**	**BBTt**	**BbTT**	**BbTt**
Bt	**BBTt**	**BBtt**	**BbTt**	**Bbtt**
bT	**BbTT**	**BbTt**	bbTT	bbTt
bt	**BbTt**	**Bbtt**	bbTt	bbtt

This is the distribution of the tall, blond couple's possible children. Nine would also be tall and blond, three would be short and blond, three would be tall and brunette, and one would be short and brunette. This perfectly follows the 9:3:3:1 ratio set out by Mendel.

Classification

Taxonomic classification is the primary method of organizing the Earth's biology. The earliest form of classification that bears any resemblance to the current system can be traced back to ancient Greece with Aristotle's organization of animals based on reproduction. The true father of modern taxonomical classification, however, is Carolus Linnaeus, who in the early 18th century developed a system of kingdoms that separated life into the categories animal, mineral and vegetable. Although Linnaeus's work lacked what would today be considered essential technologies (such as microscopes capable of imaging bacteria) and theories (such as evolution), much of his system has survived in modern classification.

With Charles Darwin's publication of On the Origin of Species in 1859 the evolutionary process became a major factor in taxonomic classification. For the first time biology could be classified by grouping the direct descendents of common ancestors rather than just grouping creatures with similar characteristics.

Today, the majority of scientists accept a hierarchical structuring of biology that begins, appropriately, with life and then goes from most general to most specific: domain, kingdom, phylum, class, order, family, genus and species. (There are sometimes smaller subcategories such as superfamily, subfamily, tribe and subspecies listed, but these are the primary eight categories.) Domain is the newest of these and is split into three primary groups: Bacteria, Archaea and Eukarya.

Each of these domains is split again with Bacteria splitting into the Kingdom Bacteria, Archaea splitting into the Kingdom Archaea and Eukarya splitting into the four kingdoms of Protista, Plantae, Fungi and finally our kingdom, Animalia. The Domain Eukarya splits so many times because eukaryotic cells are highly complex, containing such important features as cell walls and nuclei. As a result of this complexity, eukaryotic cells have gone through a much more diverse evolutionary process than prokaryotic cells such as bacteria and archaea, and thus Eukarya make up all complex life on Earth

Within each of these separate kingdoms the number of creatures is far too many to list. It is estimated that there could be as many as 100 million different species on Earth, although nowhere near that many have been physically catalogued. Of these, the majority are Bacteria and Archaea.

Since there is no way to list all of the different subdivisions of life on Earth here, we might as well focus on one specific animal: us, Homo sapiens sapiens. We are members of the Domain Eukarya, the Kingdom Animalia, the Phylum Chordata, the Class Mammalia, the Order Primates, the Family Hominidae, the Genus Homo, the Species Homo sapiens and finally the Subspecies Homo sapiens sapiens. This classification is able to demonstrate our exact biological position in relation to life on Earth.

One important thing a system like this tells us is that Homo, which is Latin for "human," is not actually our species, but our genus. This is an easy fact to forget since we are currently the only member of our genus not yet extinct. But anthropologically speaking there have been many humans including Homo habilis, Homo erectus and Homo neanderthalensis.

Furthermore, the taxonomical classification system can be seen as a map of evolution on the planet. Plants, animals and bacteria can be traced back to common ancestors and newly discovered species can be classified in relation to their ancestors, descendants and cousins. The Genus Homo, for instance, is a direct offshoot of the Tribe Hominini. (A tribe is a subcategory of the category of family, which in this case is Hominidae.) Another genus that falls under the Tribe Hominini is Pan, which houses the species Chimpanzee. This shows us that until relatively recently in the history of life, Homo sapiens and Chimpanzees were the same creature, and that Chimpanzees only split off just before Homo sapiens became fully human.

Ecology

Ecology is the scientific study of the relationship between the Earth and its life forms. Ecologists study the planet's ecosystems, the various communities of living things (biotic) and non-living structures (abiotic) that occur in localized areas throughout the world. The purpose of ecology is to understand the organizational structures that occur spontaneously in nature. Within an ecosystem there are different levels of organization that ecologists focus on and which are broken down by relative size. Each ecosystem is composed of communities of animals, and within each community exist numerous populations, or individual species groups.

Ecosystems Ecology

Ecosystems ecology studies small sections of the world that can be differentiated from neighboring areas by the types of rocks, soil and other non-living features they possess as well as by the types of plants and animals adapted to live there. A desert ecosystem may boarder an arid grassland ecosystem, which in turn may boarder a forest ecosystem. The purpose of ecosystems ecology is to analyze the system of interactions the animals and plants in a particular area have with the non-living portions environment. It also focuses heavily on local evolution, studying what traits are favored within particular ecosystems and why.

Many quantifiable factors go into making an ecosystem. Abiotic components are things such average sunlight, temperature, average rainfall and moisture levels, soil composition and other similar factors. Similarly, biotic components consist of the number and type of primary producers (generally plants), secondary producers (herbivores) and tertiary producers (carnivores and omnivores). All of this information can be quantified. For example, ecologists can calculate the amount of energy in a system by studying average amount of sunlight, the efficiency of photosynthesis in local plants, calories that exist in prey animals, nutrients absorbed by bacteria from breaking down dead predators and so on. Provided all of the factors have been accounted for, this sort of quantitative analysis of ecosystems can help ecologists determine factors such as the efficiency of the food web and the maximum supportable population. It can also help determine

 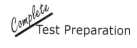

accurate ways to repair damaged ecosystems.

Community Ecology

Community ecology looks at similar regions to ecosystems ecology but focuses primarily on the biotic factors, ignoring the abiotic. In ecological terms a community describes the interactions of several species in a local area. Ecologists define these interactions between species in several ways: mutualism, interaction where both species benefit such as between bees and flowering plants; commensalism, interaction where one species benefits and the other neither notices nor minds; competition, interaction where both species are harmed; and predation or parasitism, interaction where one species is benefitted while the other is harmed such as predators attacking prey or herbivores eating plants.

All of these factors together contribute to the local food web, which in layman's terms is a graphical representation showing who eats what in nature. To ecologists, however, food webs are much more specific, showing the transfer of energy from organism to organism. Energy moves from lower trophic levels to higher ones. Trophic levels are the various positions that plants and animals occupy within the food web relative to other plants and animals that they want to eat or that want to eat them. Plants, for instance, would have a lower trophic level than grazing animals such as deer. Similarly, deer would have lower trophic levels than wolves.

Within communities species can be affected by changes either directly (such as when they are eaten by their main predator) or indirectly (such as when their main predator has its numbers diminished by a new and even bigger predator). There are also cascading effects on communities, such as when a dominant herbivorous species dies out and all of its former prey (both plant and animal) increase drastically in number.

Population Ecology

Getting even more specific is population ecology, which focuses on only one species either within a community or across a large space. The primary focuses for ecologists studying a population is its size. Population sizes can change due to an imbalance in the number of births and deaths as well as plants and animals emigrating to new areas.

Ecologists who study populations will generally model their growth rates in order to make predictions about the species. One method is the exponential growth model, which looks at current population trends and, assuming that they will remain constant, shows the increase or decrease in population over numerous generations. The other method is the logistic growth model, which slows reproduction when populations reach a certain density and increases it when they drop below a certain density to account for the increase in predators and decrease in the food supply that often follows massive population growth.

 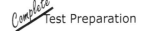

Chemistry

Chemistry is the science of matter, especially its chemical reactions, but also its composition, structure and properties. Chemistry is concerned with atoms and their interactions with other atoms, and particularly with the properties of chemical bonds.

Chemistry is sometimes called "the central science" because it connects physics with other natural sciences such as geology and biology. Chemistry is a branch of physical science but distinct from physics.

Traditional chemistry starts with the study of elementary particles, atoms, molecules, substances, metals, crystals and other aggregates of matter. in solid, liquid, and gas states, whether in isolation or combination. The interactions, reactions and transformations that are studied in chemistry are a result of interaction either between different chemical substances or between matter and energy.

A chemical reaction is a transformation of some substances into one or more other substances. It can be symbolically depicted through a chemical equation. The number of atoms on the left and the right in the equation for a chemical transformation is most often equal. The nature of chemical reactions a substance may undergo and the energy changes that may accompany it are constrained by certain basic rules, known as chemical laws.

Energy and entropy considerations are invariably important in almost all chemical studies. Chemical substances are classified in terms of their structure, phase as well as their chemical compositions. They can be analyzed using the tools of chemical analysis, e.g. spectroscopy and chromatography. Scientists engaged in chemical research are known as chemists. Most chemists specialize in one or more sub-disciplines.[7]

Basic Concepts in Chemistry

Atoms

Atoms are some of the basic building blocks of matter. Each atom is an element—an identifiable substance that cannot be further broken down into other identifiable substances—such as hydrogen, gold, or chlorine. There are just over 100 such elements, and each of them can combine with themselves and with other elements to create all the various molecules that exist in the universe. The poison gas chlorine and the explosive metal sodium, for instance, can combine at the atomic level to form sodium chloride, also known as salt.

For thousands of years atoms were thought to be the smallest thing possible. (The word "atom" comes from an ancient Greek word meaning "unbreakable.") However, experiments performed in the mid to late 19th century began to show the presence of small particles, electrons, in electric current. By the early 20th century, the electron was known to be a part of the atom that orbited a yet undefined atomic core. A few years

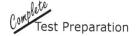

later, in 1919, the proton was discovered and found to exist in the nuclei of all atoms.

At that time it was believed that the atomic nucleus likely consisted of protons and electrons, with an orbit of electrons moving around it. However, by the 1930s the discovery of a strange sort of uncharged radiation led to the discovery of the neutron, which soon replaced electrons in the nucleus.

The protons and neutrons inside an atomic nucleus are not fundamental particles. That is, they can be divided into still smaller pieces. Protons and neutrons are known as hadrons, which is a class of particle made up of quarks. (Quarks are a fundamental particle.) There are two distinct types of hadrons, baryons and mesons, and both protons and neutrons are baryons, meaning they are both made up of a combination of three quarks. In addition to being hadrons, protons and neutrons are also known as nucleons because of their place within the nucleus. Protons have a mass of around 1.6726×10^{-27} kg and neutrons have a nearly identical mass of 1.6929×10^{-27} kg. Both particles have a ½ spin.

The number of protons inside an atomic nucleus determines what element the atom is. An element with only one proton, for instance, is hydrogen. An element with two is helium. One with three is lithium, and so on. No element (with the exception of hydrogen) can exist with only protons in its nucleus. Atoms need neutrons to bond the protons together using the strong force. In general atoms (again except for hydrogen) have an equal number of protons and neutrons in their nuclei.

This, however, does not always have to be the case. Atoms with an uneven number of protons and neutrons are called isotopes. Isotopes have all the same chemical properties as their evenly balanced counterparts, but their nuclei are not usually as stable and are more willing to react with other elements. (Two deuterium atoms, hydrogen isotopes with one proton and one neutron in their nucleus rather than only one proton, will fuse much more readily than two regular hydrogen atoms.)

Nearly all of an atoms' mass is within its nucleus. Outside of that there is a lot of empty space occupied only by a few, tiny electrons. Electrons were once viewed as orbiting an atom like planets orbit the sun. We now know that this is wrong in several ways. For one, electrons do not really "orbit" in the sense we are used to. At the quantum level no particle is really a particle, but is actually both a particle and a wave simultaneously. Heisenberg's uncertainty principle looks at this odd truth about reality and says that at no time can you watch an electron orbit the nucleus as you would watch the Earth orbit the sun. Instead, you have to observe only one of the electron's physical characteristics at a time, either viewing it as a particle in a fixed position outside the nucleus or as a wave encircling the nucleus like a halo.

Additionally, planets orbiting their stars can orbit at any distance they want. In fact, every object in our solar system has an elliptical orbit, meaning that they all move in more oval rather than circular shapes, getting closer and farther from the sun at various points. Electrons cannot do this under any circumstances.

Atoms have what are known as electron shells, which are the levels that an electron is able to occupy. Electrons cannot exist in between these shells; instead they jump from one to the next instantaneously. Each electron shell can hold a different number of atoms. When a shell fills up, additional electrons fill the outer shells. The outermost

 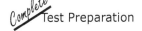

shell of any atom is called the valence shell, and it is the electrons in this shell that interact with the electrons of other atoms. The important thing about the valence shell is that each electron shell has a specific number of electrons that it can hold, and it wants to hold that many. This is important because, when atoms join together; their connecting valence electrons take up two valence shell spots, one on each atom. This means that the fewer electrons an atom has in its valence shell, the more likely it is to interact with other atoms. Conversely, the more electrons it has, the less likely it is to interact.

Electrons can also momentarily jump from one electron shell to the next if they are hit with a burst of energy from a photon. When photons hit atoms, the energy is briefly absorbed by the electrons, and this momentarily knocks them into higher "orbits." The particular "orbit" the electron is knocked into depends on the type of atom, and when the electron gives up its higher energy level it reemits a photon at a slightly different wavelength than the one it absorbed, providing a characteristic signal of that atom and showing exactly what "orbit" the electron was knocked into. This is the phenomenon responsible for spectral lines in light and is the reason we can tell what elements make up stars and planets just by looking at them.

Unlike protons and neutrons, electrons are a fundamental particle all on their own. They are known as leptons. Electrons have a negative charge that is generally balanced out by the positive charge of their atom's protons. Charged atoms, which have either gained or lost an electron for various reasons, are called ions. Ions, like isotopes, have the same properties that the regular element does; they simply have different tendencies towards reacting with other atoms. Electrons have a mass of 9.1094×10^{-31} kg and a -½ spin.

Element

The concept of chemical element is related to that of chemical substance. A chemical element is specifically a substance which is composed of a single type of atom. A chemical element is characterized by a particular number of protons in the nuclei of its atoms. This number is known as the atomic number of the element. For example, all atoms with 6 protons in their nuclei are atoms of the chemical element carbon, and all atoms with 92 protons in their nuclei are atoms of the element uranium.

Although all the nuclei of all atoms belonging to one element will have the same number of protons, they may not necessarily have the same number of neutrons; such atoms are termed isotopes. In fact several isotopes of an element may exist. Ninety–four different chemical elements or types of atoms based on the number of protons are observed on earth naturally, having at least one isotope that is stable or has a very long half-life. A further 18 elements have been recognised by IUPAC after they have been made in the laboratory.

The standard presentation of the chemical elements is in the periodic table, which orders elements by atomic number and groups them by electron configuration. Due to its arrangement, groups, or columns, and periods, or rows, of elements in the table either share several chemical properties, or follow a certain trend in characteristics such as atomic radius, electronegativity, etc. Lists of the elements by name, by symbol, and by atomic number are also available.

Compound

A compound is a substance with a particular ratio of atoms of particular chemical elements which determines its composition, and a particular organization which determines chemical properties. For example, water is a compound containing hydrogen and oxygen in the ratio of two to one, with the oxygen atom between the two hydrogen atoms, and an angle of 104.5° between them. Compounds are formed and interconverted by chemical reactions.

Substance

A chemical substance is a kind of matter with a definite composition and set of properties. Strictly speaking, a mixture of compounds, elements or compounds and elements is not a chemical substance, but it may be called a chemical. Most of the substances we encounter in our daily life are some kind of mixture; for example: air, alloys, biomass, etc.

Nomenclature of substances is a critical part of the language of chemistry. Generally it refers to a system for naming chemical compounds. Earlier in the history of chemistry substances were given names by their discoverer, which often led to some confusion and difficulty. However, today the IUPAC system of chemical nomenclature allows chemists to specify by name specific compounds amongst the vast variety of possible chemicals.

The standard nomenclature of chemical substances is set by the International Union of Pure and Applied Chemistry (IUPAC). There are well-defined systems in place for naming chemical species. Organic compounds are named according to the organic nomenclature system. Inorganic compounds are named according to the inorganic nomenclature system. In addition the Chemical Abstracts Service has devised a method to index chemical substance. In this scheme each chemical substance is identifiable by a number known as CAS registry number.

Molecule

A molecule is the smallest indivisible portion of a pure chemical substance that has its unique set of chemical properties, that is, its potential to undergo a certain set of chemical reactions with other substances. However, this definition only works well for substances that are composed of molecules, which is not true of many substances (see below). Molecules are typically a set of atoms bound together by covalent bonds, such that the structure is electrically neutral and all valence electrons are paired with other electrons either in bonds or in lone pairs.

Thus, molecules exist as electrically neutral units, unlike ions. When this rule is broken, giving the "molecule" a charge, the result is sometimes named a molecular ion or a polyatomic ion. However, the discrete and separate nature of the molecular concept usually requires that molecular ions be present only in well-separated form, such as a directed beam in a vacuum in a mass spectrograph. Charged polyatomic collections residing in solids (for example, common sulfate or nitrate ions) are generally not considered "molecules" in chemistry.

The "inert" or noble chemical elements (helium, neon, argon, krypton, xenon and ra-

 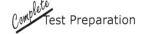

don) are composed of lone atoms as their smallest discrete unit, but the other isolated chemical elements consist of either molecules or networks of atoms bonded to each other in some way. Identifiable molecules compose familiar substances such as water, air, and many organic compounds like alcohol, sugar, gasoline, and the various pharmaceuticals.

However, not all substances or chemical compounds consist of discrete molecules, and indeed most of the solid substances that makes up the solid crust, mantle, and core of the Earth are chemical compounds without molecules. These other types of substances, such as ionic compounds and network solids, are organized in such a way as to lack the existence of identifiable molecules per se. Instead, these substances are discussed in terms of formula units or unit cells as the smallest repeating structure within the substance. Examples of such substances are mineral salts (such as table salt), solids like carbon and diamond, metals, and familiar silica and silicate minerals such as quartz and granite.

One of the main characteristic of a molecule is its geometry often called its structure. While the structure of diatomic, triatomic or tetra atomic molecules may be trivial, (linear, angular pyramidal etc.) the structure of polyatomic molecules, that are constituted of more than six atoms (of several elements) can be crucial for its chemical nature.

Ions and salts

An ion is a charged species, an atom or a molecule, that has lost or gained one or more electrons. Positively charged cations (e.g. sodium cation $Na+$) and negatively charged anions (e.g. chloride $Cl-$) can form a crystalline lattice of neutral salts (e.g. sodium chloride $NaCl$). Examples of polyatomic ions that do not split up during acid-base reactions are hydroxide ($OH-$) and phosphate ($PO43-$).

Ions in the gaseous phase are often known as plasma.

Acidity and basicity

A substance can often be classified as an acid or a base. There are several different theories which explain acid-base behavior. The simplest is Arrhenius theory, which states than an acid is a substance that produces hydronium ions when it is dissolved in water, and a base is one that produces hydroxide ions when dissolved in water. According to Brønsted–Lowry acid-base theory, acids are substances that donate a positive hydrogen ion to another substance in a chemical reaction; by extension, a base is the substance which receives that hydrogen ion.

A third common theory is Lewis acid-base theory, which is based on the formation of new chemical bonds. Lewis theory explains that an acid is a substance which is capable of accepting a pair of electrons from another substance during the process of bond formation, while a base is a substance which can provide a pair of electrons to form a new bond. According to concept as per Lewis, the crucial things being exchanged are charges. There are several other ways in which a substance may be classified as an acid or a base, as is evident in the history of this concept

Acid strength is commonly measured by two methods. One measurement, based on

 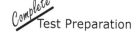

the Arrhenius definition of acidity, is pH, which is a measurement of the hydronium ion concentration in a solution, as expressed on a negative logarithmic scale. Thus, solutions that have a low pH have a high hydronium ion concentration, and can be said to be more acidic. The other measurement, based on the Brønsted–Lowry definition, is the acid dissociation constant (Ka), which measure the relative ability of a substance to act as an acid under the Brønsted–Lowry definition of an acid. That is, substances with a higher Ka are more likely to donate hydrogen ions in chemical reactions than those with lower Ka values.

Phase

In addition to the specific chemical properties that distinguish different chemical classifications, chemicals can exist in several phases. For the most part, the chemical classifications are independent of these bulk phase classifications; however, some more exotic phases are incompatible with certain chemical properties. A phase is a set of states of a chemical system that have similar bulk structural properties, over a range of conditions, such as pressure or temperature.

Physical properties, such as density and refractive index tend to fall within values characteristic of the phase. The phase of matter is defined by the phase transition, which is when energy put into or taken out of the system goes into rearranging the structure of the system, instead of changing the bulk conditions.

Sometimes the distinction between phases can be continuous instead of having a discrete boundary, in this case the matter is considered to be in a supercritical state. When three states meet based on the conditions, it is known as a triple point and since this is invariant, it is a convenient way to define a set of conditions.

The most familiar examples of phases are solids, liquids, and gases. Many substances exhibit multiple solid phases. For example, there are three phases of solid iron (alpha, gamma, and delta) that vary based on temperature and pressure. A principal difference between solid phases is the crystal structure, or arrangement, of the atoms. Another phase commonly encountered in the study of chemistry is the aqueous phase, which is the state of substances dissolved in aqueous solution (that is, in water).

Less familiar phases include plasmas, Bose-Einstein condensates and fermionic condensates and the paramagnetic and ferromagnetic phases of magnetic materials. While most familiar phases deal with three-dimensional systems, it is also possible to define analogs in two-dimensional systems, which has received attention for its relevance to systems in biology.

Redox

It is a concept related to the ability of atoms of various substances to lose or gain electrons. Substances that have the ability to oxidize other substances are said to be oxidative and are known as oxidizing agents, oxidants or oxidizers. An oxidant removes electrons from another substance. Similarly, substances that have the ability to reduce other substances are said to be reductive and are known as reducing agents, reductants, or reducers.

A reductant transfers electrons to another substance, and is thus oxidized itself. And because it "donates" electrons it is also called an electron donor. Oxidation and reduction properly refer to a change in oxidation number—the actual transfer of electrons may never occur. Thus, oxidation is better defined as an increase in oxidation number, and reduction as a decrease in oxidation number.

Bonding

Electron atomic and molecular orbitals

Atoms sticking together in molecules or crystals are said to be bonded with one another. A chemical bond may be visualized as the multipole balance between the positive charges in the nuclei and the negative charges oscillating about them. More than simple attraction and repulsion, the energies and distributions characterize the availability of an electron to bond to another atom.

A chemical bond can be a covalent bond, an ionic bond, a hydrogen bond or just because of Van der Waals force. Each of these kind of bonds is ascribed to some potential. These potentials create the interactions which hold atoms together in molecules or crystals. In many simple compounds, Valence Bond Theory, the Valence Shell Electron Pair Repulsion model (VSEPR), and the concept of oxidation number can be used to explain molecular structure and composition.

Similarly, theories from classical physics can be used to predict many ionic structures. With more complicated compounds, such as metal complexes, valence bond theory is less applicable and alternative approaches, such as the molecular orbital theory, are generally used.

Reaction

During chemical reactions, bonds between atoms break and form, resulting in different substances with different properties. In a blast furnace, iron oxide, a compound, reacts with carbon monoxide to form iron, one of the chemical elements, and carbon dioxide.

When a chemical substance is transformed as a result of its interaction with another or energy, a chemical reaction is said to have occurred. Chemical reaction is therefore a concept related to the 'reaction' of a substance when it comes in close contact with another, whether as a mixture or a solution; exposure to some form of energy, or both. It results in some energy exchange between the constituents of the reaction as well with the system environment which may be designed vessels which are often laboratory glassware.

Chemical reactions can result in the formation or dissociation of molecules, that is, molecules breaking apart to form two or more smaller molecules, or rearrangement of atoms within or across molecules. Chemical reactions usually involve the making or breaking of chemical bonds. Oxidation, reduction, dissociation, acid-base neutralization and molecular rearrangement are some of the commonly used kinds of chemical reactions.

A chemical reaction can be symbolically depicted through a chemical equation. While in a non-nuclear chemical reaction the number and kind of atoms on both sides of the equation are equal, for a nuclear reaction this holds true only for the nuclear particles viz. protons and neutrons.

The sequence of steps in which the reorganization of chemical bonds may be taking place in the course of a chemical reaction is called its mechanism. A chemical reaction can be envisioned to take place in a number of steps, each of which may have a different speed. Many reaction intermediates with variable stability can thus be envisaged during the course of a reaction. Reaction mechanisms are proposed to explain the kinetics and the relative product mix of a reaction. Many physical chemists specialize in exploring and proposing the mechanisms of various chemical reactions. Several empirical rules, like the Woodward-Hoffmann rules often come handy while proposing a mechanism for a chemical reaction.

According to the IUPAC gold book a chemical reaction is a process that results in the interconversion of chemical species". Accordingly, a chemical reaction may be an elementary reaction or a stepwise reaction. An additional caveat is made, in that this definition includes cases where the interconversion of conformers is experimentally observable. Such detectable chemical reactions normally involve sets of molecular entities as indicated by this definition, but it is often conceptually convenient to use the term also for changes involving single molecular entities (i.e. 'microscopic chemical events').

Equilibrium

Although the concept of equilibrium is widely used across sciences, in the context of chemistry, it arises whenever a number of different states of the chemical composition are possible. For example, in a mixture of several chemical compounds that can react with one another, or when a substance can be present in more than one kind of phase.

A system of chemical substances at equilibrium even though having an unchanging composition is most often not static; molecules of the substances continue to react with one another thus giving rise to a dynamic equilibrium. Thus the concept describes the state in which the parameters such as chemical composition remain unchanged over time. Chemicals present in biological systems are invariably not at equilibrium; rather they are far from equilibrium.

Energy

In the context of chemistry, energy is an attribute of a substance as a consequence of its atomic, molecular or aggregate structure. Since a chemical transformation is accompanied by a change in one or more of these kinds of structure, it is invariably accompanied by an increase or decrease of energy of the substances involved. Some energy is transferred between the surroundings and the reactants of the reaction in the form of heat or light; thus the products of a reaction may have more or less energy than the reactants.

A reaction is said to be exergonic if the final state is lower on the energy scale than the initial state; in the case of endergonic reactions the situation is the reverse. A reaction is said to be exothermic if the reaction releases heat to the surroundings; in the case of endothermic reactions, the reaction absorbs heat from the surroundings.

Chemical reactions are invariably not possible unless the reactants surmount an energy barrier known as the activation energy. The speed of a chemical reaction (at given tem-

 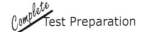

perature T) is related to the activation energy E, by the Boltzmann's population factor e − E / kT - that is the probability of molecule to have energy greater than or equal to E at the given temperature T. This exponential dependence of a reaction rate on temperature is known as the Arrhenius equation. The activation energy necessary for a chemical reaction can be in the form of heat, light, electricity or mechanical force in the form of ultrasound.

A related concept free energy, which also incorporates entropy considerations, is a very useful means for predicting the feasibility of a reaction and determining the state of equilibrium of a chemical reaction, in chemical thermodynamics. A reaction is feasible only if the total change in the Gibbs free energy is negative, if it is equal to zero the chemical reaction is said to be at equilibrium.

There exist only limited possible states of energy for electrons, atoms and molecules. These are determined by the rules of quantum mechanics, which require quantization of energy of a bound system. The atoms/molecules in a higher energy state are said to be excited. The molecules/atoms of substance in an vexcited energy state are often much more reactive; that is, more amenable to chemical reactions.

The phase of a substance is invariably determined by its energy and the energy of its surroundings. When the intermolecular forces of a substance are such that the energy of the surroundings is not sufficient to overcome them, it occurs in a more ordered phase like liquid or solid as is the case with water (H2O); a liquid at room temperature because its molecules are bound by hydrogen bonds. Whereas hydrogen sulfide (H2S) is a gas at room temperature and standard pressure, as its molecules are bound by weaker dipole-dipole interactions.

The transfer of energy from one chemical substance to another depends on the size of energy quanta emitted from one substance. However, heat energy is often transferred more easily from almost any substance to another because the phonons responsible for vibrational and rotational energy levels in a substance have much less energy than photons invoked for the electronic energy transfer. Thus, because vibrational and rotational energy levels are more closely spaced than electronic energy levels, heat is more easily transferred between substances relative to light or other forms of electronic energy. For example, ultraviolet electromagnetic radiation is not transferred with as much efficacy from one substance to another as thermal or electrical energy.

The existence of characteristic energy levels for different chemical substances is useful for their identification by the analysis of spectral lines. Different kinds of spectra are often used in chemical spectroscopy, e.g. IR, microwave, NMR, ESR, etc. Spectroscopy is also used to identify the composition of remote objects - like stars and distant galaxies - by analyzing their radiation spectra.

Energy: Kinetic Energy and Mechanical Energy

One of the most common types of energy you are exposed to is kinetic energy: energy that comes from motion. Like all forms of energy, kinetic energy is measured in joules. Kinetic energy can be imparted onto an object when a source of potential energy is

 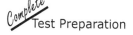

tapped to accelerate it. It can also happen when one object with kinetic energy slams into another object and kinetic energy from the first object is transferred to the second.

However it happens, imparting kinetic energy to an object causes it to accelerate. In this way movement is nothing more than an indication of the amount of kinetic energy an object has. An object will hold onto its kinetic energy until it is able to transfer it to something else, which allows it to slow down again.

As long as an object has the same level of kinetic energy, it will move at a consistent velocity forever. This is Newton's first law of motion.

The transfer of kinetic energy from one object to another can occur in many ways. It can be as simple and mundane as a baseball flying through the air—interacting with all the various molecules of oxygen, carbon dioxide, nitrogen and all the other gasses that make up our atmosphere, and transferring its kinetic energy to them—speeding them up and slowing itself down in the process. Or it can be as chaotic as a speeding truck losing control on an icy road and slamming into a wall.

The interaction between the baseball and the air and between the truck and the wall are only superficially different. One appears more chaotic than the other only because of the differences in mass between a baseball and a truck and the differences in "negative energy" possessed by free-floating air molecules compared to a solid wall. At its most basic, however, the same events are taking place in both examples. Molecules in the both wall and the air scatter when the kinetic energy they receive causes them to move, and this causes both heat and sound to be produced.

You can calculate kinetic energy with the formula $KE = \frac{1}{2}mv^2$ where m is the mass of the object in kilograms and v is its velocity in meters/second.

One important aspect of kinetic energy that makes it so potentially destructive is that the kinetic energy a moving object carries does not increase on pace with its velocity, but rather in relation to the square of its velocity. If you double an object's velocity, you will quadruple the amount of kinetic energy it possesses ($2^2 = 4$). If you quadruple the velocity, you increase the kinetic energy by sixteen times ($4^2 = 16$). This can lead to relatively small masses possessing very high kinetic energy levels when they are accelerated to only nominally high speeds. This is one reason why modern kinetic energy weapons (such as firearms) are able to cause large amounts of damage while being extremely compact.

When discussing energy it is important to take a moment to understand mechanical energy and how it relates to the objects it interacts with. Mechanical energy is not a separate type of energy in the way that potential energy and kinetic energy differ from each other. Instead mechanical energy is simply the ability of an object to do work.

Mechanical energy encompasses all of the potential energy available to an object added to all of the kinetic energy available to it, providing a total energy output. For instance, in our description of potential energy there is the example of a pole-vaulter hanging in mid-air with her pole bent at a near right angle to the ground. The bend in the pole-vaulter's pole contains elastic potential energy, which will help her clear the bar. However, that is not the only source of energy the pole-vaulter is restricted to. For anyone who has ever seen a track and field competition, you know that pole-vaulters take long, running starts before planting their poles in the ground. This imparts kinetic energy to the runners body, and it is that kinetic energy plus the pole's elastic potential energy that are added together in mid-air to impart the total mechanical energy that drives the pole-vaulter high into the air and over the bar.

Energy: Potential Energy

There are two main types of potential energy: gravitational potential energy and elastic potential energy.

Potential energy is quite simply the potential an object has to act on other objects. In the form of gravitational potential energy, the object is raised off the ground and is waiting for the force of gravity pulling at 9.8m/s2, to grab hold of it and pull it towards the Earth.

This type of energy is very common in everyday life. It describes everything from a book falling off its shelf to a child tripping on a crack in the sidewalk. Because gravitational potential energy is so common, the equation describing it PEgrav=mass*g*height should not be hard to figure out since it contains only easily observable features of matter: an object's mass, the force of gravity (g), and the object's height off the ground when it started falling.

(Note that the height does not have to be measured from the ground. Any point can be chosen—such as a table top or even a point in mid-air—provided that you are only concerned with the energy an object would have if it fell from the point it was currently at to the point you have chosen.)

If we take the example of a 1kg weight positioned at a height of 1 meter above the surface of Earth (where the gravity is 9.8m/s2—try this on Mars and you will get a different result), we end up with the equation PEgrav=1*9.8*1, which equals 9.8 joules of gravitational potential energy. A 1g weight positioned at the same height would be PEgrav=.001*9.8*1 or .0098J of potential energy, while a 1kg weight positioned a kilometer up would equal PEgrav=1*9.8*1000 or 9800J of potential energy.

From this equation you may have picked up on the fact that the height an object is raised to is directly proportional to the amount of gravitational potential energy it has. Take a 1kg object and raise it to 5m, and you get 49J of potential energy. Double that to 10m, and you get 98J. Triple it to 15m and you will get 147J—three times the original 49J.

In the form of elastic potential energy the object is stretched or compressed out of its normal "resting" shape. The amount of energy that will be released when it finally returns to rest is the amount of elastic potential energy it has while stretched or compressed. A common example of elastic potential energy is when an archer draws back the string of his bow. The farther back the bowstring is pulled, the more it will stretch. The more it stretches the more potential energy it will have waiting to send into the arrow.

In many cases the elastic potential energy of an object can be determined using Hooke's law of elasticity. Hooke's law states that F=-kx where F is the force the material will exert as it returns to its resting state measured in Newtons, x is amount of displacement the material undergoes measured in meters, and k is the spring constant and is measured in Newtons/meter.

In order to determine the potential energy of an elastic or springy material you use the equation PE=½kx2. According to this equation, an object such as a spring with a spring constant of 5N/m that is stretched 3 meters past its resting point would have a potential energy of 22.5J. That is, ½*5*32 = 2.5*9 = 22.5J.

Remember that elastic potential energy affects much more than just what you would consider elastic or springy material such as rubber bands, bungee cords and springs. There is elastic potential energy in a pole-vaulter's pole at the point where she is in the air and hanging onto a pole that is bent nearly sideways. In the next instant her forward momentum will be boosted by the conversion of her pole's potential energy into kinetic energy, pushing her over the bar. Similarly, when a hockey player shoots the puck, he drags his stick along the ice as it moves forward, bending the shaft backwards slightly. This adds extra force to the puck as the stick snaps forward back into its normal resting position.

Energy: Work and Power

In the simplest terms, Energy is the ability to do work. Energy allows objects and people to affect the physical world and displace (or move) other objects or people.

Work in the physics sense is a very specific concept. It is measured in joules, which are defined as being 1 Newton of force that displaces something by 1 meter. (J=Nm) As the mass of the object being displaced varies, the amount of work in joules required to move it a meter will vary too.

To determine the amount of work being done, you can use the equation W=F*d*cosΘ. It defines work as being the force applied, multiplied by the distance the object was displaced, multiplied by the cosine of Θ (Theta).

The force is measured in Newtons. It is covered at length in a different lesson, so there is no need to go into it here. Distance, of course, should be measured in meters. The tricky part of this equation is determining the cosine of Θ. Θ represents the difference in angle between the vector (or direction) the force is acting in and the vector the displacement is occurring. That means that there are really only three possible values for Θ.

If the force is pushing or pulling in one direction, and the object being displaced is moving in that same direction, then there is no difference in angle between the vectors and Θ=0°. This is the sort of force you get when a child pulls her sled across a snowy field. The direction the child is pulling and the direction the sled is traveling are the same. Since cos0=1 the amount of work is determined simply by multiplying the force and the displacement.

You should note that the angle of the vectors is determined by their relationship to each other and not to some sort of ideal flat surface. That is, if the child is pulling her sled up a steep hill rather than across a field, the angle of Θ is still going to be 0° since the force she exerts on the sled and the sled itself are still traveling in the same direction.

The second possibility is when the force vector acts in the opposite direction of the object's displacement. This gives you what is called "negative work" because the energy is working to hinder the object from moving rather than to help it. In this instance $\Theta=180°$ since the vector in which the force is acting and the vector in which the object is moving are opposite. This force is most commonly observed when dealing with friction. It is the reason that hockey pucks and soccer balls will not travel forever; the force of friction exerted by the ice and by the grass is acting in the opposite direction.

The final difference in vectors is when the force being exerted on an object is at a right angle to its displacement. In this case $\Theta=90°$. You can picture this as a waitress carrying a tray of drinks over to your table, and it provides for some odd conclusions. Since the force we are talking about is the force the waitress is using to hold the tray vertically, but the displacement vector of the tray is horizontally across the room, we find that the force the waitress exerts does no work at all. It is not responsible for moving the tray horizontally towards your table.

This is represented mathematically with the fact that the $\cos90=0$, meaning that the original equation $W=F*d*\cos\Theta$ would be $W=F*d*0$. Without adding any other information in, it is already obvious that work is going to equal zero joules.

A different way to imagine this is to think of cargo in the back of a truck. It took work to load the cargo up onto the truck from the ground (the force vector and the displacement vector were both pointing in the same direction), but once the cargo was loaded, no additional work was required to keep it there. The truck could drive from one end of the country to the other, but zero joules of work would be exerted keeping the cargo in place in the back of the truck.

When you add a unit of time to your calculations of work, you get a new classification: power. Power is the rate at which work is done. The equation that measures power is power=work/time. In this equation work is measured in joules, time is measured in seconds and power is measured in Watts.

Since, as we noted above, one joule is the same as one Newton multiplied by one meter, this equation can also be written as power=(force*displacement)/time where force is measured in Newtons and displacement is measured in meters. But, this opens up further possibilities. Since the math does not care whether we first multiply force with displacement before dividing the whole thing by time, or whether we divide displacement by time and then multiply the answer by force, we find the equation can also be written as power=force(displacement/time).

Given that displacement is measured in meters and the time in seconds, what we are really saying here is that power equals the amount of force applied to an object multiplied by that object's velocity (m/s).

Thus we get two equations describing power: power=work/time and power=force*velocity. By definition, power has an inverse relationship with time; the less time it takes for the work to be done, the more power is being applied. Power also has a direct relationship with force and velocity. Increase either the amount of force being applied to an object, or the speed at which it is traveling, and you have increased the power.

Force: Defining Force and Newton's Three Laws

In physics force is the term given to anything that has the power to act on an object, causing its displacement in one direction or another. Forces are a somewhat abstract concept, and it is for that reason that it took thousands of years to accurately identify and describe them. It was not until the 17th century when a man named Isaac Newton began to accurately describe the basic physical forces and show how they acted on matter.

Force is measured using the unit Newton (N). One Newton can be defined with the formula $1N=1kg(1m/s2)$. In other words, if you accelerate a kilogram of matter by one meter per second per second, you have exerted one Newton of force on it.

Newton developed three laws to explain the interactions of matter he observed. The first is often known as the "Law of Inertia." It states that an object at rest will stay at rest, and an object in motion will stay in motion, unless a force acts upon it to change its state. This means that if you fire a spaceship out into the vacuum of space, and keep it clear from planets and stars that will apply force to it, the ship will keep going at the same speed forever.

This tendency to stay moving or stay at rest is known as inertia. Inertia is directly related to an object's mass; the more mass an object has, the more inertia it will have and the harder it will be to speed it up or slow it down. This is implied by the equation defining one Newton of force, but it is also obvious in everyday life. You have to exert more force to push a box of books across the floor than you would to push a box of clothes the same size. The box of books has more mass, so it has more inertia. Similarly, a baseball player can easily catch and stop a baseball thrown at over 100km/hr. If you were to ask that same player to stop a truck traveling at 100km/hr, you would get much less pleasant results.

One important thing to remember about force is that it is a vector quantity, meaning that it points in a specific direction. Set a one kilogram object down on a table and you will have the force of gravity pulling it down at one Newton, and the force of all the atoms in the table pushing it up at one Newton. This is said to be a state of equilibrium, and it causes no change to the object's velocity.

However, if the table had been poorly built and was only capable of pushing up at .75 Newtons, the object would pull through, snapping the table at its weakest points, and fall until it found something that was capable of applying the needed force to hold it up against gravity.

As such, an object can only be at rest if it has no forces acting on it, or if it has equal and opposite forces acting on it keeping it at equilibrium. If an unopposed force acts on an object, it will move.

Newton's second law deals with what happens when you have the sort of unbalanced forces that we just described. It explains the movement of objects through the equation F=ma, where F is the force in Newtons, m is the object's mass in kilograms, and a is the object's acceleration in meters per second per second (m/s2).

Just like with Newton's first law, this equation shows that mass is a huge player when it comes to using a force to move objects. The larger the mass, the more force you will need to accelerate or decelerate it to the same velocity.

Newton's third law states simply that for every action there is an equal and opposite reaction. This means that if I pound my hand down on my desk right now, my desk will also be hitting up at my hand with the exact same force. This may sound strange, but it is the reason that pounding your hand on your desk can damage your desk and hurt your hand at the same time. It is also the reason that baseball bats can snap while imparting force onto the ball, and why a moving car hitting stationary wall will damage both.

Force: Friction

Friction is the force that resists the motion of objects in relation to other objects. When two surfaces move in relation to each other, the force of friction is what slows them down. Friction applies to all matter, whether it is a book sliding down a slanting shelf, a soccer ball rolling on the ground or a baseball flying though the air. Essentially, friction is a constant opposing force that keeps things from traveling forever.

Several laws describe how friction works. Amontons' first law of friction says that, "The force of friction is directly proportional to the applied load." His second law of friction says that, "The force of friction is independent of the apparent area of contact." Similarly, Coulomb's law of friction states that, "Kinetic friction is independent of the sliding velocity."

The two main types of Friction are static friction and kinetic friction. Static friction is what you get when one stationary object is stacked on top of another stationary object, such as a book resting on a table. The static friction between the book and the table determines how much sticking power there is between them, and at what angle you would have to tilt the table before the force of gravity overpowers the force of friction and starts the book sliding.

To figure out the maximum amount of static friction possible before the book starts sliding, you use the formula $f_s = \mu_s F_n$ where f_s is the total amount of static friction, μ_s (pronounced "mu") is the coefficient of static friction and F_n is the "normal force," the force being exerted perpendicularly through the surface into the object resting on it, keeping the object from breaking through the surface.

Another way to examine static friction is to calculate the angle the table will have to reach before the book will start sliding. This is also known as the angle of repose, and it can be calculated using the formula $\tan\theta = \mu s$ where θ (pronounced "theta") is the angle of repose and μs is the coefficient of static friction.

Aside from determining the angels that books will slide off tables, calculating static friction allows tire manufacturers to determine how "grippy" their treads are. If there were no friction, the wheel would not be a functional tool because it would not push itself against the road while moving. The higher the coefficient of friction between the tire and the road, the more grip the tire has.

Kinetic friction is sort of the inverse of static friction. It is the force that causes moving objects to slow down. Kinetic friction applies to two surfaces moving in respect to one another such as the bottom of a snowboard and the snowy ground. It can be calculated using the same basic formula used to calculate static friction: $fk = \mu kFn$ with the only differences being the sub-k marks replacing the sub-s marks of the previous equation, signifying kinetic friction.

As kinetic friction slows an object, the object's kinetic energy is transformed into heat.

We can see how both of these types of friction relate to one another by looking at a free-body diagram.

You can see the force of friction (f) pulling backwards as a negative force while F pulls forwards. (In this diagram F is either the force of gravity pulling on the resting book, or it is the velocity that the moving objects are moving in relation to each other.) Fn is the normal force pushing up on the object from the surface it is resting on. Finally, w is the weight of the object pushing down on the surface it is resting on as gravity tugs downward on the object's mass.

 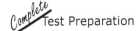

Fundamental Forces: Electromagnetism

Electromagnetism is one of the four fundamental forces. It is far more common than gravity, but only if you know where to look. Electromagnetism is responsible for nearly all interactions in which gravity plays no part. It is what holds negatively charged electrons in orbit around the positively charged protons in the nucleus of an atom. It is also the force that joins atoms to each other to create molecules.

It is also electromagnetism that is responsible for the fact that matter—which is made up of atoms and at the subatomic level is mostly empty space—feels solid. When you sit down in your chair, it is the electromagnetic attraction between the chair's atoms and between your body's atoms that keep you from falling through the chair and, conversely, that keep the chair from passing through you.

The electromagnetic force acts through a field. This sort of field can occur as a result of positively or negatively charged atoms (ions), atoms which have either more or fewer electrons than protons causing their overall charge to be unbalanced. Magnetic fields can also be created by applying electric current to conductive material (such as wire) with a conductive core (such as a nail). Electric current is nothing more than a steady flow of electrons, and by turning on the current you send electrons through the core. This aligns all the atoms in the metal so that they are parallel with each other, and this creates a magnetic field. When you turn the electric current off, the electrons stop flowing, and the atoms, no longer forced by the current to line up, cease to be magnetic.

All electromagnetic fields have a positive and a negative pole. Even the Earth's magnetic field, which is caused by the convective forces in the planet's core, sends electrons out of its negative pole (in the geographic North Pole) and reaccepts them at its positive pole (in the geographic South Pole in Antarctica). The Earth's magnetic field, like all magnetic fields, is able to affect charged particles. Additionally, magnetic fields move in one direction around the magnet. This direction is always the same in relation to the flow of current from the negative to the positive poles, and it is easy to test the direction of the field using the "right hand rule." Close your fist and make a "thumbs up" sign with your right hand. The positive pole is represented by the tip of your thumb, the negative by the other end of your hand, and the direction of the magnetic field by where your closed fingers are. Thus, if you point your thumb at yourself, your magnet has current coming out its negative pole pointed towards you and looping back around to the positive pole pointed away from you, and the field is pointed counter-clockwise, which in this case is to your left.

The effects of a magnetic field do not go on forever but follow the inverse square law. The farther you move from a magnetic field, the less its force will affect you. By moving x times away from a magnetic field, you feel $1/x2$ times less magnetism.

Closely related to the electromagnetic field is electromagnetic radiation. This radiation can take many forms, the most familiar of which being light, radio waves that carry radio and broadcast television, microwaves that cook our food, x-rays that can image the insides or our bodies, and gamma rays that come down from space and would have killed us all long ago if it were not for the Earth's magnetic field interacting with them.

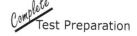

Electromagnetic radiation is created, according to James Clerk Maxwell, by the oscillations of electromagnetic fields, which create electromagnetic waves. The wave's frequency (or how energetic it is) determines what part of the electromagnetic spectrum it occupies—whether it is a gamma ray, a blue light or a radio signal. Electromagnetic radiation is the same thing as light, with what we are used to as visible light being a range of specific frequencies within the electromagnetic spectrum, so all electromagnetic radiation moves at the speed of light.

At the quantum level, the electromagnetic force has a transfer particle moving back and forth between charged atoms, attracting and repelling them. The electromagnetic transfer particle is the photon.

Fundamental Forces: Gravity

Gravity may be the most commonly, consciously experienced force. We can see its effects everyday when books fall off of shelves, when stray baseballs arc downwards and crash through windows and when Australians time and again fail to fall off the bottom of the world and out into space. Gravity is also largely responsible for the structure of the universe. Without it, stars would not ignite and begin fusion reactions, planets would not condense out of dust and metal and most matter would have no attraction to other matter in any way. Essentially, without gravity, life would not exist.

It may seem strange to learn that gravity is the weakest of all forces given that it holds the entire galaxy together. Still, even with the gravitational mass of the entire planet pulling on an object such as a ball—causing it to sit motionless on the floor rather than float aimlessly off into space—a toddler could easily pick it up and run off with it, and there would be nothing the planet could do about it. Match that with the force an electromagnet exerts on metal; there is no comparison.

The idea of gravity as a force was first formulated by Isaac Newton in the late 17th century. Newton's ideas were further elaborated on in the early 20th century by Albert Einstein, who described gravity as the effect of mass warping the fabric of space-time. This process is often portrayed as a large ball creating a divot in a flat sheet of space-time. The divot curves space-time and can catch objects that would otherwise be traveling in straight lines and redirect or even capture them.

On Earth gravity pulls objects towards the center of the planet at 9.8m/s2. The squared rate of time shows that gravity is by its nature a force causing acceleration. Every second, the force of gravity increases the speed of an object by an additional 9.8m/s, provided nothing able to resist the force gets in its way.

In Einstein's view of the universe, gravity moved in waves, which traveled through space at the speed of light. As a result he demonstrated that the force of gravity would take time to reach the object it was acting on. If, for instance, the sun were to suddenly vanish from the solar system, it would take eight minutes for the Earth to go flying off into space—the same amount of time it would take for us to stop seeing the sun's light.

 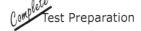

Another way to view gravity is through a series of transfer particles that interact with matter and draw it closer together. Transfer particles come into play in quantum mechanics, and they replace gravity waves as the method of spreading the force through the universe. (Actually, replace is not the right word, as quantum mechanics shows that particles and waves are really the same thing, simply looked at from different perspectives.) In quantum mechanics gravity's transfer particle is called a graviton, and it moves at the speed of light.

As you might guess from the description of gravity as a divot in space-time, its effects do not go on forever. The farther you move from a gravitational mass, the less its force will affect you. The drop in the gravitational force is governed by what is known as the inverse square law, which says that the attraction of any object drops in relation to the square of the distance you move from it. Essentially, if you are floating over the surface of the planet and then move x times away from it, you will feel $1/x^2$ times less gravity. So if you move 10 times farther away from where you were, you will feel $1/100$ the force gravity.

Fundamental Forces: The Strong and Weak Nuclear Forces

The strong and weak nuclear forces are fundamental forces, but they were discovered much later than electromagnetism and gravity primarily because they only interact with matter at a subatomic level.

The strong force is, as its name suggests, the strongest of the four fundamental forces. (It is 100 times stronger than the next strongest force, electromagnetism, and 1036 times the strength of the weakest force, gravity.) That said, for the thousands of years that people have been studying physics, it never occurred to anyone to even look for the strong force. That is because, despite the strong force's strength, it has such a limited range that it only interacts with matter across the distance of an atom's nucleus. In fact, its range is only about 10-15 meters, so small that the nuclei of the largest atoms—those filled with the highest number of protons and neutrons—are only just barely small enough for the strong force to keep working, making the nuclei of those atoms unstable.

The strong force was not discovered until the 1930s when scientists discovered the neutron. Up until that time atomic nuclei were thought to consist of a collection of protons and electrons grouped together in such a way that kept them mutually attracted to each other. With the discovery of the neutron, however, a new force was needed to hold positively charged protons together with uncharged neutrons.

The strong force actually does not interact directly with the protons and neutrons but with the fundamental particle that makes up protons and neutrons, quarks. Quarks come in three different color groupings: red, green and blue. (Quarks are not actually these colors; red, green and blue are just familiar names given to bits of matter that are utterly outside of our experience as humans, in order to make them easier to comprehend.) The different colors of quarks combine together to create protons and neutrons. Within each proton and neutron, the strong force holds the quarks together. That, in turn, bleeds out into the rest of the nucleus in a residual effect, holding the protons and neutrons together as well.

Like the other fundamental forces, the strong force is mediated at the quantum level using a transfer particle known as a gluon. However, unlike the transfer particles for gravity and electromagnetism (gravitons and photons, respectively), gluons have mass. It is the gluon's mass that limits the area where it can spread the strong force to only within the nucleus.

The other fundamental force operating inside the nucleus is the weak force. The weak force causes a specific type of radioactive decay called beta decay, so named because it causes the decaying atom to emit a beta particle, which can be either an electron or a positron (a form of anti-mater also known as an anti-electron), as a byproduct of changing into a different element.

Several things happen at once during beta decay, and we should look at each one individually. We saw while looking at the strong force that an atom's protons and neutrons are made up of smaller, fundamental particles called quarks, and it is the quarks that actually interact with the strong force. As it turns out, quarks are the only particle that interacts with all four fundamental forces, which means that inside the nucleus they are interacting with the weak force as well.

Before we get to how the weak force interacts with quarks, there is something else you should know about them. We mentioned above that quarks come in three different colors: red, blue and green. But they also can be divided into six different flavors: up, down, charm, strange, top and bottom. (This makes 18 different possible combinations of quark, each with a color and a flavor.) Of these flavors only up and down quarks are stable enough to form protons and neutrons.

What the weak force does is switch up quarks to down quarks and down quarks to up quarks. This is actually the only thing the weak force does, but it has several effects. First since quarks join together to produce protons and neutrons (two up quarks and one down quark make a proton, while two down and one up quark make a neutron), the sudden change of one type of quark to another changes that combination. β^- decay is beta decay where change of quarks causes a neutron to become a proton. This also causes the atom to emit an electron and a electron antineutrino. β^+ decay is the opposite, where a proton changes to a neutron and the atom emits a positron and an electron neutrino.

In both cases the decaying atom changes into a different kind of atom. In general, beta decay takes place in unstable isotopes (atoms that have a different number of protons and neutrons) and serves to stabilize the nucleus by equalizing the ratio of these particles. For instance, beta decay will turn the unstable plutonium 15 into a far more stable strontium.

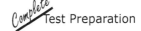

Quantum Mechanics

One of the strangest branches of modern physics is known as quantum mechanics. Quantum mechanics is usually referred to as the study of the "very small," but in a lot of ways it is more specific than that. It is the study of quanta, the most basic individual unit of any substance.

Quantum mechanics first began as a discipline within physics in 1900 when Max Planck determined that energy radiated in the form of heat could not just radiate at any old temperature it wanted, but that it could only rise and fall—and thus be emitted or absorbed—at certain, set levels. (Think of it as the difference between stairs and ramps. Stairs have set spaces where you can stand and set spaces where you cannot. Planck said that raising energy levels such as temperature was akin to climbing a set of stairs one step at a time.)

This suggested that the radiation that produced heat (and thus all electromagnetic radiation, including visible light) was made up of tiny little particles, which Planck named quanta from the Latin work "quantus," which means "how much." Planck developed an equation to describe this situation, $E=hv$ in which v stood for the already well known frequencies of electromagnetic spectrum (and which in 1900 was thought of as only acting like a wave), h stood for a number called the Planck constant that equaled 6.63×10^{-34} J s ("J s" is for Joule seconds), and E was the energy level for quanta of that frequency.

In 1905 Albert Einstein used Planck's work to define the photon, which is one quantum of electromagnetic radiation. Photons are generally thought of as light, but only some energies of photons are visible. Photons can have any energy that corresponds to electromagnetic frequency, but instead of being a continuous wave, they are thought of as individual particles.

The discovery of the particle aspect of a wave led to a realization that waves and particles were actually the same thing being looked at in different ways. This idea, called wave-particle duality, accounted for the centuries long debate between physicists over whether light was a wave or a particle, with each side producing compelling evidence to prove its thesis. As it turned out light—like everything in the universe—was both. This relationship was demonstrated by Louis de Broglie who developed the equation $p=h/\lambda$ showing that the Planck constant (h) divided by a particle's wavelength (λ, pronounced lambda) would equal its momentum (p). Since all particles are moving and have momentum, all particles have wavelengths.

One of the most important aspects of wave-particle duality comes from studying atoms. The orbits of electrons around the atomic nuclei had at one time been thought to mimic the orbits of planets around the sun. Now, however, two important factors came into play to change that view. The first was the realization that electrons could only orbit at certain distances from the nucleus. When changing from one electron shell to the next, an electron would not take a gradual trajectory to its new home in the way a spaceship from Earth to Mars might. The electron would simply vanish from one shell and appear instantaneously at the next. In essence, electrons could also only display certain quanta of energy. They could have one energy level or another, but they could not exist

 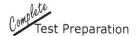

in between.

The second important thing that quantum mechanics showed physicists about the orbit of electrons was that the word "orbit" was in no senses an accurate description of what was happening, and was little more than a symbolic way to describe electrons. Since all particles are also waves, an electron could not simply be in one place at one time but had to exist as across a range of areas as a frequency which described its momentum.

This seemingly nonsensical idea was explained mathematically though the Heisenberg uncertainty principle, which stated that it was possible to measure the exact position of a particle, and it was possible to measure the exact velocity of a particle, but you could not know both factors at once. In other words, measuring one would make it impossible to measure the other. This was an unavoidable fact of reality given de Broglie's equation; if you were moving you were spread out like a wave.

A strange side effect of this was it meant that no particles in the universe could be said to have definite positions in space. Instead, everything had a likely position given its velocity. Matter could not be said to exist at certain points in space, it could merely have certain probabilities of existing at those points.

These realizations have made quantum theory an indispensable part of modern physics. However, the theory still has one major problem: gravity. The 21st century understanding of gravity comes from Einstein's work on Special and General Relativity. The various predictions made by Einstein's theories have been proven correct experimentally on numerous occasions, and there is no doubt that his ideas accurately explain reality. But they do not mix with quantum mechanics.

It is possible to look at physics and think of there as being three distinct zones: relativity, which describes the very big and the very fast; quantum mechanics, which describes the very small; and Newtonian physics, which describes everything in between. But Newtonian physics easily unifies with quantum theory since the chaos and weirdness at the individual wave-particle level smoothes out as you add more and more particles together, which is what we see when we look at the macro world in which we live. (That is, when you look at an object in front of you, you see it existing in a definite point in space because so many particles make it up the probability that they will all end up suddenly existing elsewhere—the way individual particles can—drops to nearly zero.) Additionally, three of the four fundamental forces, electromagnetism, the strong force and the weak force, can all be explained through quantum mechanics using their three transfer particles; photons, gluons and bosons. Essentially, they have been unified.

But the use of a gravity transfer particle, the graviton, in models has been less successful at bringing the experimentally accurate predictions of relativity in line with the functioning of reality at the quantum level.

 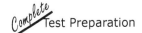

States of Matter

Matter on Earth can exist in three main states or phases: solid, liquid and gas. There is also a fourth phase, plasma, that occurs when matter is superheated. The primary difference between the different phases of matter is the behaviour of molecules in relation to the temperature the matter is exposed to. The lower the temperature, the closer together and more locked together the molecules are. The higher the temperature, the farther apart the molecules are and the more they move relative to one another.

Solid

Solid matter exists in a state where its molecules are locked together in a rigid structure preventing them from moving and, as a result, solid matter is held together in a specific shape. There are two primary types of solids, each defined by the structures in which their molecules are held. When the molecules in solid matter maintain a uniform organization they form a polycrystalline structure. This is how molecules in metal, ice and salt are organized. Polycrystalline structures are generally a result of the molecules' ionic properties. Water molecules, for instance, are formed in such a way that there are distinct ends, one with two hydrogen atoms and one with a single oxygen atom. The structure of the atoms within a water molecule means these ends are charged, giving it what amount to poles and causing water molecules to join together only in specific patterns. Under a microscope polycrystalline solids are generally described as resembling lattice work or a chain link fence, with the same pattern of molecules from one end to the other.

When molecules electromagnetic properties do not incline them to form into particular structures, they glob together in whatever patterns they can. This produces amorphous solids, most notably foams, glass and many types of plastic. Amorphous solids have no regular pattern throughout their structure and, as a result, are poor conductors of heat and electricity.

Liquid

When solids are heated past a certain point, the electromagnetic bonds holding their molecules together loosen, and the molecules are able to move more freely. While the temperatures required for this to happen can vary widely, the particular physical qualities of a liquid are always the same. Liquids are considered to be fluids, which differ from solids primarily in their ability to take the shape of any container they are held in. This is the result of a less intense electromagnetic connection between the molecules than there is in solids; however, there is still enough that liquids still want to stay all in the same place. This is why liquids still maintain a low density that is nearly identical to their densities in solid form, and why they will maintain a constant volume rather than just drift off the way gasses do.

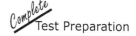

Liquids also have a property known as viscosity, which describes their willingness to flow over and away from themselves. Liquids such as water and honey have a constant viscosity and are known as Newtonian fluids. Non-Newtonian fluids, such as a goopy mixture of water and cornstarch can change their viscosities.

GAS

The third state of matter that is commonly found on Earth is gas. Gasses are formed when matter is heated beyond its liquid state so that the electromagnetic bonds holding its molecules together are severed almost completely. Gasses are also considered fluids and like liquids have no definite shape. But unlike liquids they also lack a definite volume and have an extremely low density compared to their solid forms.

Since gasses lack both a shape and a volume, they will expand to fill any container they are placed in. Left unbounded they will expand forever. Conversely, gasses are perfectly happy to compress together in an enclosed space. (However, the more molecules of a gas that are enclosed in a space together, the higher the gas's pressure—the force exerted by the molecules on the container's surface—will be.) One interesting thing about this expansion and compression is that it will always be homogeneous, meaning that as a gas expands to fill a container, there will never be pockets of a higher density of molecules in some areas with a lower density of molecules in others. The molecules will expand to fill the container equally.

PLASMA

A final state of matter is called plasma. Although plasma is rarely found on Earth, it is the most common state of matter throughout the universe. (It is the primary state of matter in stars, for instance.) Plasma is the next step up from a gas; it is when a gas's molecules become super heated to the point where the molecular bonds themselves break down and the atoms begin shedding their electrons. This gives plasma some unique characteristics, not the least of which is that it is ionized, or electrically charged. In many ways plasma acts like a gas. It lacks any definite shape or volume, and it will homogeneously fill any container. But it is can also be manipulated by electromagnetic fields, which can be used to alter its shape or contain it. Essentially, plasma is a super-heated, magnetically charged gas.

 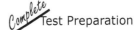

Anatomy and Physiology
Self-Assessment and Tutorials

THIS SECTION CONTAINS AN ANATOMY AND PHYSIOLOGY SELF-ASSESSMENT AND TUTORIALS. The Tutorials are designed to familiarize general principals and the Self-Assessment contains general questions similar to the questions likely to be on the HESI exam, but are not intended to be identical to the exam questions. Many Universities recommend that students take an introductory Science courses before taking the HESI Exam. The tutorials are not designed to be a complete math course, and it is assumed that students have some familiarity with Anatomy and Physiology. If you do not understand parts of the tutorial, or find the tutorial difficult, it is recommended that you seek out additional instruction.

The purpose of the self-assessment is:

- Identify your strengths and weaknesses.

- Develop your personalized study plan (above)

- Get accustomed to the HESI format

- Extra practice – the self-assessment is a 3rd test!

Since this is a self-assessment, and depending on how confident you are with Anatomy and Physiology, timing yourself is optional. There are a total of 25 questions which must be answered in 25 minutes. The self-assessment has 15 questions, so allow 15 minutes to complete this assessment.

NOTE: The Anatomy and Physiology section is an optional module that not all schools include. We strongly suggest that you check with your school for the HESI A2 exam details. It is always a good idea to give the materials you receive when you register to take the HESI a careful review.

The questions below are not exactly the same as you will find on the HESI - that would be too easy! And nobody knows what the questions will be and they change all the time. Below are general Anatomy and Physiology questions that cover the same areas as the HESI. So while the format and exact wording of the questions may differ slightly, and change from year to year, if you can answer the questions below, you will have no problem with the Anatomy and Physiology section of the HESI.

The self-assessment is designed to give you a baseline score in the different areas covered. Here is a brief outline of how your score on the self-assessment relates to your understanding of the material.

75% - 100%	Excellent – you have mastered the content
50 – 75%	Good. You have a working knowledge. Even though you can just pass this section, you may want to review the Tutorials and do some extra practice to see if you can improve your mark.
25% - 50%	Below Average. You do not understand the content. Review the tutorials, and retake this quiz again in a few days, before proceeding to the rest of the Practice Test Course.
Less than 25%	Poor. You have a very limited understanding. Please review the Tutorials, and retake this quiz again in a few days, before proceeding to the rest of the course.

Anatomy and Physiology

1. Anatomy breaks the human abdomen down into segments called _____.

    a. Regions

    b. Districts

    c. Quadrants

    d. Areas

2. The quadrant that is largely responsible for digestion is _____

    a. Left Upper

    b. Right Upper

    c. Right Left

    d. Left Lower

3. The body organ that is NOT located within the Right Upper Quadrant is _____

    a. Liver

    b. Gall Bladder

    c. Duodenum

    d. Sigmoid colon

4. The organ that is located in the Right Lower Quadrant is _____

    a. Appendix

    b. Heart

    c. Left lung

    d. Trachea

5. One reason that medical professionals should know the names and locations of the Quadrant is _____.

    a. To keep the patient's condition a secret from him.

    b. To communicate about patients' conditions with other doctors and medical professionals.

    c. For insurance purposes.

    d. Not knowing the quadrants almost always results in death for the patient.

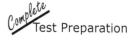

6. The stomach and colon are both in the _____.

   a. Left Upper Quadrant

   b. Right Upper Quadrant

   c. Right Lower Quadrant

   d. Left Lower Quadrant

7. Commonly used abbreviations for the Quadrants of the abdomen are _____.

   a. QUR, QUL, QLR, QLL

   b. ABC, DEF, GHI, JKL

   c. RUQ, LUQ, RLQ, LLQ

   d. RR, LL, QQ, RQ

8. The intestines are located in _____.

   a. LUQ

   b. LLQ

   c. RLQ

   d. All of the above

9. The stomach is located in _____.

   a. LLQ

   b. LUQ

   c. RUQ

   d. RLQ

10. The gallbladder is located in _____.

   a. RUQ

   b. LUQ

   c. LLQ

   d. RLQ

11. An example of human homeostasis is _____.

   a. Metabolism

   b. Adrenalin

   c. Hormones

   d. Fluid Balance

12. Human homeostasis is the ability of the body to regulate its _____ in response to fluctuations in the environment outside the body.

    a. Inner environment

    b. Outer environment

    c. Temperature

    d. Metabolism

13. The amount of energy / calories that your body requires to maintain itself is known as _____.

    a. Temperature

    b. Fluid balance

    c. Botulism

    d. Metabolism

14. An example of a person whose metabolism has lowered is _____.

    a. A woman who is in her teens and quite athletic

    b. A man who is past 30 and whose body is losing muscle.

    c. A man who is past 30 and works out daily.

    d. A man who is past 30 and eats a low-fat diet.

15. An example of something that increases a person's metabolism is _____.

    a. Aerobic exercise

    b. Mental exercise

    c. Eating a fatty diet

    d. Reading

Anatomy and Physiology

1. C
Anatomy breaks the human abdomen down into segments called **quadrants.**

2. A
The Left upper quadrant of the abdomen, is often abbreviated as LUQ, contains the stomach, spleen, left lobe of the liver, body of the pancreas, left kidney and adrenal gland.

3. D
The right upper quadrant of the abdomen, often abbreviated as RUQ, contains the liver, gall bladder, duodenum and head of the pancreas.

4. A
The Right lower quadrant of the human abdomen, often abbreviated as RLQ, contains the appendix and ascending colon.

5. B
Medical personnel divide the abdomen into smaller regions to facilitate study and discussion.

6. A
The stomach and colon are both in the Left Upper Quadrant, together with, liver, spleen, left kidney, pancreas and large intestine.

7. C
The commonly used abbreviations for the Quadrants are, Right Upper Quadrant, RUQ, Left Upper Quadrant, LUQ, Right Lower Quadrant, RLQ, Left Lower Quadrant, LLQ.

8. D
All of the above. The Large Intestine passes through all of the quadrants.

9. B
The stomach and colon are both in the Left Upper Quadrant, together with, liver, spleen, left kidney, pancreas and large intestine.

10. A
The gallbladder is located in the Right Upper Quadrant together with the liver, right kidney, colon, pancreas and large intestine.

11. D
The human body manages a multitude of highly complex interactions to maintain balance within a normal range. The kidneys are responsible for regulating blood water levels, re-absorption of substances into the blood, maintenance of salt and ion levels in the blood, regulation of blood pH, and excretion of urea and other wastes.[8]

12. A
Human homeostasis is the ability of the body to regulate its **inner environment** in re-

sponse to fluctuations in the environment outside the body.

13. D

The amount of energy / calories that your body requires to maintain itself is known as metabolism.

14. B

Exercise and low fat diets will increase metabolism. Choice B, **a man who is past 30 and whose body is losing muscle** is the only choice.

15. A

Exercise will increase metabolism, so Choice A **aerobic exercise**.

Anatomy and Physiology Tutorials

Circulatory System

Tour of the System

The easiest way to see how the circulatory system works is by taking a tour with erythrocytes (red blood cells) through the system:

The erythrocytes start in the *left ventricle* of the heart.

They then move through the *aortic valve* into the *aorta.*

As the aorta branches into smaller arteries, the erythrocytes move into an *artery* then split into smaller blood vessels known as *arterioles.*

From arterioles, the erythrocytes pass into a capillary, or capillary bed.

Capillaries are tiny blood vessels and it is in these vessels that the exchange of oxygen, nutrients and carbon dioxide takes place.

After this exchange, the erythrocytes are de-oxygenated (oxygen has been removed from the erythrocyte).

Blood that contains these de-oxygenated erythrocytes is also known as *venous blood.*

The erythrocytes, which now contain carbon dioxide and other waste products, pass from the capillaries into *venules.*

Venules come together to form veins.

From the veins, the erythrocytes flow into the superior vena cava, and into the right atrium. They pass through the tricuspid valve into the right ventricle.

The erythrocytes pass through the pulmonary valve and into the pulmonary artery on their way to the lungs. The pulmonary artery is the only artery that carries deoxygenated blood.

In the lungs, the erythrocytes give up their carbon dioxide and absorb oxygen. Now the blood goes back to the left atrium, through the mitral valve and into the left ventricle, ready to start its journey once again.

The movement of the blood to and from the heart is the systemic circulation and the movement of the blood from the heart to the lungs and back again is the pulmonary circulation.

The blood pressure in arteries is regulated by muscular contraction or expansion of the arterial walls, according to need.

The circulatory system also consists of the lymphatic system, which has the job of distributing lymph throughout the body. This is how lymph moves through the system:

In capillaries, the serum, or the liquid part of the blood, seeps through the tissues.

If tissues are inflamed, the capillaries are more permeable and so seepage is faster.

This serum is called lymph.

Lymph makes its way through tissues, until it collects in the lymphatic ducts.

Once in the ducts, lymph begins to make its way back to the venous blood stream.

As lymph moves, it is filtered by lymph nodes.

These lymph nodes contain **leukocytes** (white blood cells) which are ready to attack bacteria or viruses.

Functions

The circulatory system has a number of key functions, including:

- Controlling the movement of blood and lymph through the body

- Exchanging gases (oxygen and carbon dioxide) with other cells and tissues in the body

- Exchanging nutrients (such as amino acids and electrolytes) with other cells and tissues

- Assisting with immune responses

- Assisting with clotting

- Assisting in the maintenance of body temperature and pH (maintaining homeostasis)

Components

Heart: This is what pumps blood around the body. Because the heart is a muscle, it also needs oxygen, so it has its own circulatory system known as the *coronary circulation*, which takes blood to and from the heart.

Aorta: This is the main artery that receives blood from the heart. It is a very tough, muscular artery.

Arteries: These blood vessels also contain muscle to make them elastic. This helps to move the blood along.

Arterioles: Also muscular these smaller vessels contract to deliver blood to the capillaries.

Capillaries: These are the diameter of a single cell, making exchange of gases and other products from erythrocytes easy.

Venules: Many of these small blood vessels come together to form a vein.

Veins: Unlike arteries, these do not contract. With a tube-like structure, they contain valves to prevent blood from flowing backwards.

Lymph ducts: These empty lymph into the veins.

Lymph nodes: These act as filters for the lymph and are very important in the immune system. Inflammation of these usually indicates infection in the body.

Common Diseases and Disorders

Angina: Is a type of chest pain that often radiates down the arm. Angina is caused when the heart cannot receive the blood and oxygen that it needs (usually because the coronary arteries are blocked with plaque).

Cardiac Arrest: The heart stops pumping blood around the body. Unlike a heart attack, this can happen suddenly without a known cause (such as coronary heart disease).

Coronary heart disease: Coronary arteries (which supply the heart with blood) are narrowed because of plaque deposits on their walls. These deposits prevent enough oxygen from reaching the heart.

Heart Attack or Myocardial Infarction: When the coronary arteries (which supply blood the heart muscle with blood) become blocked with plaque, blood flow to the heart muscles is reduced. This causes damage to the heart muscle as well as increasing the risk of part of the heart muscle dying.

Phlebitis: This is inflammation of a vein. A common place is in the legs, where the veins swell and block the blood, so the leg swells markedly.

Varicose veins: Unnaturally swollen veins caused by faulty valves. These are usually in the legs.

 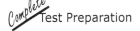

Medical Terminology

Blood pressure: This is how much pressure there is against the walls of the main arteries. The systolic pressure is when the ventricles of the heart contract and the diastolic pressure is when ventricles relax and refill. The classic blood pressure measurement is 120/80 (120 is the systole value and 80 is the diastole value).

Erythrocytes: These red blood cells carry oxygen, carbon dioxide and other products through the circulatory system.

Hypertension: High blood pressure

Hypotension: Low blood pressure

Leukocytes: There are several different kinds of white blood cells and they play a key role in the immune system.

Platelets: Platelets are cell fragments found in the blood. They are essential for blood clotting.

Pulse rate/heart rate: The number of times the heart beats per minute.

The circulatory system is also important when *assessing a person's color*. The color changes when more or less blood diverts to the skin, so color is a good indicator of health.

Terms to denote a lack of color include: pale, ashen, pallid, sallow, white, colorless, white as a ghost, blanched.

Terms to denote too much color include: florid, flushed, crimson, ruddy, feverish.

There are also *trauma terms* for the circulatory system:

Bleeding: Blood coming from a lesion. Internal bleeding is bleeding inside the body, often caused by an injury or disease. Blood may sometimes leak from an opening such as the mouth or anus.

Bleeding nose (Epistaxis): Blood coming from the nose, usually due to trauma. A bleeding nose can sometimes start spontaneously due to increased blood pressure.

Bruised: Discolored due to a blow. Usually the skin is not broken (a bruise is also called a contusion).

Cut or Incision: A clean-cut wound or slit such as one caused by a knife.

Crush: Caused by pressure a crush is a contusion or bruise, indicating internal bleeding.

Gash or laceration: A wound that is torn or ragged.

Scrape: An abrasion or graze caused by scraping off the upper tissues of the skin.

Swollen: Bigger than usual, often through accumulation of fluid.

Throbbing: When used with pain, it means that the pain gets worse in a rhythmic pattern (with the heartbeat).

Other miscellaneous medical and trauma terms include:

Blood blister: A dark swelling of the skin caused by pinching, which breaks a small blood vessel. The skin remains unbroken.

Blood tests: A variety of tests carried out with a blood sample. A blood test can check for many disorders including anemia, infections or even liver damage.

Blood in the urine: Indicates problems with the bladder, kidneys or prostate gland.

Hemangioma (blood spot or birthmark): Is a dark red discoloration of the skin.

Occult blood: "Occult" means hidden. To detect colon cancer, feces is checked for occult blood.

Palpitations or bumping: This refers to an irregular heartbeat, often experienced by the patient as a "bumping in the chest."

Tarry stools: These are feces that dark in color, like tar, caused by old blood in the digestive tract. Tarry stools can indicate internal bleeding.

Transfusion: Transfusing, or giving of blood taken from a blood donor.

The Digestive System

Tour of the System

The digestive system is an extensive system that begins at the lips and ends at the anus. The easiest way to explore the digestive system is on a journey with a peanut butter and jelly sandwich (PB&J):

The PB&J passes through the lips and into the mouth (oral cavity).

The oral cavity contains teeth and the tongue. Beneath the tongue is the floor of the mouth and above the tongue, the hard palate.

The soft palate (which does not contain bone) is at the back of the mouth.

The PB&J is *masticated* (chewed) by the teeth.

There are normally 32 teeth and in each arch there are:

- 4 incisors

- 2 cuspids (or canines - they resemble the long cuspids that dogs have)

- 4 premolars or bicuspids

- 6 molars. The last molar is the "wisdom tooth".

Chewing the PB&J also requires assistance from the muscular tongue.

Chewing stimulates the release of saliva from the salivary glands in the mouth to moisten the sandwich. Saliva contains enzymes that help to break down carbohydrates.

The PB&J is now a homogeneous smooth mass called a bolus.

Swallowing or deglutition is a complex process controlled by the nervous system.

The lingual nerve in the tongue determines when the bolus is 'ready' for swallowing.

Once the bolus is pushed to the back of the tongue, receptors initiate the pharyngeal phase of swallowing.

This phase is when breathing chewing, coughing and other activities stop.

The bolus passes the tonsils, the pharynx and goes into the esophagus to the stomach.

The stomach is located just below the diaphragm and when empty it has a volume of around 45ml. When full, it can extend to hold as much as three liters of food.

In the stomach, the bolus mixes with liquids, acid and digestive juices.

These break the bolus down into simpler chemical substances so they can be absorbed into the blood more easily.

After some hours, the semi-liquid mass, now called chyme, passes into the small intestine.

In the first part of the small intestine, called the duodenum, bile from the liver emulsifies fats. Pancreatic juice and enzymes also break down materials further.

Broken down materials are absorbed into the bloodstream and taken to the liver for filtration, toxin removal and further processing.

Anything remaining in the small intestine moves to the large intestine via peristalsis.

Fermentation, aided by gut bacteria left in the chyme, breaks down some of the remaining substances.

The chyme moves into the cecum, which is a pouch that connects the last part of the small intestine (ileum) with the first part of the large intestine.

Attached to the cecum is the appendix. In humans, the appendix is vestigial, which means it has no known function.

The large intestine takes around 16 hours to complete the digestive processes.

Digested matter moves from the cecum to the colon.

The colon is able to absorb vitamins (including vitamin K) produced by the bacteria which inhabit the colon (colonic bacteria).

The colon also absorbs salts and water and stores feces until defecation.

Feces move along the colon by peristalsis to the last part of the large intestine, the rectum.

From here, defecation, the final process of digestion occurs.

This whole process of digestion takes between 24 and 72 hours.

Functions

The main function of the digestive system is to digest, or break down food into smaller chemical components (also called *catabolism*).

 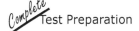

Components

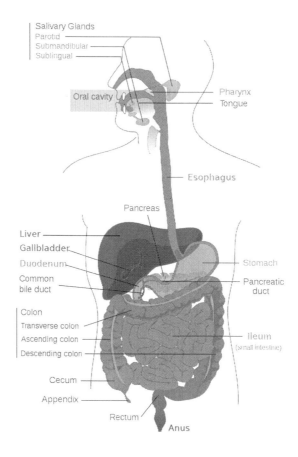

Salivary Glands
Parotid
Submandibular
Sublingual

Oral cavity

Pharynx
Tongue

Esophagus

Pancreas

Liver
Gallbladder
Duodenum
Common
bile duct

Stomach
Pancreatic
duct

Colon
Transverse colon
Ascending colon
Descending colon

Ileum
(small intestine)

Cecum

Appendix

Rectum
Anus

1

Pharynx

This is the part of the throat located behind the mouth and nasal cavity.

Tongue

This muscle is used to manipulate food during chewing (mastication). The tongue also contains taste buds.

Esophagus

This is a muscular tube connecting the pharynx to the stomach. A bolus moves through the esophagus via peristalsis.

Epiglottis

This is a cartilage flap attached at the entrance to the voice box (larynx). When this is closed, it prevents food from entering the trachea (windpipe).

Large intestine

This starts at the cecum, contains the colon and ends at the rectum. It is involved in absorbing some nutrients but primarily water and salts.

Small intestine

The majority of digestion and absorption occurs in the small intestine and this is why this organ is very long, offering the maximum surface area for its digestive functions.

Stomach

This is J shaped and connects the esophagus to the small intestine. As well as a food mixing and processing area, the stomach also 'holds' food until it is ready to move into the small intestine. The stomach is acidic as its enzymes work best at a low pH.

Liver

This produces a number of chemicals needed for digestion. It is also able to store some nutrients such as vitamins.

Pancreas

This produces a number of digestive juices to assist in digestion.

Gallbladder

This produces and stores bile until required by the small intestine.

Rectum

The final part of the large intestine it temporarily stores feces.

Common Diseases and Disorders

Appendicitis: This is inflammation or infection of the appendix. If infected the appendix can swell and burst. Also called peritonitis, this is very serious because then the contents of the intestines spill into the abdominal cavity.

Colon cancer: This can develop without symptoms, which is why doctors often take an occult blood sample every two years. This test detects small amounts of blood in the feces, which can be a symptom of colon cancer.

Constipation: Refers to infrequent or difficult evacuation of the feces.

Diarrhea: Is abnormal frequency and liquidity of feces.

Diverticulosis: As people age, the large intestine sometimes forms small pouches.

Sometimes sharp foods like seeds or grains lodge in these pouches and cause inflammation or infection. This is diverticulitis.

Gallstones: These are hard stones created from a buildup of bile in the gall bladder. They cause acute pain but are often able to be removed with a catheter and ultrasound.

Perforated ulcer: A stomach ulcer has broken through the stomach wall is now perforated. This allows the contents of the stomach to move into the abdominal cavity and can be very serious.

A 'sore mouth' could mean one of many things, including cold sores (herpes simplex), mouth ulcers (aphthous ulcers) or lesions of the teeth and gums.

Sore throats are another common problem, usually due to infection in the tonsils, or an inflamed pharynx.

Stomach ulcers: Prolonged chronic stress is often the main cause of stomach ulcers. Because the stomach produces too much stomach acid, it damages the mucosal covering of the stomach, causing a lesion.

Medical Terminology

GI tract: Gastrointestinal or GI tract can sometimes include all structures from the mouth to the anus, but medically it is often differentiated between the upper and lower GI tracts.

Lower GI: The lower gastrointestinal tract includes the large intestine, small intestine and anus.

Peristalsis: This is a very strong, rhythmic contraction and relaxation of muscles throughout the digestive system that push the contents along.

Upper GI: The upper GI or gastrointestinal tract generally refers to the esophagus, stomach and duodenum.

The Endocrine System

Tour of the System

The endocrine system is an amazingly complex system with many important roles throughout the body. It works alongside the nervous system to coordinate functions of all of the different body systems.

The endocrine system contains endocrine glands that release their products (known as hormones) directly into the bloodstream.

Hormones are substances that arouse the body into activity. Hormones are often dependent upon one another in their action. That is, the secretion of one hormone will often excite another gland to produce its hormone too. The balance that the body strikes with these hormones is unique for each individual.

Although hormones travel around the body in the bloodstream, they only affect certain cells, which are their target cells. Only target cells will contain the correct molecular information that will allow a hormone to bind to that particular cell.

How cells respond to hormones depends on the cell itself as well as the hormone. One hormone may synthesize (make) a product in one type of cell and make a completely different product in another type of cell.

One of the easiest ways when touring this complex system is to look at where endocrine glands are and what hormones they secrete.

The diagrams below show endocrine glands and their hormones.

Hormones produced in the head and neck

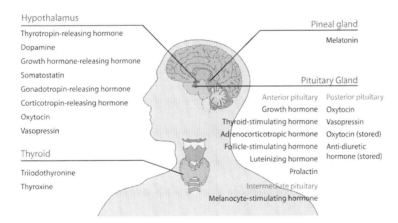

2

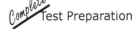

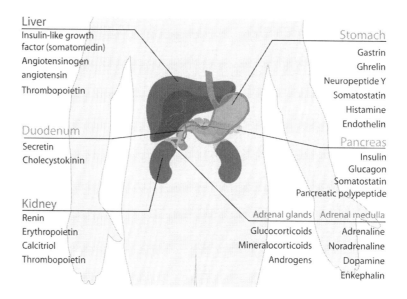

Liver
Insulin-like growth
factor (somatomedin)
Angiotensinogen
angiotensin
Thrombopoietin

Stomach
Gastrin
Ghrelin
Neuropeptide Y
Somatostatin
Histamine
Endothelin

Duodenum
Secretin
Cholecystokinin

Pancreas
Insulin
Glucagon
Somatostatin
Pancreatic polypeptide

Kidney
Renin
Erythropoietin
Calcitriol
Thrombopoietin

Adrenal glands | Adrenal medulla
Glucocorticoids | Adrenaline
Mineralocorticoids | Noradrenaline
Androgens | Dopamine
Enkephalin

2

Functions

The endocrine system secretes hormones into the bloodstream to regulate the body, helping to maintain homeostasis.

Components

Hypothalamus

This is the 'master' endocrine gland, located in the brain. The hypothalamus links the endocrine and nervous system. The hypothalamus receives information about pain, stress etc. It also regulates the autonomic nervous system that controls body temperature, hunger, thirst etc. The hypothalamus regulates release of a number of hormones that act on other glands.

The pituitary gland

The pituitary gland is in the center of the skull, attached to the hypothalamus. The release or suppression of pituitary hormones is controlled by the hypothalamus. As well as having its own unique effects, it can influence the performance of the other endocrine glands.

It has two parts, a posterior pituitary gland and the anterior pituitary gland.

The posterior pituitary gland tends to store oxytocin, used for uterine contractions and anti-diuretic hormone (ADH), which stimulates water retention.

Hormones released from the *anterior pituitary gland*

Hormone group	Function	Example	How it works
Somatotrophs	Stimulate the thyroid gland.	Growth hormone (GH)	If growth hormone is produced for too long, gigantism occurs. If growth hormone is produced after the epiphyseal disks have calcified in the skeleton, acromegaly occurs, causing abnormally large hands, feet and mandible (jaw). If not enough growth hormone is produced, the child will not grow and artificial growth hormone is usually administered to correct this.
Thyrotrophs	These hormones stimulate activity in other glands.	Thyroid-stimu-lating hormone (TSH)	This controls secretion of other hormones in the thyroid gland.
Gonadotrophs	These are involved in ovulation, although they are present in both males and females.	Follicle stimulating hormone (FSH) and luteinizing hormone (LH)	FSH and LH are needed to secrete estrogens and progesterone and assist in reproduction,
Lactotrophs	Lactotrophs are involved in growth and regulation of mammary glands.	Prolactin	Initiate milk production in mammary glands
Corticotrophs	Synthesize ACTH	Adreno-corticot-rophin (ACTH)	ACTH stimulates the adrenal cortex to produce glucocorticoids (required in glucose metabolism).

 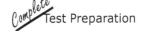

There are also a number of other hormones secreted from the pituitary gland.

The Thyroid gland

Situated at the base of the larynx, its middle part, the isthmus, covers the second and third cartilaginous rings of the trachea.

It secretes the thyroid hormones thyroxin and triiodothyronine. These have an important role in controlling metabolism (including energy or ATP production) throughout the body.

It also secretes calcitonin that alters calcium levels in the blood.

The Parathyroid glands

There are usually four parathyroid glands, two on each side of the thyroid gland. Although they are very small, they control the amount of calcium and magnesium in the blood stream.

Without them, there is not enough calcium in the blood for the nervous system to function properly. Those who have *hyperparathyroidism* have bones that are de-mineralized and the calcium in their bones is literally urinated away.

Adrenal or Suprarenal glands

These are located on the top of the kidneys. The adrenal glands essentially produce three types of steroids. *Steroid* hormones are fat (lipid) hormones.

The outside of the adrenal glands (*adrenal cortex*) produces three types of hormones:

1. Mineralocorticoids - control sodium and potassium levels in the body

2. Glucocorticoids – involved in metabolism and resistance to stress. One of these is cortisone, a hormone that has a variety of functions in the body.

Androgens – These have little effect on the body as significant amounts of androgens are produced in the testes. In women, these contribute to sex drive.

The inner of the adrenal glands, the *adrenal medulla* produces **epinephrine** and **norepinephrine** (noradrenalin). These hormones prepare the body to either "fight or flight". Epinephrine (adrenalin) increases the heart rate and breathing rate, adjusts blood supply to the extremities and causes the blood to clot more readily. Therefore, if you are suddenly startled, you notice these changes in the body.

Pancreas

The pancreas contains special cells called *islets of Langerhans*. These secrete a number of hormones:

Insulin - controls the amount of glucose in the blood stream. Insulin causes removal and storage of glucose from the blood.

Glucagon – Raises blood sugar levels by breaking down glycogen in the liver. This causes the release of glucose into the blood.

The other two hormones, **somatostatin** and **pancreatic polypeptides** assist insulin and glucagon with their actions.

Pineal gland

This gland is located in the brain and secretes **melatonin,** a hormone that plays an important role in the sleep and wake cycle. The cause of jetlag is through melatonin disruption.

Thymus gland

This plays a key role in immunity, helping white blood cells to mature.

There are also hormones produced throughout other tissues and organs in the body, including erythropoietin from the kidney, which helps to increase the rate of erythrocyte (red blood cell) production.

Common Diseases and Disorders

Cretinism: This is caused by a lack of thyroid hormones produced during development. The severe hormone deficiency causes a hard form of edema, called myxedema.

Diabetes: An insufficiency of insulin production causes diabetes. For those who suffer with type 1 diabetes, it means that the cells in their pancreas have stopped producing insulin, or produce very little. Those with Type 2 diabetes are able to produce some insulin, but not enough to regulate blood glucose levels. Type 2 diabetes is often seen in obese patients.

Goiter: This is an enlargement of the thyroid gland, often caused by iodine deficiency.

Hyperthyroidism: Is caused by too much thyroxin, resulting in a higher than normal metabolic rate.

Hypothyroidism: Is a lack of thyroxin.

Polycystic ovary syndrome: This is a common female endocrine disorder. Although it may have genetic causes, hormone imbalances play a key role in this syndrome.

Medical Terminology

Autonomic nervous system: This is part of the nervous system. It helps to control the body. It is usually unconscious and controls actions such as the heart rate, digestion

 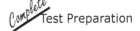

and respiratory rate.

Endocrinology: Is the study of the endocrine system and the resulting hormone balance.

Homeostasis: This is the ability of the human body to maintain a stable internal environment, when dealing with both internal and external environmental changes.

Negative feedback: This helps to maintain homeostasis in the body. If a gland is producing too much of one hormone, signals are sent to the brain and an opposing hormone is released. This reduces the levels of the first hormone. An example of this is glucagon and insulin, regulating blood glucose levels.

Positive feedback: Rarely seen in the body, a positive feedback loop is the secretion of oxytocin during delivery. This increases contractions to allow delivery of the baby.

The Integumentary System

Tour of the System

The integumentary system is composed of the skin, hair and nails. It has a variety of functions, but one of the main ones is to protect the body. It is the largest organ system in the body, consisting of around 15% of the total body weight.

The skin is a key indicator of an individual's health status. It is readily visible, without any intrusive procedures. The skin of the face and hands can reveal a lot about the circulatory system, the lifestyle of the patient and their general health. Those who have yellowing skin are usually suffering with jaundice whereas those who have a blue-grey tint are suffering with cyanosis. A deep red hue can indicate hypertension (high blood pressure) or white skin can be an indicator of medical shock. How skin feels can also indicate disease or trauma. Skin may feel cold, clammy, hot or dry.

Functions

The skin **protects internal tissues and organs.**

The skin **prevents organisms** (such as bacteria or viruses) from entering the body.

The skin **protects the body from dehydrating.**

The skin **acts as a waterproof barrier**. It allows a wet body to exist in dry air, allows immersion in fresh water without swelling with water, or immersion in salt water without becoming desiccated.

The skin **protects the body from sudden temperature changes** (maintains homeostasis). On hot days, the skin helps regulate body temperature in three main ways:

Arterioles vasodilate and send more blood to superficial capillaries in the skin. This allows heat loss.

The hairs on the skin remain flat, preventing insulating air from trapping between the hairs and the skin.

Sweating or perspiration is also essential for cooling the body, through the process of evaporation.

The skin **protects the body from UV damage** by secreting melanin. Pigmented or freckled skin is an adaptation to intense sunlight.

The skin **excretes waste materials**, such as salts and urea, through perspiration.

The skin **stores a variety of substances** include water, fat, glucose and vitamin D.

The skin **produces Vitamin D** from UV exposure. An absence of Vitamin D causes rickets.

The skin **forms new skin cells** to repair skin damage.

The skin **maintains the form** of the body.

The **skin acts as a receptor** for:

- touch

- pressure

- pain

- heat

- cold

These receptors are also part of the *somatosensory system.* Because the skin receives many stimuli, it plays a major role in man's adaptation to his environment. In particular, the skin acts as an early warning system for unhealthy conditions.

Components

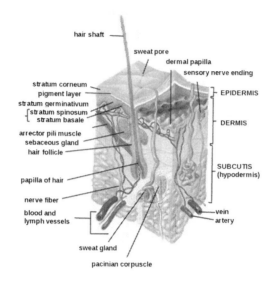

hair shaft

sweat pore

dermal papilla

sensory nerve ending

stratum corneum

pigment layer

stratum germinativum

{ stratum spinosum

stratum basale

arrector pili muscle

sebaceous gland

hair follicle

papilla of hair

nerve fiber

blood and lymph vessels

sweat gland

pacinian corpuscle

EPIDERMIS

DERMIS

SUBCUTIS (hypodermis)

vein

artery

3

Skin consists of two main layers, the epidermis and the dermis and these contain a number of other components:

The Epidermis

This is the top layer of skin made up of epithelial cells.

The cells lower in the epidermis are responsible for the growth of this layer. As mitosis (cell division) occurs at the *basale layer,* cells move up through the strata (thin layer), pushed upwards by the dividing cells below.

The epidermis does not contain blood vessels.

There are a number of different types of cell found in the epidermis, including keratinocytes and melanocytes.

Keratinocytes are the most common cell found in the epidermis.

Keratinocytes mainly act as a barrier cell. They also produce a protein known as *keratin.*

Keratin makes the top layer strong and water resistant.

As production of keratin increases, the keratinocytes die. This process is *cornification.*

These cornified keratinocytes are then lost (or shed) from the surface of the skin and replaced with new cells.

Renewal of the epidermis, also known as the process of maturation and desquamation takes around 21 days.

Nails develop in the epidermis and extend down into the dermis.

The Dermis

This contains a variety of connective tissues such as collagen and elastin that give skin stretch and flexibility.

The dermis helps cushion the body from stresses.

Ends of blood vessels and nerves are located in the dermis.

The blood vessels nourish and remove waste from the dermis and the basale layer of the epidermis.

The base of sweat glands and sebaceous glands are also located in the dermis.

Hair follicles may extend down into the underlying connective tissue, but they originally arise from the epidermis.

Sweat glands

Sweat glands are small tubular structures of the skin that produce sweat.

Eccrine sweat glands are all over the body. These play a key role in perspiring and cooling the skin

Apocrine sweat glands are larger and limited to the armpits and perianal areas. These become active during puberty and secrete odorous sweat.

Hair

The functions of hair include warmth and protection. In animals, hair has many other important functions such as camouflage.

Hair develops from keratin and it grows from the hair follicles that arise from the epidermis.

Once hair leaves the follicle, it is 'dead'.

Attached to the hair follicle is a sebaceous gland that lubricates the hair and the *erector pili* muscle that causes hair to stand up (goose bumps).

Nails

The main function of nails is to protect the delicate fingertip from injury and assist with delicate finger movements.

The condition of nails is also a good indicator of general health.

A nail consists of a nail plate, nail matrix and nail bed.

Nail plate cells grow in the *cell matrix* and push older nail plate cells forward.

The nail plate is the actual nail and this is made of keratin, forming a strong flexible material composed of layers of dead cells.

The *nail bed* is similar in structure to the skin, containing a dermis and epidermis.

Hypodermis

The *hypodermis* or *subcutaneous layer* is often associated with the skin. Its main function is to attach the skin to bone and muscle and supply the skin with blood vessels and nerves.

The main cells contained within the hypodermis are fibroblasts, macrophages and adipocytes (fat cells).

The hypodermis contains 50% of body fat and is essential as padding and insulation for the body.

Common Diseases and Disorders

Allergic reactions: The skin will often respond with a red rash due to exposure to an allergen. An allergen can be swallowed, inhaled, injected or even touched. Common allergens include stings and animal fur.

Boil: A boil or furuncle develops from bacterial infection of the hair follicle.

Carcinomas: This is the medical term for cancer and the skin is subject to several kinds of carcinomas: basal cell, squamous cell carcinomas, as well as melanomas.

- Basal cell carcinoma is the most common type of skin cancer. Although it rarely kills, it is considered malignant as it can cause a lot of damage as it invades surrounding tissues.

- Squamous cell carcinoma is also a common cancer and can develop on the skin and other parts of the body. The cells involved in this type of carcinoma continue to divide uncontrollably.

A melanoma is a malignant tumor made up of melanocyte cells (which produce the pigment melanin). Many melanomas are visible as changes to existing moles or the appearance of a new lesion on the skin.

Cysts: If a sebaceous gland is blocked, a cyst can form. Because a cyst is enclosed, when it grows it displaces other structures around it. It does not invade other tissues (non-invasive).

Dermatitis: Sometimes used interchangeably with eczema. Dermatitis is inflammation of the skin of which there are a number of causes. Contact dermatitis often occurs on the hands as a reaction to latex gloves or chemicals.

Eczema: This condition has scaly, itchy patches with blisters.

Impetigo: A contagious bacterial infection of the skin that is very common amongst children

Pimples: When sebaceous glands are blocked, their oily discharge (sebum) accumulates under the skin, causing a small swelling. These often become infected.

Psoriasis: This is a skin disorder characterized by scaly red patches of the skin. When this disorder affects the fingers, it can cause nails to become deformed.

Pustules: These are common in acne. Pustules are small, inflamed and pus-filled lesions on the surface of the skin. They can occur anywhere on the body but are common on the face, shoulders and back.

Rash: Allergic reactions and a number of illnesses manifest with a skin rash. Nearly all "childhood diseases" such as measles and chicken pox have a skin rash. With these types of disease, often the rash provides the final diagnosis, even before the bacterial analyses are completed.

Medical Terminology

Basale layer: The lowest layer of the epidermis, this is the layer where epidermal cell division occurs.

Cyanosis: Translates as 'blue disease'. This skin discoloration occurs with low oxygen levels in tissues near to the surface of the skin.

Homeostasis: This is the ability of the human body to maintain a stable internal environment, when dealing with both internal and external environmental changes.

Keratin: This protein has a number of functions in the skin, including waterproofing.

Keratinocytes: These cells produce keratin.

Melanin: The pigment found in skin and hair that are the primary determinant of color.

Melanocytes: These cells produce melanin.

Vasodilation: This is when smooth muscle, found in arteries, arterioles and large veins relaxes to allow an increased flow of blood through. This plays an important role in controlling body temperature.

Vasoconstriction: The opposite of vasodilation, this occurs when blood vessels narrow, restricting the amount of blood that can flow through these vessels.

 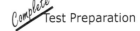

The Reproductive System

Tour of the System

Reproduction is any type of reproduction that conceives a child and the reproductive systems of both males and females are required for conception to occur.

Under normal circumstances, an embryo will form when a spermatozoa (gamete) fertilizes a female ovum (a gamete). Gametes are different to other cells in the body because they only contain half of the usual numbers of chromosomes (which contain the genetic information). Each gamete contains 23 chromosomes (including sex chromosomes) and when they join a zygote is formed, containing 46 (or 23 pairs) of chromosomes. This zygote then develops into an embryo.

Because the ovum always contains one female sex (X) chromosome, the spermatozoa dictates the sex of the unborn child. The sperm cell may contain another X chromosome (producing a girl) or a Y chromosome that will produce a male child.

The fundamental organ of both reproductive systems is the gonad. In adult females, these are the ovaries and in adult males, the testes.

In the embryo, the gonads are at first undifferentiated and it is impossible to see whether it is male or female. With time, the gonads differentiate and certain features develop, while other features are suppressed. This is probably due to the influence of environmental conditions such as hormone production.

Hormones are critical for development and regulation of the reproductive system and there are many different types of hormones involved. During puberty in girls, the pituitary gland (located at the back of the brain) releases various hormones. These hormones signal the ovaries to release an ovum every twenty-eight days as well as inducing the ovary to start functioning as an endocrine (hormone releasing) gland itself.

The first hormone the ovaries produce is estrogen. Estrogen induces the development of the secondary sexual characteristics (growth of breasts, change of body shape etc.). A second hormone, progesterone, produced by the corpus luteum encourages the endometrium to thicken, so that if fertilization occurs, the ovum will have optimal conditions to grow there.

There is a similar development process in boys. The hormones released from the pituitary gland cause development of secondary sexual characteristics (facial hair, pubic hair, penis growth etc.) and development of the reproductive organs. The key male androgen is testosterone and this is important for normal sperm development as well as physical and mental well-being in men.

Female Reproductive System

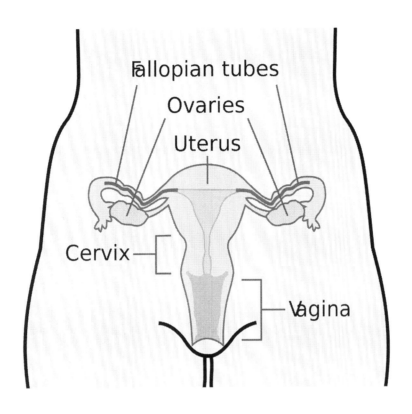

4

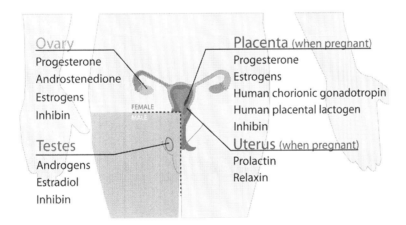

When the ovum (or gamete) develops in the ovary, it is in an ovarian follicle (sac).

The ovum moves along the fallopian tube towards the uterus with the help of contractions.

As the ovum matures, the follicular sac ruptures. The ruptured sac closes after releasing the egg and forms the corpus luteum. This produces the hormone progesterone.

The corpus luteum grows for about two weeks and then dies, unless it receives a different hormone from a developing embryo.

In pregnancy, however, the corpus luteum develops for several months and becomes quite large until the placenta takes over its job.

If during this journey, the ovum meets a sperm, fertilization may occur.

Fertilization often occurs in the fallopian tube although it can be in the uterus.

Once an ovum is fertilized, it is a zygote.

The zygote usually makes its way into the uterus and attaches to the special lining of the uterus called the endometrium and begins to develop into an embryo.

In a sexually mature woman, (before the menopause), this lining thickens up, becomes engorged with blood and is shed every twenty-eight days through menstruation.

The key time for fertilization is around halfway through the ovulation cycle and menstruation cannot occur if fertilization has occurred.

Male Reproductive System

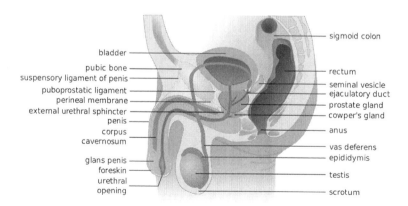

The male reproductive system consists of two main organs, the testes and the penis. There are also various glands and complicated tubal systems.

The testes make and store sperm cells (spermatozoa).

Three main glands lubricate the male reproductive system and nourish the spermatozoa.

One of these, the seminal vesicle produces the energy source that spermatozoa require for movement (motility).

The second, the bulbourethral glands produce a fluid released into the urethra. This assists in nourishing the spermatozoa.

Spermatozoa move to the third and final gland, the prostate gland, which produces the fluid vehicle (semen).

Semen is a mix of sperm cells, prostate fluid and seminal fluid. It also contains an enzyme, hyaluronidase, which assists the spermatozoa with penetrating the outer covering of the ovum.

From the prostate gland, semen moves into the urethra for expulsion during ejaculation.

Once ejaculation has occurred, sperm then travels through the vagina, towards the cervix and into the uterus or fallopian tubes to fertilize the ovum.

Functions

The function of the reproductive system is reproduction. Because there are differences between males and females, reproduction creates a greater combination of genetic material in the offspring (child).

Female Components

Fallopian tube (or oviducts)

The two fallopian tubes connect to the uterus. They also have special properties that assist ova to move towards the uterus.

Uterus

This is the organ in which the embryo and then fetus develops during gestation. The uterus stays in place with the help of ligaments. The cervix of the uterus protrudes into the vagina. The uterus also plays an important part in the female sexual response, by diverting blood to the external genitalia.

 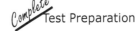

Ovary

The ovaries produce the ovum (or gametes). Females have two, although they function independently. Ligaments attach the ovaries to the uterus, rather than to the fallopian tubes.

Vagina

The vagina is a flattened tube and serves as a sheath for the male organ in sexual intercourse. It opens to the exterior through two folds of skin, the labia majora, and the labia minora. At the anterior end of these folds is the clitoris, which is analogous to the head of the male penis. In fact, it has a common embryonic origin.

Male Components

Testes

These have two functions, production of spermatozoa and production of the male sex hormone, testosterone. The release of other hormones stimulates the production of both of these. The scrotum protects the testes and these are outside the body as spermatozoa function better at a temperature slightly lower than normal body temperature.

Penis

One of the main male sex organs it also carries urine from the bladder. The penis contains erectile tissue so that when it fills with blood an erection can occur. The penis needs to be erect for ejaculation to occur.

Common Diseases and Disorders

Amenorrhea: Is an absence of the menstrual cycle, caused by starvation, stress, major illness, as well as pregnancy.

Dysmenorrhea: These are severe symptoms of menstruation. During menstruation, it is usual for a woman to have stomach cramps, headaches and salt retention and if these affect daily living, it becomes dysmenorrhea.

Ectopic pregnancy: This is when a zygote attaches to the wall of the fallopian tube and begins to develop. It can also occur in the cervix, ovaries or abdomen.

Prostate cancer: This is one of the most common types of cancer in men, often diagnosed when men have difficulties with urinating.

Medical Terminology

Andrology: This is the branch of medicine for male reproductive health and urology.

Androgen: An androgen is any hormone that stimulates or maintains male characteristics, such as testosterone.

Artificial insemination (AI) or **Assisted Reproductive Technology**: This allows conception of a child without sexual intercourse/natural insemination.

Gestation: This is the length of time from fertilization of an ovum until birth, around forty weeks in humans.

Menopause: This is when the ovaries no longer release ova and neither does menstruation occur. This cessation is hormone-regulated. The formal date of menopause is from the time of the last menstruation, or period.

Obstetrics: This is the branch of medical care specifically for the female reproductive system, including pregnancy, birth and after birth (antenatal).

Ovulation: The point at which the ovum is released from the follicle sac.

Urethra: In men, the urethra carries both semen and urine out through the penis and in women; it carries urine from the bladder to the body exit.

The Respiratory System

Tour of the System

Life itself depends upon the ability of the blood to deliver oxygen to and remove carbon dioxide from every cell, tissue and organ of the body. This is the responsibility of the respiratory system. This system also works very closely with other body systems, including the circulatory system.

Breathing rate is regulated by the medulla in the brain, based largely on the carbon dioxide content of the blood. Breathing is automatic, although under 'normal' conditions, there is the ability to alter the breathing rate consciously. The respiratory system consists of two main processes, **inhalation** and **exhalation,** which occurs in the **thoracic cavity**.

There is around 21% oxygen inhaled from the air and around 16% oxygen exhaled; this is why resuscitation can be effective in saving lives.

Inhalation

The diaphragm (located at the base of the ribcage) contracts, ribs move outwards and upwards, creating more space in the pleural cavity (space between the lining and covering of the lung).This changes the air pressure via a vacuum mechanism, forcing air into the lungs.

The air enters the nose through the *nostrils* (nares).

In the nasal cavity, air passes through *nasal conchae*.

The nasal conchae are mucosal tissues in the nose. As well as directing the movement of air, they heat, moisten and filter the air.

The air then passes through the *pharynx*, *larynx* and into the *trachea*.

The trachea is *ciliated* and secretes *mucus*.

Mucus is required to keep the airways lubricated and trap foreign particles, such as bacteria.

The cilia move mucus steadily upwards, until it can be swallowed and pass through the digestive system.

As the trachea moves towards the lungs, it divides into two main branches, the *primary bronchi*.

The bronchi enter the lung with blood vessels, lymphatics and nerves at a point known as the *root of the lung*.

The bronchi branch repeatedly, until the branches are very small.

These small branches are *bronchioles*.

Bronchioles eventually end at the very thin walled *alveoli* of the lungs.

Gas exchange

Red blood cells (erythrocytes) enter the lungs to rid themselves of carbon dioxide and pick up oxygen. The blood vessels keep getting smaller until they are very small capillaries in the walls of the alveoli. As the blood passes through these capillaries, the exchange of gases takes place in a split second.

Because the alveoli are very thin and cover a surface area of around 75 meters squared they provide the maximum surface area for the exchange of oxygen and carbon dioxide. This exchange or diffusion takes place through changes in pressure.

Exhalation

This is the reverse of inhalation. Air is pushed out of the lungs as the rib cage is lowered and pulled in. The diaphragm also relaxes. Exhaled air is rich in carbon dioxide, which is the main waste product from cellular respiration (energy production) in the body.

Functions

The respiratory system brings oxygen into the body, performs gas exchange in the lungs and removes waste carbon dioxide from the body.

Components

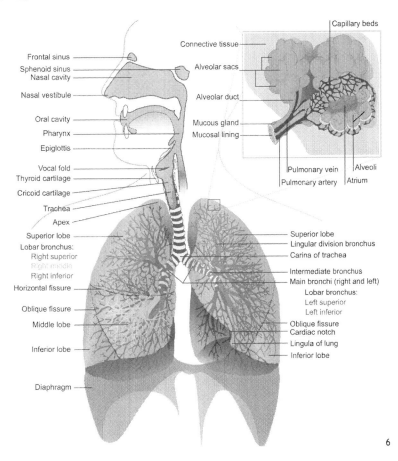

6

Pharynx

This is the part of the throat located behind the mouth and nasal cavity and is important in the digestive system.

Epiglottis

Complete Test Preparation

This is a cartilage flap at the entrance to the voice box (larynx). When this is closed, food cannot enter the trachea (windpipe), or 'go down the wrong way'.

Larynx

The larynx or voice box allows the generation of sound with the help of varying pressures in the lungs.

Trachea

The trachea or windpipe connects the larynx to the lungs, allowing air to move between the two. It also contains goblet cells, which produce mucus.

Bronchi

These passages (singular is broncus) connect the trachea to the bronchioles.

Bronchiole

Bronchioles end at the alveoli. They are typically less than 1 mm in diameter and they are able to change diameter to decrease or increase airflow.

Lungs

These are the main respiratory organs. They transport oxygen into the blood stream and release carbon dioxide. They contain many alveoli. The right lung has three lobes (sections) and the left lung is slightly smaller with two lobes, to leave room for the heart. They are composed of a variety of different tissues, including smooth muscle. The lungs of an average male can hold 6 liters of air and a woman's lungs can hold around 4 liters of air.

Ribcage

The 12 sets of ribs that make up the ribcage protect the lungs and assist in the process of respiration. Between the ribs are *intercostal muscles* that move the rib cage during the respiratory cycle.

Diaphragm

This is a sheet of skeletal muscle found at the bottom of the ribcage. It separates the thoracic cavity (lungs, ribs and heart) from the abdominal cavity. The diaphragm is also essential in altering pressure in the thoracic cavity during respiration.

Alveoli

The alveoli (singular is alveolus) are the site of gas exchange in the lungs.

Common Diseases and Disorders

Asthma: The airways constrict in this chronic disease and symptoms include shortness of breath, wheezing and coughing.

Bronchitis: Infection of the bronchial tubes.

Cold/Common Cold: A cold is characterized by a sore throat, cough and runny nose. A virus from the Rhinovirus family often causes colds.

Emphysema: With exposure to heavy air pollution, often through smoking, the walls of the alveoli break down. When this occurs, the alveoli double in size and fill with fluid. Because this puts further pressure on the walls of the alveoli, they continue to break and allow fluid to accumulate. This repeats itself and destroys the lungs, impairing body function.

Flu or influenza: A virus from the influenza (Orthomyxoviridae) group of viruses causes flu. Not only is it highly infectious, flu can also cause severe illness.

Laryngitis: When people "lose their voice"; this is through infection or inflammation of the larynx. Sounds are created when air pushes by the vocal chords in the larynx. If these vocal chords are inflamed, they are unable to vibrate properly.

Pneumonia: This is infection of the lungs. Pneumonia caused by bacteria is easier to treat than infection caused by a virus. Viral pneumonia can be very serious in medically compromised people or the elderly.

Pleurisy: If the pleural cavity around the lungs becomes infected, fluid starts to accumulate. Not only does this hamper breathing, it is also very painful.

Medical Terminology

Bronchodilation: The process by which the bronchioles dilate, allowing more air to the alveoli.

Bronchoconstriction: A decrease in the diameter of bronchioles, reducing air flow.

Cilia: These are hair-like projections found on many lining cells in the body. They play an important role in moving substances along.

Coughing: This is essential to keep the lungs clear from debris such as mucus and dust.

Diffusion: This is the movement of molecules from an area of high concentration to an area of low concentration through a membrane. Diffusion allows gas exchange at the alveoli.

Mucus: Produced by certain cells, mucus often lines surfaces in the body. There are different types of mucus, but their main role is protection.

Pulmo: Any word beginning with *pulmo* relates to the lung.

Pulmonology: The branch of internal medicine that cares for respiratory disorders.

Vital capacity: This is the maximum amount of air exhaled after a maximum inspiration. This measurement is taken with a spirometer and is a frequent measure of respiratory health.

The Skeletal System

Tour of the System

The early skeleton forms during gestation and continues to develop for a number of years after birth through a process called endochondral ossification.

A baby has more than 300 bones, whereas an adult only has 206. This is because a number of bones fuse together during growth.

There are different cells involved in producing bone and these cells are located in the matrix of the bone. This matrix also contains a variety of substances and collagen. As this matrix hardens, bone forms. Formation, re-formation and repair of bones takes place over a long period of time.

Muscles, tendons, ligaments and cartilage support the skeleton and together these are the musculoskeletal system. There are a number of differences between male and female skeletons, including the pelvis, which has to allow for childbirth.

Functions

The skeleton has a number of key functions:

It supports the body and maintains the shape of the body.

The joints between the bones allow movement.

It protects organs, such as the skull protecting the brain, eyes and inner ears.

It produces cells in its bone marrow (hematopoiesis).

The skeleton stores a variety of substances including calcium and iron.

It is also involved in regulation of blood sugar levels and fat deposits through release of a hormone called oseteocalcin.

Components

Skeleton

The skeleton consists of the axial skeleton and the appendicular skeleton:

The axial skeleton is central bones including the skull, vertebrae and ribcage.

The appendicular skeleton consists of the pelvis, upper and lower limbs.

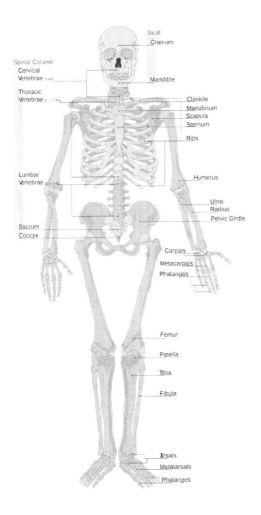

7

Bone

Two types of bone structure make up the skeleton:

Compact or dense bone is most of the adult skeleton. This has a smooth, white appearance.

Cancellous or *trabecular bone* is the spongy bone tissue found inside compact bone. This contains room for blood vessels and marrow.

As well as the two types of bone structure, there are also five types of bone in the human body:

Type	Description	Example
Long bones	The shaft (or diaphysis) is longer than its width	Femur, tibia, radius
Short bones	Cube shaped	Wrist bones, ankle bones
Flat bones	Thin and curved	Skull, sternum
Irregular bones	Irregular and complicated shape	Hip, spinal bones
Sesamoid bones	Found embedded in tendon	Patella (kneecap)

Joints

Joints or *articulation*s are:

- where bone meets bone

- bone meets cartilage

- bone meets teeth

Joints are key components of the skeletal system. Diseases of the joints constitute the single greatest cause of disability in the civilized world.

How joints move can categorize them:

- Synarthosis: An immoveable joint
- Amphiarthosis: A slightly moveable joint
- Diarthosis: Freely moveable joint

The group known as synarthoses (immoveable joints) contain three joints:

1. **Suture:** This is a connective tissue joint, joining the bones of the skull. Some sutures are also present in the skeletons of children until replaced with bone. This type of temporary suture is a synostosis.

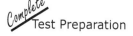

2. **Gomphosis:** A peg fits into a socket. These joints are the roots of teeth and their connection with the skull and jawbone.

3. **Synchondrosis:** This is a cartilage joint found where a bone joins to another bone with cartilage. An example is the sternocostal joints, where costal cartilage attached the ribs to the sternum (breastbone). These joints also occur in the epiphyseal (growth) plate of long bones during development. This joint eventually becomes bone.

Amphiarthoses (slightly moveable joints) contain only two sub-types of joint:

1. **Syndesmosis:** Is a fibrous joint that contains more connective tissue than a suture. An example of this joint is between the tibia and fibula.

2. **Symphasis:** This joint contains a flat disc of cartilage. The main examples are the spine and hipbones.

Diarthoses or freely moveable joints (also called synovial joints) all contain a space called a synovial cavity. This cavity contains synovial fluid that lubricates and prevents friction in joints. These joints also contain cartilage that covers the ends of the bones.

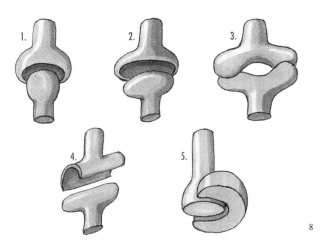

1. Ball and socket joint
2. Condyloid joint
3. Saddle joint
4. Hinge joint
5. Pivot joint

8

1. A ball and socket joint consists of the ball shaped end of one bone, fitting into the depression of another bone. These joints allow a variety of movement. The shoulder and hip joints are the only two ball and socket joints.
2. A condyloid joint allows side-to-side and backward and forwards movement. The joint at the wrist is a condyloid joint.
3. A saddle joint is similar to a condyloid joint, but allows more movement. The

thumb is a saddle joint.

4. A hinge joint allows flexion and extension because a convex surface of one bone fits into the concave surface of another. Examples include the knee, elbow and ankle.

5. A pivot joint allows rotation of a bone. The pivot joint found at the end of the radius and ulna allows the hand to turn upwards and downwards.

6. A gliding joint allows side-to-side and backwards and forwards movement. An example is the clavicle (collarbone) gliding on the sternum (breastbone) and scapula (shoulder blade).

Muscles

Muscles assist the skeleton with movement and this skeletal muscle attaches to the bones with tendons.

Tendons

Tendons are fibrous connective tissues that connect bone to muscle. These work with muscles for movement.

Ligaments

Ligaments connect bone to bone, such as the cruciate ligaments in the knee.

Cartilage

There are different types of cartilage in the body, some of which is at the joints of moveable bones, helping joints to move freely. Cartilage can also act as a shock absorber for the skeleton.

Common Diseases and Disorders

Dislocation: A dislocation or luxation occurs when bones displace at the joint. Sudden trauma, such as a fall can cause a dislocation.

Fractures: These occur when there is a break in the bone. A closed (or simple fracture) means that the skin is unbroken, whereas an open fracture has a wound at the fracture site.

Osteoporosis: This is a condition where there is a reduction in bone density, increasing the chance of fractures. This is more common in post-menopausal women, due to hormone changes.

Osteoarthritis: This is degeneration of the joints. Eventually cartilage at the end of the bones is lost

Osteomyelitis: This is infection of either the bone or its marrow.

Spur: Spurs or osteophytes form on bone as it ages, often caused with the onset of arthritis.

Medical Terminology

Collagen: This is part of connective tissue. There are many different types of collagen, found in scar tissue, skin, hair, cartilage, ligaments, bone and many other body tissues.

Connective tissue: This is a fibrous tissue with many structural roles, found in tendons, bone, cartilage and ligaments.

Endochondral ossification: Is the name for the development of the skeleton after birth.

Greenstick fracture: This fracture only occurs in children when the bones are still soft.

Haematopoiesis: The name given to the process by which different components of the blood develop in bone marrow. This includes erythrocytes, white blood cells and platelets. These all develop from stem cells.

Orthopedic: Branch of surgery concerned with the musculoskeletal system.

Strain: This occurs when a muscle is torn. It can affect also affect tendons.

Sprain: Similar to a strain, but occurs when a ligament has been over-stretched.

The Nervous System

Tour of the System

The nervous system is an incredibly complex system and along with the endocrine system, it has responsibility for maintaining homeostasis in the body. By doing this, it also controls other body systems in their functions.

The nervous system contains two main parts, the central nervous system and the peripheral nervous system:

The central nervous system (CNS) is the brain and spinal cord. This analyzes incoming sensory information, generates thoughts and emotions and also creates and stores memories.

The peripheral nervous system (PNS) contains cranial nerves that come from the brain and spinal nerves that come from the spinal cord, or any other part of the nervous sys-

 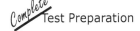

tem that does not lie within the CNS. This can further be divided into two systems:

The sensory, or afferent (which means towards) component of the PNS takes information from nerve cells throughout the body to the CNS.

The motor, or efferent (which means away from) component of the PNS takes information from the CNS to nerve cells. There are two components to this, the somatic nervous system and the autonomic nervous system (ANS):

The somatic nervous system is voluntary. This controls information to muscles that are under voluntary control. This system is in use when we pick up a pen to start writing.

The autonomic nervous system is more complicated as it is an involuntary system. This controls information to muscles that are not under voluntary control, such as the cardiac muscle and endocrine glands. This system is controlling our heart rate, or releasing epinephrine in the body.

The key cells involved in the nervous system are nerve cells, or neurons.

Information in the nervous system is created and communicated in the form of electrical signals, created by chemical changes in neurons. These signals are nerve impulses.

This useful diagram summarizes the nervous system. The blue arrows represent information going into the nervous system (input) and the red arrows represent information going out (output) of the nervous system.

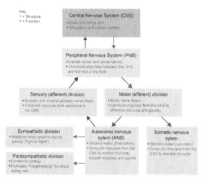

9

Functions

There are three main functions:

- The nervous system senses changes in the internal or external environment (changes are stimuli).

Complete Test Preparation

- The nervous system analyses the stimuli, stores some information about it and uses the remaining information to make decisions.

- The nervous system often responds to stimuli by initiating gland secretions or muscle movements.

Components

Brain

The brain is the most complex organ in the body and not only does it control other body systems, it allows us to think, communicate and feel emotions. The brain contains mostly neurons and neuroglia cells. Tissues called meninges (inflammation of this causes meningitis) and cerebrospinal fluid help to protect the brain.

Spinal cord

This extends from the *medulla oblongata* in the brain. The vertebrae of the spine protect the spinal cord. Information passes through the spinal cord to and from the brain and it is the main pathway connecting the brain and PNS.

Nerves within the spinal cord can communicate information extremely quickly and like the brain, it is protected by meninges and cerebrospinal fluid.

There are 33 nerve segments in the spine, most of which emerge from above their corresponding vertebrae:

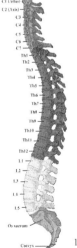

- Cervical nerve segments, identified as C1 to C8
- Thoracic nerve segments, identified as T1 to T12
- Lumbar nerve segments, identified as L1 to L5
- Sacral nerve segments, identified as S1 to S5

 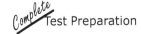

The spinal cord also has a special nervous response, called a reflex arc. This is when information does not enter the brain first (as there is not enough time), instead it enters the spinal cord and the spinal cord sends a message to the muscles to act.

A reflex arc occurs is when we touch something hot and we have already moved our hand away before we have 'realized' that it is hot. This response assists us to survive.

Neurons

These vary in size from being tiny to the longest cells in the body. There are also different types of neuron, although the two main types are:

Motor neurons that communicate and control muscles.

Sensory neurons receive information from stimuli and pass this information to the CNS.

A neuron contains a cell body. This, like other cells contains the nucleus and other cell components. It also contains dendrites that extend from the cell body. These are where information (nerve impulses) enters the neuron.

The long axon allows nerve impulses to pass from the cell body to the terminal of the axon, located at the opposite end of the cell.

At the axon terminal are neurotransmitters. These molecules pass on nerve impulses to the dendrites of other neurons as well as muscles or glands.

Covering the axon is a special insulating sheath called a myelin sheath. This works like a cable covering, preventing information from being lost along the way. Breakdown of this myelin sheath causes disorders such as multiple sclerosis.

The diagram below shows how a neuron connects to its neighbors and shows where neurotransmitters are located at the axon terminals (in structures called synapses).

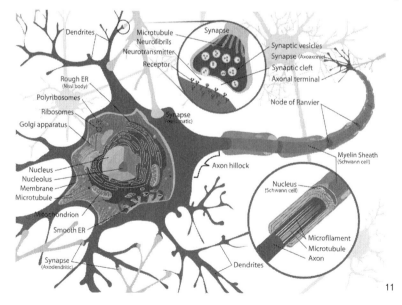

Neuroglia

Neuroglia or glia cells are not nerve cells, but they form myelin sheath for the neurons and also support and protect neurons. There are more of these than there are neurons.

Common Diseases and Disorders

Alzheimer's disease: Although the exact causes of Alzheimer's remain unknown, a breakdown of nervous tissue in the brain is involved. Neuroscientists suggest that keeping the brain active can help to delay some of the onset of Alzheimer's.

Epilepsy: Seizures are caused by abnormal electrical signals in the brain.

Multiple sclerosis (MS): This occurs with destruction of myelin sheaths of CNS neurons. This destruction prevents nerve impulses moving through the body properly.

Parkinson's disease (PD): Usually affects people around 60 years of age and causes problems with the neurotransmitters. This results in involuntary muscle movements, such as hand tremors.

Stroke: A stroke or cerebrovascular accident (CVA) occurs when blood flow to the brain is disturbed. This creates damage to the nervous tissue in the affected part of the brain. Symptoms such as slurred speech and lack of movement in one side of the body occur because of damage to the nervous tissues.

Medical Terminology

EEG (Electroencephalogram): This shows brain waves. The brain waves are the nerve impulses generated by the nervous system. These appear as electrical information.

Epidural: This is anesthetic placed in the epidural space (just inside the vertebrae) with the use of a catheter.

General anesthesia: This removes all sensations including pain and causes unconsciousness.

Homeostasis: This is the ability of the human body to maintain a stable internal environment, when dealing with both internal and external environmental changes.

Local anesthetic: Novocain and lidocaine prevents nerve impulses passing to other neurons.

Lumber puncture: Cerebrospinal fluid (CSF) is drawn from the lumber region of the spine using a needle. Often used to diagnose in disease diagnosis.

 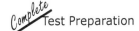

Neurology: This is the branch of medicine for nervous system function and disorders.

Spinal anesthesia: This blocks nerve impulses from a certain point in the spine downwards. This is different to an epidural.

The Urinary System

Tour of the System

The urinary system removes waste by products of metabolism. It is a very complicated system and works closely with the endocrine and cardiovascular system.

Waste products such as urea and ammonia seep from cells and tissues into the blood stream.

If these waste molecules remain in the bloodstream, they can accumulate to toxic levels in a very short time.

This liquid waste enters the kidneys through the renal arteries, from the abdominal aorta.

Around 1200 ml of blood can enter the kidneys per minute.

The renal artery entering each kidney branches into segmental arteries.

These branch into interlobar arteries.

Eventually the blood vessels become arterioles that supply the glomeruli.

The glomerulus is a ball-shaped tangled network of capillaries and is part of a nephron - the main structural and functional unit of the kidney.

Below the glomeruli is space, called the interstitium. Any fluid for reabsorption recovered from urine passes into here.

There are two main sections in the kidney, the renal cortex and renal medulla.

In the diagram below, the renal cortex is where the blood vessels are around the kidney and the renal medulla is the area between the renal pyramids.

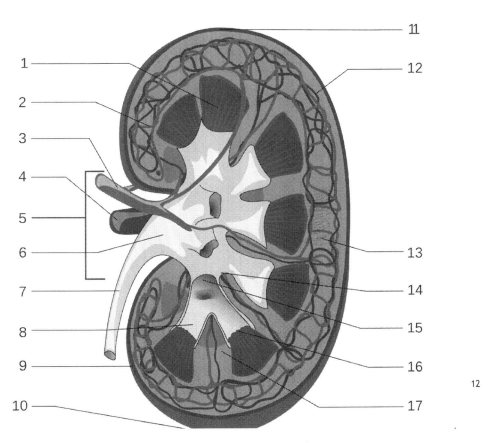

1. Renal pyramid

2. Interlobular artery

3. Renal artery

4. Renal vein

5. Renal hilum

6. Renal pelvis

7. Ureter

8. Minor calyx

9. Renal capsule

10. Inferior renal capsule

11. Superior renal capsule

12. Interlobular vein

13. Nephron

14. Minor calyx

15. Major calyx

16. Renal papilla

17. Renal column

Nephrons are located throughout the kidney and the first part of the nephron is located in the cortex. This part of the nephron, the renal corpuscle filters urine.

Nephrons have a thin wall that allows fluid to pass from the glomeruli into them.

Blood eventually drains out of nephrons into peritubular capillaries.

These then become venules and veins until filtered blood leaves the kidney through the renal vein.

Urine filtered from the blood through the nephrons passes through the renal tubule and through various tubes and processes.

It eventually reaches minor calyces and then major calyces.

The urine then enters the renal pelvis that becomes the ureter.

The ureter passes urine to the bladder.

The body makes about a liter of urine a day and this is stored in the bladder until emptying.

Urine exits the body through the urethra.

Because about one fifth of the body's supply of blood passes through the kidneys at any given time, they are terribly vulnerable to damage by toxins.

Functions

The functions of the urinary system are to help maintain **homeostasis** by:

- Producing urine

- Storing urine

- Eliminating urine

Components

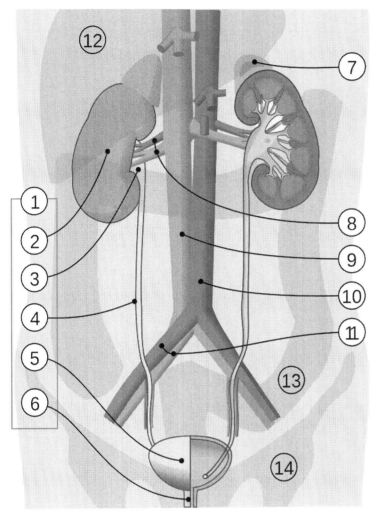

1. *Human urinary system*

2. Kidney

3. Renal pelvis

4. Ureter

5. Urinary bladder

6. Urethra. (Left side with frontal section)

7. Adrenal gland

Vessels:

8. Renal artery and vein

9. Inferior vena cava

10. Abdominal aorta

11. Common iliac artery and vein

12. Liver

13. Large intestine

14. Pelvis

13

Kidneys

These are approximately 10-12 cm wide. As well as assisting with the urinary system, kidneys also have other important functions.

They help maintain homeostasis in the body, by helping to control the composition, the volume and the pressure of blood.

Kidneys also help to control blood pH and contribute to metabolic processes such as helping the body to produce vitamin D. They also play an important role in hormone secretion.

Kidneys contain over one million nephrons and roughly 1700 liters of blood pass through these in a day. From this, 170 liters of filtrate is formed. As the filtrate passes along the nephrons, 169 liters of filtrate is reabsorbed back into the blood stream. The remaining one liter is urine.

Ureters

These two muscular tubes move urine from the kidney to the bladder. These are around 25-30 cm long and 4 mm in diameter.

Bladder

This organ collects urine from the kidneys. It is a muscular organ under both voluntary and involuntary control. As the bladder wall stretches, the nervous system contracts the detrusor muscle. This encourages urine to enter the urethra. Urine can only enter the urethra if the external sphincter, controlled voluntarily, is open.

The urge to urinate usually occurs when around 25% of the bladder is full. If the bladder reaches 100% volume then the bladder will just empty. Micturition is another name for urination.

Urethra

This allows urine to exit the body. In males, the urethra also carries semen.

Testing urine can identify abnormal components that should not be in the urine, such as glucose or erythrocytes.

Common Diseases and Disorders

Acute renal failure (ARF): this is when glomerular filtration either reduces or stops. When this occurs, urine production stops. Causes include circulatory problems or kidney stones.

Chronic renal failure (CRF): This is a progressive and usually irreversible decline in filtration. This is when dialysis and a kidney transplant may be required. Kidney transplants are quite successful, with the donor living with one kidney and the recipient maintaining a normal life.

Cystitis: Is a common UTI, especially in women. Cystitis is often called a bladder infection. Symptoms include a constant urge to urinate and burning when urinating.

Diabetes insipidus (DI): Is when there is a very large volume of dilute urine excreted. This is usually associated with kidney disease and is a different disorder to diabetes mellitus.

Incontinence: This usually arises from problems between voluntary and involuntary controlled muscles in the bladder.

Kidney infection: Also called pyelonephritis or pyelitis, this is a UTI that has reached the kidneys. This type of infection can be life threatening.

Kidney stones: Also known as renal calculus, these are a solid mass formed in the kidneys from minerals, such as calcium. Kidney stones can pass though the urinary system without any damage, but if they continue to grow, the ureter becomes blocked causing immense pain.

UTI or Urinary tract infection: This is any bacterial infection affecting any part of the urinary system.

Medical Terminology

Diuresis: Increased urine excretion, diuresis can be induced with diuretics, used frequently in medicine.

Homeostasis: This is the ability of the human body to maintain a stable internal environment, when dealing with both internal and external environmental changes.

Nephrology: Specialized branch of medicine dealing with the kidneys.

Polyuria: Excessive formation of urine.

Urology: Branch of medicine dealing with the urinary systems.

Practice Test Questions Set 1

Section I – Reading Comprehension

Questions: 45
Time: 45 Minutes

Section II – Mathematics

Questions: 50
Time: 60 Minutes

Section III – Part 1 - English Grammar (optional)

Questions: 50
Time: 50 Minutes

Section III - Part II – Vocabulary

Questions: 50
Time: 50 Minutes

Section IV – Part I – Science (optional)

Questions: 50
Time: 50 minutes

Section IV – Part II – Anatomy & Physiology (optional)

Questions: 50
Time: 50 minutes

The questions below are not exactly the same as you will find on the HESI - that would be too easy! And nobody knows what the questions will be and they change all the time. Below are general questions that cover the same subject areas as the HESI. So while the format and exact wording of the questions may differ slightly, and change from year to year, if you can answer the questions below, you will have no problem with the HESI.

For the best results, take this Practice Test as if it were the real exam. Set aside time when you will not be disturbed, and a location that is quiet and free of distractions. Read the instructions carefully, read each question carefully, and answer to the best of your ability.

Use the bubble answer sheets provided. When you have completed the Practice Test, check your answer against the Answer Key and read the explanation provided.

NOTE: The Science, Anatomy and Physiology and English sections are optional. Check with your school for exam details.

 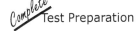

Answer Sheet – Section 1 - Reading Comprehension

1. Ⓐ Ⓑ Ⓒ Ⓓ
2. Ⓐ Ⓑ Ⓒ Ⓓ
3. Ⓐ Ⓑ Ⓒ Ⓓ
4. Ⓐ Ⓑ Ⓒ Ⓓ
5. Ⓐ Ⓑ Ⓒ Ⓓ
6. Ⓐ Ⓑ Ⓒ Ⓓ
7. Ⓐ Ⓑ Ⓒ Ⓓ
8. Ⓐ Ⓑ Ⓒ Ⓓ
9. Ⓐ Ⓑ Ⓒ Ⓓ
10. Ⓐ Ⓑ Ⓒ Ⓓ
11. Ⓐ Ⓑ Ⓒ Ⓓ
12. Ⓐ Ⓑ Ⓒ Ⓓ
13. Ⓐ Ⓑ Ⓒ Ⓓ
14. Ⓐ Ⓑ Ⓒ Ⓓ
15. Ⓐ Ⓑ Ⓒ Ⓓ
16. Ⓐ Ⓑ Ⓒ Ⓓ
17. Ⓐ Ⓑ Ⓒ Ⓓ

18. Ⓐ Ⓑ Ⓒ Ⓓ
19. Ⓐ Ⓑ Ⓒ Ⓓ
20. Ⓐ Ⓑ Ⓒ Ⓓ
21. Ⓐ Ⓑ Ⓒ Ⓓ
22. Ⓐ Ⓑ Ⓒ Ⓓ
23. Ⓐ Ⓑ Ⓒ Ⓓ
24. Ⓐ Ⓑ Ⓒ Ⓓ
25. Ⓐ Ⓑ Ⓒ Ⓓ
26. Ⓐ Ⓑ Ⓒ Ⓓ
27. Ⓐ Ⓑ Ⓒ Ⓓ
28. Ⓐ Ⓑ Ⓒ Ⓓ
29. Ⓐ Ⓑ Ⓒ Ⓓ
30. Ⓐ Ⓑ Ⓒ Ⓓ
31. Ⓐ Ⓑ Ⓒ Ⓓ
32. Ⓐ Ⓑ Ⓒ Ⓓ
33. Ⓐ Ⓑ Ⓒ Ⓓ
34. Ⓐ Ⓑ Ⓒ Ⓓ

35. Ⓐ Ⓑ Ⓒ Ⓓ
36. Ⓐ Ⓑ Ⓒ Ⓓ
37. Ⓐ Ⓑ Ⓒ Ⓓ
38. Ⓐ Ⓑ Ⓒ Ⓓ
39. Ⓐ Ⓑ Ⓒ Ⓓ
40. Ⓐ Ⓑ Ⓒ Ⓓ
41. Ⓐ Ⓑ Ⓒ Ⓓ
42. Ⓐ Ⓑ Ⓒ Ⓓ
43. Ⓐ Ⓑ Ⓒ Ⓓ
44. Ⓐ Ⓑ Ⓒ Ⓓ
45. Ⓐ Ⓑ Ⓒ Ⓓ
46. Ⓐ Ⓑ Ⓒ Ⓓ
47. Ⓐ Ⓑ Ⓒ Ⓓ
48. Ⓐ Ⓑ Ⓒ Ⓓ
49. Ⓐ Ⓑ Ⓒ Ⓓ
50. Ⓐ Ⓑ Ⓒ Ⓓ

Complete Test Preparation

Answer Sheet – Section II - Math

1. Ⓐ Ⓑ Ⓒ Ⓓ   18. Ⓐ Ⓑ Ⓒ Ⓓ   35. Ⓐ Ⓑ Ⓒ Ⓓ

2. Ⓐ Ⓑ Ⓒ Ⓓ   19. Ⓐ Ⓑ Ⓒ Ⓓ   36. Ⓐ Ⓑ Ⓒ Ⓓ

3. Ⓐ Ⓑ Ⓒ Ⓓ   20. Ⓐ Ⓑ Ⓒ Ⓓ   37. Ⓐ Ⓑ Ⓒ Ⓓ

4. Ⓐ Ⓑ Ⓒ Ⓓ   21. Ⓐ Ⓑ Ⓒ Ⓓ   38. Ⓐ Ⓑ Ⓒ Ⓓ

5. Ⓐ Ⓑ Ⓒ Ⓓ   22. Ⓐ Ⓑ Ⓒ Ⓓ   39. Ⓐ Ⓑ Ⓒ Ⓓ

6. Ⓐ Ⓑ Ⓒ Ⓓ   23. Ⓐ Ⓑ Ⓒ Ⓓ   40. Ⓐ Ⓑ Ⓒ Ⓓ

7. Ⓐ Ⓑ Ⓒ Ⓓ   24. Ⓐ Ⓑ Ⓒ Ⓓ   41. Ⓐ Ⓑ Ⓒ Ⓓ

8. Ⓐ Ⓑ Ⓒ Ⓓ   25. Ⓐ Ⓑ Ⓒ Ⓓ   42. Ⓐ Ⓑ Ⓒ Ⓓ

9. Ⓐ Ⓑ Ⓒ Ⓓ   26. Ⓐ Ⓑ Ⓒ Ⓓ   43. Ⓐ Ⓑ Ⓒ Ⓓ

10. Ⓐ Ⓑ Ⓒ Ⓓ   27. Ⓐ Ⓑ Ⓒ Ⓓ   44. Ⓐ Ⓑ Ⓒ Ⓓ

11. Ⓐ Ⓑ Ⓒ Ⓓ   28. Ⓐ Ⓑ Ⓒ Ⓓ   45. Ⓐ Ⓑ Ⓒ Ⓓ

12. Ⓐ Ⓑ Ⓒ Ⓓ   29. Ⓐ Ⓑ Ⓒ Ⓓ   46. Ⓐ Ⓑ Ⓒ Ⓓ

13. Ⓐ Ⓑ Ⓒ Ⓓ   30. Ⓐ Ⓑ Ⓒ Ⓓ   47. Ⓐ Ⓑ Ⓒ Ⓓ

14. Ⓐ Ⓑ Ⓒ Ⓓ   31. Ⓐ Ⓑ Ⓒ Ⓓ   48. Ⓐ Ⓑ Ⓒ Ⓓ

15. Ⓐ Ⓑ Ⓒ Ⓓ   32. Ⓐ Ⓑ Ⓒ Ⓓ   49. Ⓐ Ⓑ Ⓒ Ⓓ

16. Ⓐ Ⓑ Ⓒ Ⓓ   33. Ⓐ Ⓑ Ⓒ Ⓓ   50. Ⓐ Ⓑ Ⓒ Ⓓ

17. Ⓐ Ⓑ Ⓒ Ⓓ   34. Ⓐ Ⓑ Ⓒ Ⓓ

Answer Sheet – Section III Part I - English Grammar

1. Ⓐ Ⓑ Ⓒ Ⓓ	18. Ⓐ Ⓑ Ⓒ Ⓓ	35. Ⓐ Ⓑ Ⓒ Ⓓ
2. Ⓐ Ⓑ Ⓒ Ⓓ	19. Ⓐ Ⓑ Ⓒ Ⓓ	36. Ⓐ Ⓑ Ⓒ Ⓓ
3. Ⓐ Ⓑ Ⓒ Ⓓ	20. Ⓐ Ⓑ Ⓒ Ⓓ	37. Ⓐ Ⓑ Ⓒ Ⓓ
4. Ⓐ Ⓑ Ⓒ Ⓓ	21. Ⓐ Ⓑ Ⓒ Ⓓ	38. Ⓐ Ⓑ Ⓒ Ⓓ
5. Ⓐ Ⓑ Ⓒ Ⓓ	22. Ⓐ Ⓑ Ⓒ Ⓓ	39. Ⓐ Ⓑ Ⓒ Ⓓ
6. Ⓐ Ⓑ Ⓒ Ⓓ	23. Ⓐ Ⓑ Ⓒ Ⓓ	40. Ⓐ Ⓑ Ⓒ Ⓓ
7. Ⓐ Ⓑ Ⓒ Ⓓ	24. Ⓐ Ⓑ Ⓒ Ⓓ	41. Ⓐ Ⓑ Ⓒ Ⓓ
8. Ⓐ Ⓑ Ⓒ Ⓓ	25. Ⓐ Ⓑ Ⓒ Ⓓ	42. Ⓐ Ⓑ Ⓒ Ⓓ
9. Ⓐ Ⓑ Ⓒ Ⓓ	26. Ⓐ Ⓑ Ⓒ Ⓓ	43. Ⓐ Ⓑ Ⓒ Ⓓ
10. Ⓐ Ⓑ Ⓒ Ⓓ	27. Ⓐ Ⓑ Ⓒ Ⓓ	44. Ⓐ Ⓑ Ⓒ Ⓓ
11. Ⓐ Ⓑ Ⓒ Ⓓ	28. Ⓐ Ⓑ Ⓒ Ⓓ	45. Ⓐ Ⓑ Ⓒ Ⓓ
12. Ⓐ Ⓑ Ⓒ Ⓓ	29. Ⓐ Ⓑ Ⓒ Ⓓ	46. Ⓐ Ⓑ Ⓒ Ⓓ
13. Ⓐ Ⓑ Ⓒ Ⓓ	30. Ⓐ Ⓑ Ⓒ Ⓓ	47. Ⓐ Ⓑ Ⓒ Ⓓ
14. Ⓐ Ⓑ Ⓒ Ⓓ	31. Ⓐ Ⓑ Ⓒ Ⓓ	48. Ⓐ Ⓑ Ⓒ Ⓓ
15. Ⓐ Ⓑ Ⓒ Ⓓ	32. Ⓐ Ⓑ Ⓒ Ⓓ	49. Ⓐ Ⓑ Ⓒ Ⓓ
16. Ⓐ Ⓑ Ⓒ Ⓓ	33. Ⓐ Ⓑ Ⓒ Ⓓ	50. Ⓐ Ⓑ Ⓒ Ⓓ
17. Ⓐ Ⓑ Ⓒ Ⓓ	34. Ⓐ Ⓑ Ⓒ Ⓓ	

Answer Sheet – Section III Part I – Vocabulary

1. (A) (B) (C) (D)
2. (A) (B) (C) (D)
3. (A) (B) (C) (D)
4. (A) (B) (C) (D)
5. (A) (B) (C) (D)
6. (A) (B) (C) (D)
7. (A) (B) (C) (D)
8. (A) (B) (C) (D)
9. (A) (B) (C) (D)
10. (A) (B) (C) (D)
11. (A) (B) (C) (D)
12. (A) (B) (C) (D)
13. (A) (B) (C) (D)
14. (A) (B) (C) (D)
15. (A) (B) (C) (D)
16. (A) (B) (C) (D)
17. (A) (B) (C) (D)

18. (A) (B) (C) (D)
19. (A) (B) (C) (D)
20. (A) (B) (C) (D)
21. (A) (B) (C) (D)
22. (A) (B) (C) (D)
23. (A) (B) (C) (D)
24. (A) (B) (C) (D)
25. (A) (B) (C) (D)
26. (A) (B) (C) (D)
27. (A) (B) (C) (D)
28. (A) (B) (C) (D)
29. (A) (B) (C) (D)
30. (A) (B) (C) (D)
31. (A) (B) (C) (D)
32. (A) (B) (C) (D)
33. (A) (B) (C) (D)
34. (A) (B) (C) (D)

35. (A) (B) (C) (D)
36. (A) (B) (C) (D)
37. (A) (B) (C) (D)
38. (A) (B) (C) (D)
39. (A) (B) (C) (D)
40. (A) (B) (C) (D)
41. (A) (B) (C) (D)
42. (A) (B) (C) (D)
43. (A) (B) (C) (D)
44. (A) (B) (C) (D)
45. (A) (B) (C) (D)
46. (A) (B) (C) (D)
47. (A) (B) (C) (D)
48. (A) (B) (C) (D)
49. (A) (B) (C) (D)
50. (A) (B) (C) (D)

Answer Sheet – Section IV Part I – Biology and Chemistry

1. (A) (B) (C) (D)   18. (A) (B) (C) (D)   35. (A) (B) (C) (D)
2. (A) (B) (C) (D)   19. (A) (B) (C) (D)   36. (A) (B) (C) (D)
3. (A) (B) (C) (D)   20. (A) (B) (C) (D)   37. (A) (B) (C) (D)
4. (A) (B) (C) (D)   21. (A) (B) (C) (D)   38. (A) (B) (C) (D)
5. (A) (B) (C) (D)   22. (A) (B) (C) (D)   39. (A) (B) (C) (D)
6. (A) (B) (C) (D)   23. (A) (B) (C) (D)   40. (A) (B) (C) (D)
7. (A) (B) (C) (D)   24. (A) (B) (C) (D)   41. (A) (B) (C) (D)
8. (A) (B) (C) (D)   25. (A) (B) (C) (D)   42. (A) (B) (C) (D)
9. (A) (B) (C) (D)   26. (A) (B) (C) (D)   43. (A) (B) (C) (D)
10. (A) (B) (C) (D)   27. (A) (B) (C) (D)   44. (A) (B) (C) (D)
11. (A) (B) (C) (D)   28. (A) (B) (C) (D)   45. (A) (B) (C) (D)
12. (A) (B) (C) (D)   29. (A) (B) (C) (D)   46. (A) (B) (C) (D)
13. (A) (B) (C) (D)   30. (A) (B) (C) (D)   47. (A) (B) (C) (D)
14. (A) (B) (C) (D)   31. (A) (B) (C) (D)   48. (A) (B) (C) (D)
15. (A) (B) (C) (D)   32. (A) (B) (C) (D)   49. (A) (B) (C) (D)
16. (A) (B) (C) (D)   33. (A) (B) (C) (D)   50. (A) (B) (C) (D)
17. (A) (B) (C) (D)   34. (A) (B) (C) (D)

Answer Sheet – Section IV Part I – Anatomy and Physiology

1. Ⓐ Ⓑ Ⓒ Ⓓ
2. Ⓐ Ⓑ Ⓒ Ⓓ
3. Ⓐ Ⓑ Ⓒ Ⓓ
4. Ⓐ Ⓑ Ⓒ Ⓓ
5. Ⓐ Ⓑ Ⓒ Ⓓ
6. Ⓐ Ⓑ Ⓒ Ⓓ
7. Ⓐ Ⓑ Ⓒ Ⓓ
8. Ⓐ Ⓑ Ⓒ Ⓓ
9. Ⓐ Ⓑ Ⓒ Ⓓ
10. Ⓐ Ⓑ Ⓒ Ⓓ
11. Ⓐ Ⓑ Ⓒ Ⓓ
12. Ⓐ Ⓑ Ⓒ Ⓓ
13. Ⓐ Ⓑ Ⓒ Ⓓ
14. Ⓐ Ⓑ Ⓒ Ⓓ
15. Ⓐ Ⓑ Ⓒ Ⓓ
16. Ⓐ Ⓑ Ⓒ Ⓓ
17. Ⓐ Ⓑ Ⓒ Ⓓ
18. Ⓐ Ⓑ Ⓒ Ⓓ
19. Ⓐ Ⓑ Ⓒ Ⓓ
20. Ⓐ Ⓑ Ⓒ Ⓓ
21. Ⓐ Ⓑ Ⓒ Ⓓ
22. Ⓐ Ⓑ Ⓒ Ⓓ
23. Ⓐ Ⓑ Ⓒ Ⓓ
24. Ⓐ Ⓑ Ⓒ Ⓓ
25. Ⓐ Ⓑ Ⓒ Ⓓ
26. Ⓐ Ⓑ Ⓒ Ⓓ
27. Ⓐ Ⓑ Ⓒ Ⓓ
28. Ⓐ Ⓑ Ⓒ Ⓓ
29. Ⓐ Ⓑ Ⓒ Ⓓ
30. Ⓐ Ⓑ Ⓒ Ⓓ
31. Ⓐ Ⓑ Ⓒ Ⓓ
32. Ⓐ Ⓑ Ⓒ Ⓓ
33. Ⓐ Ⓑ Ⓒ Ⓓ
34. Ⓐ Ⓑ Ⓒ Ⓓ
35. Ⓐ Ⓑ Ⓒ Ⓓ
36. Ⓐ Ⓑ Ⓒ Ⓓ
37. Ⓐ Ⓑ Ⓒ Ⓓ
38. Ⓐ Ⓑ Ⓒ Ⓓ
39. Ⓐ Ⓑ Ⓒ Ⓓ
40. Ⓐ Ⓑ Ⓒ Ⓓ
41. Ⓐ Ⓑ Ⓒ Ⓓ
42. Ⓐ Ⓑ Ⓒ Ⓓ
43. Ⓐ Ⓑ Ⓒ Ⓓ
44. Ⓐ Ⓑ Ⓒ Ⓓ
45. Ⓐ Ⓑ Ⓒ Ⓓ
46. Ⓐ Ⓑ Ⓒ Ⓓ
47. Ⓐ Ⓑ Ⓒ Ⓓ
48. Ⓐ Ⓑ Ⓒ Ⓓ
49. Ⓐ Ⓑ Ⓒ Ⓓ
50. Ⓐ Ⓑ Ⓒ Ⓓ

SECTION I - READING COMPREHENSION.

Directions: The following questions are based on a number of reading passages. Each passage is followed by a series of questions. Read each passage carefully, and then answer the questions based on it. You may reread the passage as often as you wish. When you have finished answering the questions based on one passage, go right on to the next passage. Choose the best answer based on the information given and implied.

Questions 1 – 4 refer to the following passage.

Passage 1 - Infectious Disease

An infectious disease is a clinically evident illness resulting from the presence of pathogenic agents, such as viruses, bacteria, fungi, protozoa, multi cellular parasites, and unusual proteins known as prions. Infectious pathologies are also called communicable diseases or transmissible diseases, due to their potential of transmission from one person or species to another by a replicating agent (as opposed to a toxin).

Transmission of an infectious disease can occur in many different ways. Physical contact, liquids, food, body fluids, contaminated objects, and airborne inhalation can all transmit infecting agents.

Transmissible diseases that occur through contact with an ill person, or objects touched by them, are especially infective, and are sometimes referred to as contagious diseases. Communicable diseases that require a more specialized route of infection, such as through blood or needle transmission, or sexual transmission, are usually not regarded as contagious.

The term infectivity describes the ability of an organism to enter, survive and multiply in the host, while the infectiousness of a disease indicates the comparative ease with which the disease is transmitted. An infection however, is not synonymous with an infectious disease, as an infection may not cause important clinical symptoms. [9]

1. What can we infer from the first paragraph in this passage?

a. Sickness from a toxin can be easily transmitted from one person to another.

b. Sickness from an infectious disease can be easily transmitted from one person to another.

c. Few sicknesses are transmitted from one person to another.

d. Infectious diseases are easily treated.

2. What are two other names for infections' pathologies?

a. Communicable diseases or transmissible diseases

b. Communicable diseases or terminal diseases

c. Transmissible diseases or preventable diseases

d. Communicative diseases or unstable diseases

3. What does infectivity describe?

a. The inability of an organism to multiply in the host

b. The inability of an organism to reproduce

c. The ability of an organism to enter, survive and multiply in the host

d. The ability of an organism to reproduce in the host

4. How do we know an infection is not synonymous with an infectious disease?

a. Because an infectious disease destroys infections with enough time.

b. Because an infection may not cause important clinical symptoms or impair host function.

c. We do not. The two are synonymous.

d. Because an infection is too fatal to be an infectious disease.

Questions 5 – 8 refer to the following passage.

Passage 2 - Viruses

A virus (from the Latin virus meaning toxin or poison) is a small infectious agent that can replicate only inside the living cells of other organisms. Most viruses are too small to be seen directly with a microscope. Viruses infect all types of organisms, from animals and plants to bacteria and single-celled organisms.

Unlike prions and viroids, viruses consist of two or three parts: all viruses have genes made from either DNA or RNA, all have a protein coat that protects these genes, and some have an envelope of fat that surrounds them when they are outside a cell. (Viroids do not have a protein coat and prions contain no RNA or DNA.) Viruses vary from simple to very complex structures. Most viruses are about one hundred times smaller than an average bacterium. The origins of viruses in the evolutionary history of life are unclear: some may have evolved from plasmids—pieces of DNA that can move between cells—while others may have evolved from bacteria.

Viruses spread in many ways; plant viruses are often transmitted from plant to plant by insects that feed on sap, such as aphids, while animal viruses can be carried by blood-sucking insects. These disease-bearing organisms are known as vectors. Influenza viruses are spread by coughing and sneezing. HIV is one of several viruses transmit-

 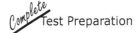

ted through sexual contact and by exposure to infected blood. Viruses can infect only a limited range of host cells called the "host range". This can be broad as when a virus is capable of infecting many species or narrow. [10]

5. What can we infer from the first paragraph in this selection?

    a. A virus is the same as bacterium

    b. A person with excellent vision can see a virus with the naked eye

    c. A virus cannot be seen with the naked eye

    d. Not all viruses are dangerous

6. What types of organisms do viruses infect?

    a. Only plants and humans

    b. Only animals and humans

    c. Only disease-prone humans

    d. All types of organisms

7. How many parts do prions and viroids consist of?

    a. Two

    b. Three

    c. Either less than two or more than three

    d. Less than two

8. What is one common virus spread by coughing and sneezing?

    a. AIDS

    b. Influenza

    c. Herpes

    d. Tuberculosis

Questions 9 – 11 refer to the following passage.

Passage 3 – Clouds

The first stage of a thunderstorm is the cumulus stage, or developing stage. In this stage, masses of moisture are lifted upwards into the atmosphere. The trigger for this lift can be insulation heating the ground producing thermals, areas where two winds converge, forcing air upwards, or where winds blow over terrain of increasing elevation. Moisture in the air rapidly cools into liquid drops of water, which appears as cumulus clouds.

As the water vapor condenses into liquid, latent heat is released which warms the air, causing it to become less dense than the surrounding dry air. The warm air rises in an updraft through the process of convection (hence the term convective precipitation). This creates a low-pressure zone beneath the forming thunderstorm. In a typical thunderstorm, approximately 5×10^8 kg of water vapor is lifted, and the amount of energy released when this condenses is about equal to the energy used by a city of 100,000 in a month. [11]

9. The cumulus stage of a thunderstorm is the

    a. The last stage of the storm

    b. The middle stage of the storm formation

    c. The beginning of the thunderstorm

    d. The period after the thunderstorm has ended

10. One of the ways the air is warmed is

    a. Air moving downwards, which creates a high-pressure zone

    b. Air cooling and becoming less dense, causing it to rise

    c. Moisture moving downward toward the earth

    d. Heat created by water vapor condensing into liquid

11. Identify the correct sequence of events

    a. Warm air rises, water droplets condense, creating more heat, and the air rises further.

    b. Warm air rises and cools, water droplets condense, causing low pressure.

    c. Warm air rises and collects water vapor, the water vapor condenses as the air rises, which creates heat, and causes the air to rise further.

    d. None of the above.

Questions 12 – 14 refer to the following passage.

Passage 4 – US Weather Service

The United States National Weather Service classifies thunderstorms as severe when they reach a predetermined level. Usually, this means the storm is strong enough to inflict wind or hail damage. In most of the United States, a storm is considered severe if winds reach over 50 knots (58 mph or 93 km/h), hail is ¾ inch (2 cm) diameter or larger, or if meteorologists report funnel clouds or tornadoes. In the Central Region of the United States National Weather Service, the hail threshold for a severe thunderstorm is 1 inch (2.5 cm) in diameter. Though a funnel cloud or tornado indicates the presence

 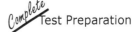

of a severe thunderstorm, the various meteorological agencies would issue a tornado warning rather than a severe thunderstorm warning in this case.

Meteorologists in Canada define a severe thunderstorm as either having tornadoes, wind gusts of 90 km/h or greater, hail 2 centimeters in diameter or greater, rainfall more than 50 millimeters in 1 hour, or 75 millimeters in 3 hours.

Severe thunderstorms can develop from any type of thunderstorm. [11]

12. What is the purpose of this passage?

   a. Explaining when a thunderstorm turns into a tornado

   b. Explaining who issues storm warnings, and when these warnings should be issued

   c. Explaining when meteorologists consider a thunderstorm severe

   d. None of the above

13. It is possible to infer from this passage that

   a. Different areas and countries have different criteria for determining a severe storm

   b. Thunderstorms can include lightning and tornadoes, as well as violent winds and large hail

   c. If someone spots both a thunderstorm and a tornado, meteorological agencies will immediately issue a severe storm warning

   d. Canada has a much different alert system for severe storms, with criteria that are far less

14. What would the Central Region of the United States National Weather Service do if hail was 2.7 cm in diameter?

   a. Not issue a severe thunderstorm warning.

   b. Issue a tornado warning.

   c. Issue a severe thunderstorm warning.

   d. Sleet must also accompany the hail before the Weather Service will issue a storm warning.

Questions 15 – 18 refer to the following passage.

Passage 5 – Clouds

A cloud is a visible mass of droplets or frozen crystals floating in the atmosphere above the surface of the Earth or other planetary bodies. Another type of cloud is a mass of material in space, attracted by gravity, called interstellar clouds and nebulae. The branch of meteorology which studies clouds is called nephrology. When we are speaking of Earth clouds, water vapor is usually the condensing substance, which forms small droplets or ice crystal. These crystals are typically 0.01 mm in diameter. Dense, deep clouds reflect most light, so they appear white, at least from the top. Cloud droplets scatter light very efficiently, so the further into a cloud light travels, the weaker it gets. This accounts for the gray or dark appearance at the base of large clouds. Thin clouds may appear to have acquired the color of their environment or background. [12]

15. What are clouds made of?

    a. Water droplets.

    b. Ice crystals.

    c. Ice crystals and water droplets.

    d. Clouds on Earth are made of ice crystals and water droplets.

16. The main idea of this passage is

    a. Condensation occurs in clouds, having an intense effect on the weather on the surface of the earth.

    b. Atmospheric gases are responsible for the gray color of clouds just before a severe storm happens.

    c. A cloud is a visible mass of droplets or frozen crystals floating in the atmosphere above the surface of the Earth or other planetary body.

    d. Clouds reflect light in varying amounts and degrees, depending on the size and concentration of the water droplets.

17. The branch of meteorology that studies clouds is called

    a. Convection

    b. Thermal meteorology

    c. Nephology

    d. Nephelometry

18. Why are clouds white on top and grey on the bottom?

a. Because water droplets inside the cloud do not reflect light, it appears white, and the further into the cloud the light travels, the less light is reflected making the bottom appear dark.

b. Because water droplets outside the cloud reflect light, it appears dark, and the further into the cloud the light travels, the more light is reflected making the bottom appear white.

c. Because water droplets inside the cloud reflects light, making it appear white, and the further into the cloud the light travels, the more light is reflected making the bottom appear dark.

d. None of the above.

Questions 19 - 22 refer to the following recipe.

Chocolate Chip Cookies

3/4 cup sugar
3/4 cup packed brown sugar
1 cup butter, softened
2 large eggs, beaten
1 teaspoon vanilla extract
2 1/4 cups all-purpose flour
1 teaspoon baking soda
3/4 teaspoon salt
2 cups semisweet chocolate chips

If desired, 1 cup chopped pecans, or chopped walnuts.
Preheat oven to 375 degrees.

Mix sugar, brown sugar, butter, vanilla and eggs in a large bowl. Stir in flour, baking soda, and salt. The dough will be very stiff.

Stir in chocolate chips by hand with a sturdy wooden spoon. Add the pecans, or other nuts, if desired. Stir until the chocolate chips and nuts are evenly dispersed.

Drop dough by rounded tablespoonfuls 2 inches apart onto a cookie sheet.

Bake 8 to 10 minutes or until light brown. Cookies may look underdone, but they will finish cooking after you take them out of the oven.

 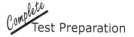

19. What is the correct order for adding these ingredients?

    a. Brown sugar, baking soda, chocolate chips

    b. Baking soda, brown sugar, chocolate chips

    c. Chocolate chips, baking soda, brown sugar

    d. Baking soda, chocolate chips, brown sugar

20. What does sturdy mean?

    a. Long

    b. Strong

    c. Short

    d. Wide

21. What does disperse mean?

    a. Scatter

    b. To form a ball

    c. To stir

    d. To beat

22. When can you stop stirring the nuts?

    a. When the cookies are cooked.

    b. When the nuts are evenly distributed.

    c. As soon as the nuts are added.

    d. After the chocolate chips are added.

Questions 23 – 25 refer to the following passage.

Passage 7 – Caterpillars

Butterfly larvae, or caterpillars, eat enormous quantities of leaves and spend practically all their time in search of food. Although most caterpillars are herbivorous, a few species eat other insects. Some larvae form mutual associations with ants. They communicate with ants using vibrations transmitted through the soil, as well as with chemical signals. The ants provide some degree of protection to the larvae and they in turn gather honeydew secretions. [13]

 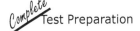

23. What do most larvae spend their time looking for?

   a. Leaves

   b. Insects

   c. Leaves and insects

   d. Honeydew secretions

24. What benefit do larvae get from association with ants?

   a. They do not receive any benefit

   b. Ants give them protection

   c. Ants give them food

   d. Ants give them honeydew secretions

25. Do ants or larvae benefit most from association?

   a. Ants benefit most.

   b. Larvae benefit most.

   c. Both benefit the same.

   d. Neither benefits.

Questions 26 – 30 refer to the following passage.

Passage 8 – Navy Seals

The United States Navy's Sea, Air and Land Teams, commonly known as Navy SEALs, are the U.S. Navy's principal special operations force, and a part of the Naval Special Warfare Command (NSWC) as well as the maritime component of the United States Special Operations Command (USSOCOM).

The unit's acronym ("SEAL") comes from their capacity to operate at sea, in the air, and on land – but it is their ability to work underwater that separates SEALs from most other military units in the world. Navy SEALs are trained and have been deployed in a wide variety of missions, including direct action and special reconnaissance operations, unconventional warfare, foreign internal defence, hostage rescue, counter-terrorism and other missions. All SEALs are members of either the United States Navy or the United States Coast Guard.

In the early morning of May 2, 2011 local time, a team of 40 CIA-led Navy SEALs completed an operation to kill Osama bin Laden in Abbottabad, Pakistan about 35 miles (56 km) from Islamabad, the country's capital. The Navy SEALs were part of the Naval Special Warfare Development Group, previously called "Team 6". President Barack Obama later confirmed the death of bin Laden. The unprecedented media coverage raised the public profile of the SEAL community, particularly the counter-terrorism specialists commonly known as SEAL Team 6. [14]

26. Are Navy SEALs part of USSOCOM?

   a. Yes
   b. No
   c. Only for special operations
   d. No, they are part of the US Navy

27. What separates Navy SEALs from other military units?

   a. Belonging to NSWC
   b. Direct action and special reconnaissance operations
   c. Working underwater
   d. Working for other military units in the world

28. What other military organizations do SEALs belong to?

   a. The US Navy
   b. The Coast Guard
   c. The US Army
   d. The Navy and the Coast Guard

29. What other organization participated in the Bin Laden raid?

   a. The CIA
   b. The US Military
   c. Counter-terrorism specialists
   d. None of the above

30. What is the new name for Team 6?

   a. They were always called Team 6
   b. The counter-terrorism specialists
   c. The Naval Special Warfare Development Group
   d. None of the above

 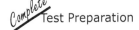

Questions 31 – 34 refer to the following passage.

Passage 9 - Gardening

Gardening for food extends far into prehistory. Ornamental gardens were known in ancient times, a famous example being the Hanging Gardens of Babylon, while ancient Rome had dozens of gardens.

The earliest forms of gardens emerged from the people's need to grow herbs and vegetables. It was only later that rich individuals created gardens for purely decorative purposes.

In ancient Egypt, rich people created ornamental gardens to relax in the shade of the trees. Egyptians believed that gods liked gardens. Commonly, walls surrounded ancient Egyptian gardens with trees planted in rows.

The most popular tree species were date palms, sycamores, fig trees, nut trees, and willows. In addition to ornamental gardens, wealthy Egyptians kept vineyards to produce wine.

The Assyrians are also known for their beautiful gardens in what we know today as Iraq. Assyrian gardens were very large, with some of them used for hunting and others as leisure gardens. Cypress and palm were the most popular trees in Assyrian gardens. [13]

31. Why did wealthy people in Egypt have gardens?

    a. For food.
    b. To relax in the shade.
    c. For ornamentation.
    d. For hunting.

32. What did the Egyptians believe about gardens?

    a. They believed gods loved gardens.
    b. They believed gods hated gardens.
    c. The didn't have any beliefs about gods and Gardens.
    d. They believed gods hated trees.

33. What kinds of trees did the Assyrians like?

    a. The Assyrians liked date palms, sycamores, fig trees, nut trees, and willows.

    b. The Assyrians liked Cypresses and palms.

    c. The Assyrians didn't like trees.

    d. The Assyrians liked hedges and vines.

34. Which came first, gardening for vegetables or ornamental gardens?

    a. Ornamental gardens came before vegetable gardens.

    b. Vegetable gardens came before ornamental gardens.

    c. Vegetable and ornamental gardens appeared at the same time.

    d. The passage does not give enough information.

Questions 35 – 38 refer to the following passage.

Passage 10 - Gardens

Ancient Roman gardens are known for their statues and sculptures, which were never missing from the lives of Romans. Romans designed their gardens with hedges and vines as well as a wide variety of flowers, including acanthus, cornflowers and crocus, cyclamen, hyacinth, iris and ivy, lavender, lilies, myrtle, narcissus, poppy, rosemary and violet. Flower beds were popular in the courtyards of the rich Romans.

The Middle Ages was a period of decline in gardening. After the fall of Rome, gardening was only for the purpose of growing medicinal herbs and decorating church altars.

Islamic gardens were built after the model of Persian gardens, with enclosed walls and watercourses dividing the garden into four. Commonly, the center of the garden would have a pool or pavilion. Mosaics and glazed tiles used to decorate elaborate fountains are specific to Islamic gardens. [15]

35. What is a characteristic feature of Roman gardens?

    a. Statues and Sculptures.

    b. Flower beds.

    c. Medicinal Herbs.

    d. Courtyard gardens.

 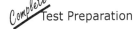

36. When did gardening decline?

a. Before the Fall of Rome.

b. Gardening did not decline.

c. Before the Middle Ages.

d. After the Fall of Rome.

37. What kind of gardening was done during the Middle Ages?

a. Gardening with hedges and vines.

b. Gardening with a wide variety of flowers.

c. Gardening for herbs and church alters.

d. Gardening divided by watercourses.

38. What is a characteristic feature of Islamic Gardens?

a. Statues and Sculptures.

b. Decorative tiles and fountains.

c. Herbs.

d. Flower beds.

Questions 39 – 42 refer to the following passage.

Passage 11 - Coral Reefs

Coral reefs are underwater structures made from calcium carbonate secreted by corals. Corals are colonies of tiny animals found in marine waters that contain few nutrients. Most coral reefs are built from a type of coral called stony corals or Scleractinia, which in turn consist of polyps that cluster in groups. The polyps are like tiny sea anemones, which they are closely related. But unlike sea anemones, coral polyps secrete hard carbonate exoskeletons which support and protect their bodies. Reefs grow best in warm, shallow, clear, sunny and agitated waters. They are most commonly found in shallow tropical waters, but deep water and cold water corals also exist on smaller scales in other areas.

Often called "rainforests of the sea", coral reefs form some of the most diverse ecosystems on Earth. They occupy less than one tenth of one percent of the world's ocean surface, about half the area of France, yet they provide a home for twenty-five percent of all marine species.

Paradoxically, coral reefs flourish even though they are surrounded by ocean waters that provide few nutrients. [16]

Complete Test Preparation

39. Why are coral reefs called rainforests of the sea?

    a. Because they are so colorful.

    b. Because they are a diverse ecosystem.

    c. Because they look like rainforests.

    d. Because occupy less than one tenth of one percent of the world's ocean surface.

40. What marine animal are corals closely related to?

    a. Sea Anemones.

    b. Polyps.

    c. Sea Polyps.

    d. Anemones and Polyps.

41. Where are coral reefs found?

    a. In freshwater with few nutrients.

    b. In marine water with a lot of nutrients.

    c. In marine waters with few nutrients.

    d. In marine water with no nutrients.

42. Where do corals reefs grow?

    a. Hot deep water.

    b. Clear, warm still water.

    c. Warm agitated water.

    d. Warm, clear, shallow and agitated water.

Questions 43 – 45 refer to the following passage.

Coral Reefs II

Most coral reefs were formed after the last glacial period 10,000 years ago when melting ice caused the sea level to rise and flood the continental shelves. As communities established themselves on the shelves, the reefs grew upwards, pacing the rising sea levels. Reefs that rose too slowly became drowned reefs, covered by so much water there was insufficient light.

Different types of coral reefs grow in the deep sea away from the continental shelves, around oceanic islands and as atolls. The vast majority of these islands are volcanic in origin. The few exceptions have tectonic origins where plate movements have lifted the deep ocean floor on the surface. [16]

43. When did most coral reefs form?

    a. Before the last glacial period.

    b. After the last glacial period.

    c. Before the sea level rose.

    d. When the sea level rose.

44. What can you say about how fast coral reefs grew?

    a. They grew at the same rate as the rising sea levels.

    b. They grew faster than the rising sea levels.

    c. They grew slower than the rising sea levels.

    d. They grew before the sea levels rose.

45. What happened to the coral reefs that did grow at the proper rate?

    a. They died due to lack of light.

    b. They died due to lack of water.

    c. They didn't die.

    d. They adapted to grow faster.

Section II – Math

1. What is 1/3 of 3/4?

    a.   1/4

    b.   1/3

    c.   2/3

    d.   3/4

2. What fraction of $1500 is $75?

    a. 1/14

    b. 3/5

    c. 7/10

    d. 1/20

3. 3.14 + 2.73 + 23.7 =

 a. 28.57
 b. 30.57
 c. 29.56
 d. 29.57

4. A woman spent 15% of her income on an item and ends up with $120. What percentage of her income is left?

 a. 12%
 b. 85%
 c. 75%
 d. 95%

5. Express 0.27 + 0.33 as a fraction.

 a. 3/6
 b. 4/7
 c. 3/5
 d. 2/7

6. What is (3.13 + 7.87) X 5?

 a. 65
 b. 50
 c. 45
 d. 55

7. Reduce 2/4 X 3/4 to lowest terms.

 a. 6/12
 b. 3/8
 c. 6/16
 d. 3/4

8. 2/3 – 2/5 =

 a. 4/10
 b. 1/15
 c. 3/7
 d. 4/15

9. 2/7 + 2/3 =

    a. 12/23
    b. 5/10
    c. 20/21
    d. 6/21

10. 2/3 of 60 + 1/5 of 75 =

    a. 45
    b. 55
    c. 15
    d. 50

11. 8 is what percent of 40?

    a. 10%
    b. 15%
    c. 20%
    d. 25%

12. 9 is what percent of 36?

    a. 10%
    b. 15%
    c. 20%
    d. 25%

13. Three tenths of 90 equals:

    a. 18
    b. 45
    c. 27
    d. 36

14. .4% of 36 is

    a. 1.44
    b. .144
    c. 14.4
    d. 144

15. The physician ordered 5 mg Coumadin; 10 mg/tablet is on hand. How many tablets will you give?

    a. .5 tablets

    b. 1 tablet

    c. .75 tablets

    d. 1.5 tablets

16. The physician ordered 20 mg Tylenol/kg of body weight; on hand is 80 mg/ tablet. The child weighs 12 kg. How many tablets will you give?

    a. 1 tablet

    b. 3 tablets

    c. 2 tablets

    d. 4 tablets

17. The physician ordered 20 mg Tylenol/kg of body weight; on hand is 80 mg/ tablet. The child weighs 44 lb. How many tablets will you give?

    a. 5 tablets

    b. 5.5 tablets

    c. 4.5 tablets

    d. 3 tablets

18. The physician ordered 3,000 units of heparin; 5,000 U/mL is on hand. How many milliliters will you give?

    a. 0.5 ml

    b. 0.6 ml

    c. 0.75 ml

    d. 0.8 ml

19. The physician orders 60 mg Augmentin; 80 mg/mL is on hand. How many milliliters will you give?

    a. 1 ml

    b. 0.5 ml

    c. 0.75 ml

    d. 0.95 ml

 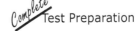

20. The physician ordered 16 mg Ibuprofen/kg of body weight; on hand is 80 mg/ tablet. The child weighs 15 kg. How many tablets will you give?

    a. 3 tablets

    b. 2 tablets

    c. 1 tablet

    d. 2.5 tablets

21. The physician orders 1000 mg Benbadryl liquid; 1 g/tsp is on hand. How many teaspoons will you give?

    a. .75 tsp

    b. 1.5 tsp

    c. 1 tsp

    d. 1.25 tsp

22. The physician ordered 10 units of regular insulin and 200 U/mL is on hand. How many milliliters will you give?

    a. .45 ml

    b. .75 ml

    c. .25 ml

    d. .05 ml

23. If y = 4 and x = 3, solve yx^3

    a. -108

    b. 108

    c. 27

    d. 4

24. Convert 0.007 kilograms to grams

    a. 7 grams

    b. 70 grams

    c. 0.07 grams

    d. 0.70 grams

25. Convert 16 quarts to gallons

    a. 1 gallons

    b. 8 gallons

    c. 4 gallons

    d. 4.5 gallons

26. Convert 2 teaspoons to milliliters.

    a. 4.3 milliliters

    b. 9 milliliters

    c. 9.86 milliliters

    d. 4 milliliters

27. Convert 200 meters to kilometers

    a. 50 kilometers

    b. 20 kilometers

    c. 12 kilometers

    d. 0.2 kilometers

28. Convert 72 inches to feet

    a. 12 feet

    b. 6 feet

    c. 4 feet

    d. 17 feet

29. Convert 3 yards to feet

    a. 18 feet

    b. 12 feet

    c. 9 feet

    d. 27 feet

30. Convert 45 kg. to pounds.

    a. 10 pounds

    b. 100 pounds

    c. 1,000 pounds

    d. 110 pounds

31. Convert 0.63 grams to mg.

    a. 630 g.

    b. 63 mg.

    c. 630 mg.

    d. 603 mg.

32. 5x + 3 = 7x -1. Find x

    a. 1/3

    b. ½

    c. 1

    d. 2

33. 5x+2(x+7) = 14x – 7. Find x

    a. 1

    b. 2

    c. 3

    d. 4

34. 12t -10 = 14t + 2. Find t

    a. -6

    b. -4

    c. 4

    d. 6

35. 5(z+1) = 3(z+2) + 11. Z=?

    a. 2

    b. 4

    c. 6

    d. 12

36. The price of a book went up from \$20 to \$25. What percent did the price increase?

    a. 5%

    b. 10%

    c. 20%

    d. 25%

37. The price of a book decreased from \$25 to \$20. What percent did the price decrease?

    a. 5%

    b. 10%

    c. 20%

    d. 25%

38. After taking several practice tests, Brian improved the results of his GRE test by 30%. Given that the first time he took the test Brian answered 150 questions correctly, how many questions did he answer correctly on the second test?

    a. 105

    b. 120

    c. 180

    d. 195

39. In local baseball team, 4 players (or 12.5% of the team) have long hair and the rest have short hair. How many short-haired players are there on the team?

    a. 24

    b. 28

    c. 32

    d. 50

40. In the time required to serve 43 customers, a server breaks 2 glasses and slips 5 times. The next day, the same server breaks 10 glasses. How many customers did she serve?

    a. 25

    b. 43

    c. 86

    d. 215

41. A square lawn has an area of 62,500 square meters. What will is the cost of building fence around it at a rate of $5.5 per meter?

    a. $4000

    b. $4500

    c. $5000

    d. $5500

42. Mr. Brown bought 5 cheese burgers, 3 drinks, and 4 fries for his family, and a cookie pack for his dog. If the price of all single items is the same at $1.30 and a 3.5% tax is added, what is the total cost of dinner for Mr. Brown?

    a. $16

    b. $16.9

    c. $17

    d. $17.5

43. The length of a rectangle is twice of its width and its area is equal to the area of a square with 12 cm. sides. What will be the perimeter of the rectangle to the nearest whole number?

    a. 36 cm

    b. 46 cm

    c. 51 cm

    d. 56 cm

44. There are 15 yellow and 35 orange balls in a basket. How many more yellow balls must be added to make the yellow balls 65%?

    a. 35

    b. 50

    c. 65

    d. 70

45. A farmer wants to plant 65,536 trees in such a way that number of rows must be equal to the number of plants in a row. How many trees should he plant in a row?

    a. 1684

    b. 1268

    c. 668

    d. 256

46. A distributor purchased 550 kilograms of potatoes for $165. He distributed these at a rate of $6.4 per 20 kilograms to 15 shops, $3.4 per 10 kilograms to 12 shops and the remainder at $1.8. If his distribution cost is $10, what will be his profit?

    a. $10.4

    b. $24.60

    c. $14.9

    d. $23.4

47. A farmer wants to plant trees around the outside boundaries of his rectangular field of dimensions 650 meters × 780 meters. Each tree requires 5 meters of free space all around it from the stem. How many trees can he plant?

    a. 572

    b. 568

    c. 286

    d. 282

48. A farmer wants to plant trees at the outside boundaries of his rectangular field of dimensions 650 meters × 780 meters. Each tree requires 5 meter of free space all around it from the stem. How much free area will be left?

    a. 478,800 m^2

    b. 492,800 m^2

    c. 507,625 m^2

    d. 518,256 m^2

49. How much pay does Mr. Johnson receive if he gives half of his pay to his family, $250 to his landlord, and has exactly 3/7 of his pay left over?

    a. $3600

    b. $3500

    c. $2800

    d. $1750

50. A boy has 4 red, 5 green and 2 yellow balls. He chooses two balls randomly. What is the probability that one is red and other is green?

    a. 2/11

    b. 19/22

    c. 20/121

    d. 9/11

Section III – Part 1 - English

1. Choose the sentence with the correct grammar.

a. Don would never have thought of that book, but you could have reminded him.

b. Don would never of thought of that book, but you could have reminded him.

c. Don would never have thought of that book, but you could of have reminded him.

d. Don would never of thought of that book, but you could of reminded him.

2. Choose the sentence with the correct grammar.

a. The mother would not of punished her daughter if she could have avoided it.

b. The mother would not have punished her daughter if she could of avoided it.

c. The mother would not of punished her daughter if she could of avoided it.

d. The mother would not have punished her daughter if she could have avoided it.

3. Choose the sentence with the correct grammar.

a. There was scarcely no food in the pantry, because nobody ate at home.

b. There was scarcely any food in the pantry, because nobody ate at home.

c. There was scarcely any food in the pantry, because not nobody ate at home.

d. There was scarcely no food in the pantry, because not nobody ate at home.

4. Choose the sentence with the correct grammar.

a. Although you may not see nobody in the dark, it does not mean that nobody is there.

b. Although you may not see anyone in the dark, it does not mean that not nobody is there.

c. Although you may not see anyone in the dark, it does not mean that no one is there.

d. Although you may not see nobody in the dark, it does not mean that not nobody is there.

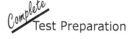

5. Choose the sentence with the correct grammar.

a. Michael has lived in that house for forty years, while I has owned this one for only six weeks.

b. Michael have lived in that house for forty years, while I have owned this one for only six weeks.

c. Michael have lived in that house for forty years, while I has owned this one for only six weeks.

d. Michael has lived in that house for forty years, while I have owned this one for only six weeks.

6. Choose the sentence with the correct grammar.

a. The older children have already eat their dinner, but the baby has not yet eaten anything.

b. The older children have already eaten their dinner, but the baby has not yet ate anything.

c. The older children have already eaten their dinner, but the baby has not yet eaten anything.

d. The older children have already eat their dinner, but the baby has not yet ate anything.

7. Choose the sentence with the correct grammar.

a. If they had gone to the party, he would have gone, too.

b. If they had went to the party, he would have gone, too.

c. If they had gone to the party, he would have went, too.

d. If they had went to the party, he would have went, too.

8. Choose the sentence with the correct grammar.

a. He should have went to the appointment; instead, he went to the beach.

b. He should have gone to the appointment; instead, he went to the beach.

c. He should have went to the appointment; instead, he gone to the beach.

d. He should have gone to the appointment; instead, he gone to the beach.

9. Choose the sentence with the correct grammar.

a. Lee pronounced it's name incorrectly; it's an impatiens, not an impatience.

b. Lee pronounced its name incorrectly; its an impatiens, not an impatience.

c. Lee pronounced it's name incorrectly; its an impatiens, not an impatience.

d. Lee pronounced its name incorrectly; it's an impatiens, not an impatience.

 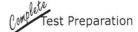

10. Choose the sentence with the correct grammar.

a. Its important for you to know its official name; its called the Confederate Museum.

b. It's important for you to know it's official name; it's called the Confederate Museum.

c. It's important for you to know its official name; it's called the Confederate Museum.

d. Its important for you to know it's official name; it's called the Confederate Museum.

11. The Ford Motor Company was named for Henry Ford, _____.

a. which had founded the company.

b. who founded the company.

c. whose had founded the company.

d. whom had founded the company.

12. Thomas Edison _____ since he invented the light bulb, television, motion pictures, and phonograph.

a. has always been known as the greatest inventor

b. was always been known as the greatest inventor

c. must have had been always known as the greatest inventor

d. will had been known as the greatest inventor

13. The weatherman on Channel 6 said that this has been the _____.

a. most hottest summer on record

b. most hottest summer on record

c. hottest summer on record

d. hotter summer on record

14. Although Joe is tall for his age, his brother Elliot is _____ of the two.

a. the tallest

b. more tallest

c. the tall

d. the taller

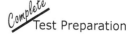

15. When KISS came to town, all of the tickets _____ before I could buy one.

    a. will be sold out

    b. had been sold out

    c. were being sold out

    d. was sold out

16. The rules of most sports _____ more complicated than we often realize.

    a. are

    b. is

    c. was

    d. has been

17. Neither of the Wright Brothers _____ that they would be successful with their flying machine.

    a. have any doubts

    b. has any doubts

    c. had any doubts

    d. will have any doubts

18. The Titanic _____ mere days into its maiden voyage.

    a. has already sunk

    b. will already sunk

    c. already sank

    d. sank

19. _____ won first place in the Western Division?

    a. Who

    b. Whom

    c. Which

    d. What

20. There are now several ways to listen to music, including radio, CDs, and Mp3 files _____ you can download onto an MP3 player.

    a. on which

    b. who

    c. whom

    d. which

21. As the tallest monument in the United States, the St. Louis Arch _____.

    a. has rose to an impressive 630 feet.

    b. is risen to an impressive 630 feet.

    c. rises to an impressive 630 feet.

    d. was rose to an impressive 630 feet.

22. The tired, old woman should _____ on the sofa.

    a. lie

    b. lays

    c. laid

    d. lain

23. Did the students understand that Thanksgiving always _____ on the fourth Thursday in November?

    a. fallen

    b. falling

    c. has fell

    d. falls

24. Collecting stamps, _____ and listening to shortwave radio were Rick's main hobbies.

    a. building models,

    b. to build models,

    c. having built models,

    d. build models,

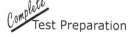

25. Choose the sentence with the correct usage.

a. The ceremony had an emotional effect on the groom, but the bride was not affected.

b. The ceremony had an emotional affect on the groom, but the bride was not affected.

c. The ceremony had an emotional effect on the groom, but the bride was not effected.

d. The ceremony had an emotional affect on the groom, but the bride was not affected.

26. Choose the sentence with the correct usage.

a. Anna was taller then Luis, but then he grew four inches in three months.

b. Anna was taller then Luis, but than he grew four inches in three months.

c. Anna was taller than Luis, but than he grew four inches in three months.

d. Anna was taller than Luis, but then he grew four inches in three months.

27. Choose the sentence with the correct usage.

a. Their second home is in Boca Raton, but there not their for most of the year.

b. They're second home is in Boca Raton, but they're not there for most of the year.

c. Their second home is in Boca Raton, but they're not there for most of the year.

d. There second home is in Boca Raton, but they're not there for most of the year.

28. Choose the sentence with the correct usage.

a. They're going to graduate in June; after that, their best option will be to go there.

b. There going to graduate in June; after that, their best option will be to go there.

c. They're going to graduate in June; after that, there best option will be to go their.

d. Their going to graduate in June; after that, their best option will be to go there

29. Choose the sentence with the correct usage.

a. You're mistaken; that is not you're book.

b. Your mistaken; that is not your book.

c. You're mistaken; that is not your book.

d. Your mistaken; that is not you're book.

30. Choose the sentence with the correct usage.

    a. You're classes are on the west side of campus, but you're living on the east side.

    b. Your classes are on the west side of campus, but your living on the east side.

    c. Your classes are on the west side of campus, but you're living on the east side.

    d. You're classes are on the west side of campus, but you're living on the east side.

31. Choose the sentence with the correct usage.

    a. Disease is highly prevalent in poorer nations; the most dominant disease is malaria.

    b. Disease are highly prevalent in poorer nations; the most dominant disease is malaria.

    c. Disease is highly prevalent in poorer nations; the most dominant disease are malaria.

    d. Disease are highly prevalent in poorer nations; the most dominant disease are malaria.

32. Choose the sentence with the correct usage.

    a. Although I would prefer to have dog, I actually own a cat.

    b. Although I would prefer to have a dog, I actually own cat.

    c. Although I would prefer to have a dog, I actually own a cat.

    d. Although I would prefer to have dog, I actually own cat.

33. Choose the sentence with the correct usage.

    a. The principal of the school lived by one principle: always do your best.

    b. The principle of the school lived by one principle: always do your best.

    c. The principal of the school lived by one principal: always do your best.

    d. The principle of the school lived by one principal: always do your best.

34. Choose the sentence with the correct usage.

    a. Even with an speed limit sign clearly posted, an inattentive driver may drive too fast.

    b. Even with a speed limit sign clearly posted, a inattentive driver may drive too fast.

    c. Even with an speed limit sign clearly posted, a inattentive driver may drive too fast.

    d. Even with a speed limit sign clearly posted, an inattentive driver may drive too fast.

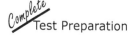

35. Choose the sentence with the correct usage.

    a. Except for the roses, she did not accept John's frequent gifts.

    b. Accept for the roses, she did not except John's frequent gifts.

    c. Accept for the roses, she did not accept John's frequent gifts.

    d. Except for the roses, she did not except John's frequent gifts.

36. Choose the sentence with the correct usage.

    a. Although he continued to advise me, I no longer took his advice.

    b. Although he continued to advice me, I no longer took his advise.

    c. Although he continued to advise me, I no longer took his advise.

    d. Although he continued to advice me, I no longer took his advise.

37. Choose the sentence with the correct usage.

    a. In order to adopt to the climate, we had to adopt a different style of clothing.

    b. In order to adapt to the climate, we had to adapt a different style of clothing.

    c. In order to adapt to the climate, we had to adopt a different style of clothing.

    d. In order to adapt to the climate, we had to adapt a different style of clothing.

38. Choose the sentence with the correct usage.

    a. When he's between friends, Robert seems confident, but between you and me, he is really very shy.

    b. When he's among friends, Robert seems confident, but among you and me, he is really very shy.

    c. When he's between friends, Robert seems confident, but among you and me, he is really very shy.

    d. When he's among friends, Robert seems confident, but between you and me, he is really very shy.

39. Choose the sentence with the correct usage.

    a. I will be finished at ten in the morning, and will be arriving at home at about 6:30.

    b. I will be finished at about ten in the morning, and will be arriving at home at 6:30.

    c. I will be finished at about ten in the morning, and will be arriving at home at about 6:30.

    d. I will be finished at ten in the morning, and will be arriving at home at 6:30.

 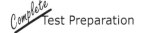

40. Choose the sentence with the correct usage.

   a. Beside the red curtains and pillows, there was a red rug beside the couch.

   b. Besides the red curtains and pillows, there was a red rug beside the couch.

   c. Besides the red curtains and pillows, there was a red rug besides the couch.

   d. Beside the red curtains and pillows, there was a red rug besides the couch.

41. Choose the sentence with the correct usage.

   a. Although John can swim very well, the lifeguard may not allow him to swim in the pool.

   b. Although John may swim very well, the lifeguard may not allow him to swim in the pool.

   c. Although John can swim very well, the lifeguard cannot allow him to swim in the pool.

   d. Although John may swim very well, the lifeguard may not allow him to swim in the pool.

42. Choose the sentence with the correct usage.

   a. Her continuous absences caused a continual disruption at the office.

   b. Her continual absences caused a continuous disruption at the office.

   c. Her continual absences caused a continual disruption at the office.

   d. Her continuous absences caused a continuous disruption at the office.

43. Choose the sentence with the correct usage.

   a. During the famine, the Irish people had to emigrate to other countries; many of them immigrated to the United States.

   b. During the famine, the Irish people had to immigrate to other countries; many of them immigrated to the United States.

   c. During the famine, the Irish people had to emigrate to other countries; many of them emigrated to the United States.

   d. During the famine, the Irish people had to immigrate to other countries; many of them emigrated to the United States.

44. Choose the sentence with the correct usage.

   a. His home was farther than we expected; farther, the roads were very bad.

   b. His home was farther than we expected; further, the roads were very bad.

   c. His home was further than we expected; further, the roads were very bad.

   d. His home was further than we expected; farther, the roads were very bad.

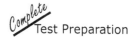

45. Choose the sentence with the correct usage.

  a. The volunteers brought groceries and toys to the homeless shelter; the latter were given to the staff, while the former were given directly to the children.

  b. The volunteers brought groceries and toys to the homeless shelter; the former was given to the staff, while the latter was given directly to the children.

  c. The volunteers brought groceries and toys to the homeless shelter; the groceries were given to the staff, while the former was given directly to the children.

  d. The volunteers brought groceries and toys to the homeless shelter; the latter was given to the staff, while the groceries were given directly to the children.

46. Choose the sentence with the correct usage.

  a. Vegetables are a healthy food; eating them can make you more healthful.

  b. Vegetables are a healthful food; eating them can make you more healthful.

  c. Vegetables are a healthy food; eating them can make you more healthy.

  d. Vegetables are a healthful food; eating them can make you more healthy.

47. Choose the sentence with the correct usage.

  a. After you lay the books on the counter, you may lay down for a nap.

  b. After you lie the books on the counter, you may lay down for a nap.

  c. After you lay the books on the counter, you may lie down for a nap.

  d. After you lay the books on the counter, you may lay down for a nap.

48. Choose the sentence with the correct usage.

  a. After you lay the books on the counter, you may lay down for a nap.

  b. After you lie the books on the counter, you may lay down for a nap.

  c. After you lay the books on the counter, you may lie down for a nap.

  d. After you lay the books on the counter, you may lay down for a nap.

49. Choose the sentence with the correct usage.

  a. Once the chickens had layed their eggs, they lay on their nests to hatch them.

  b. Once the chickens had lay their eggs, they lay on their nests to hatch them.

  c. Once the chickens had laid their eggs, they lay on their nests to hatch them.

  d. Once the chickens had laid their eggs, they laid on their nests to hatch them.

50. Choose the sentence with the correct usage.

    a. Mrs. Foster taught me many things, but I learned the most from Mr. Wallace.

    b. Mrs. Foster learned me many things, but I was taught the most by Mr. Wallace.

    c. Mrs. Foster learned me many things, but I learned the most from Mr. Wallace.

    d. Mrs. Foster taught me many things, but I was learned the most from Mr. Wallace.

Section III – Part II – Vocabulary

Choose the word that matches the given definition.

1. VERB To build up or strengthen in relation to morals or religion.

    a. Sanctify

    b. Amplify

    c. Edify

    d. Wry

2. NOUN Exit or way out.

    a. Door-jamb

    b. Egress

    c. Regress

    d. Furtherance

3. ADJECTIVE Private, personal.

    a. Confidential

    b. Hysteric

    c. Simplistic

    d. Promissory

4. NOUN Serious criminal offence that is punishable by death or imprisonment above a year.

- a. Trespass
- b. Hampers
- c. Felony
- d. Obligatory

5. VERB To encourage or incite troublesome acts.

- a. Comment
- b. Foment
- c. Integument
- d. Atonement

6. ADJECTIVE Dignified, solemn that is appropriate for a funeral.

- a. Funereal
- b. Prediction
- c. Wailing
- d. Vociferous

7. NOUN Warmth and kindness of disposition.

- a. Seethe
- b. Geniality
- c. Desists
- d. Predicate

8. ADJECTIVE Polite and well mannered.

- a. Chivalrous
- b. Hilarious
- c. Genteel
- d. Governance

9. VERB To encourage, stimulate or incite and provoke.

- a. Push
- b. Force
- c. Threaten
- d. Goad

10. ADJECTIVE Shocking, terrible or wicked.

    a. Pleasantries

    b. Heinous

    c. Shrewd

    d. Provencal

11. NOUN A person of thing that tells or announces the coming of someone or something.

    a. Harbinger

    b. Evasion

    c. Apostate

    d. Coquette

12. ADJECTIVE Similar or identical.

    a. Soluble

    b. Assembly

    c. Conclave

    d. Homologous

13. ADJECTIVE Common, not honorable or noble.

    a. Princely

    b. Ignoble

    c. Shameful

    d. Sham

14. ADJECTIVE Irrelevant not having substance or matter.

    a. Immaterial

    b. Prohibition

    c. Prediction

    d. Brokerage

15. ADJECTIVE Perfect, no faults or errors.

    a. Impeccable

    b. Formidable

    c. Genteel

    d. Disputation

16. VERB Place side by side for contrast or comparison.

    a. Peccadillo

    b. Fallible

    c. Congeal

    d. Juxtapose

17. NOUN Ruling council of a military government.

    a. Sophist

    b. Counsel

    c. Virago

    d. Junta

18. NOUN Someone who takes more time than necessary.

    a. Demagogue

    b. Haggard

    c. Laggard

    d. Investiture

19. ADJECTIVE Lacking enthusiasm, strength or energy.

    a. Hapless

    b. Languid

    c. Ubiquitous

    d. Promiscuous

20. NOUN A person of influence, rank or distinction.

    a. Consummate

    b. Sinister

    c. Accolade

    d. Magnate

21. NOUN A lingering disease or ailment of the human body.

    a. Treatment

    b. Frontal

    c. Malady

    d. Assiduous

22. ADJECTIVE Quick and light in movement.

    a. Quickest

    b. Nimble

    c. Rapacious

    d. Perspicuities

23. ADJECTIVE A loud unpleasant noise.

    a. Nosy

    b. Racket

    c. Ravage

    d. Noisome

24. ADJECTIVE Relating to a wedding or marriage.

    a. Nefarious

    b. Fluctuate

    c. Nuptial

    d. Flatulence

25. ADJECTIVE Open display or apparent.

    a. Ostensible

    b. Complacent

    c. Revealing

    d. Harrowing

26. NOUN A sheet of paper that can be folded into 8 leaves.

    a. Octagon

    b. Harangue

    c. Octavo

    d. Wreckage

27. ADJECTIVE Appearing weak or pale.

    a. Pallid

    b. Palliative

    c. Deviant

    d. Expatiate

28. NOUN A picture or series of pictures representing a continuous scene.

a. Accolade

b. Obdurate

c. Panorama

d. Personification

29. NOUN A self contradictory statement that can only be true if its false and vice versa.

a. Inbred

b. Paradox

c. Attribute

d. Fealty

30. ADJECTIVE Often complaining.

a. Querulous

b. Complaint

c. Compound

d. Vestige

31. Choose the best definition of mollify.

a. To anger

b. To modify

c. To irritate

d. To soothe

32. Choose the best definition of redundant.

a. Backup

b. Necessary repetition

c. Unnecessary repetition

d. No repetition

33. Choose the best definition of bicker.

a. Chat

b. Discuss

c. Argue

d. Debate

34. Choose the best definition of sombre.

    a. Gothic

    b. Black

    c. Serious

    d. Evil

35. Choose the best definition of maverick.

    a. Rebel

    b. Conformist

    c. Unconventional

    d. Conventional

36. Choose the best definition of tenuous.

    a. Strong

    b. Tense

    c. Firm

    d. Weak

37. Choose the best definition of pandemonium.

    a. Chaos

    b. Orderly

    c. Quiet

    d. Noisy

38. Choose the best definition of perpetual.

    a. Continuous

    b. Slowly

    c. Over a very long time

    d. Motion

39. Choose the best definition of denigrate.

    a. Compliment

    b. Belittle

    c. Praise

    d. Admire

40. Choose the best definition of mundane.

    a. Exciting

    b. Continuous

    c. Unforgiving

    d. Ordinary

41. Choose the best definition of importune.

    a. To find an opportunity

    b. To ask all the time.

    c. Cannot find an opportunity

    d. None of the above

42. Choose the best definition of volatile.

    a. Not explosive

    b. Catches fire easily

    c. Does not catch fire

    d. Explosive

43. Choose the best definition of plaintive.

    a. Happy

    b. Mournful

    c. Faint

    d. Plain

44. Choose the best definition of nexus.

    a. A connection

    b. A telephone switch

    c. Part of a computer

    d. None of the above

45. Choose the best definition of conjoin.

    a. A connection

    b. To marry

    c. Weld together

    d. To join together

46. Choose the best definition of petrify.

 a. Turn into a fossil

 b. Turn to stone

 c. Turn into wood

 d. Turn into glass

47. Choose the best definition of inherent.

 a. To receive money in a will

 b. An essential part of

 c. To receive money from a will

 d. None of the above

48. Choose the best definition of torpid.

 a. Fast

 b. Rapid

 c. Sluggish

 d. Violent

49. Choose the best definition of gregarious.

 a. Sociable

 b. Introverted

 c. Large

 d. Solitary

50. Choose the best definition of alloy.

 a. To mix with something superior

 b. To mix

 c. To mix with something inferior

 d. To purify

Section III – Science

1. Electricity is a general term encompassing a variety of phenomena resulting from the presence and flow of electric charge. Which of the following statements about electricity is/are true?

    a. Electrically charged matter is influenced by, and produces, electromagnetic fields.

    b. Electric current is a movement or flow of electrically charged particles.

    c. Electric potential is a fundamental interaction between the magnetic field and the presence and motion of an electric charge.

    d. An influence produced by an electric charge on other charges in its vicinity is an electric field.

2. Which of the following is/are not included in Ohm's Law?

    a. Ohm's Law defines the relationships between (P) power, (E) voltage, (I) current, and (R) resistance.

    b. One ohm is the resistance value through which one volt will maintain a current of one ampere.

    c. Using Ohm's Law, voltage is determined using V = IR, with I equaling current and R equaling resistance.

    d. An ohm (Ω) is a unit of electrical voltage.

3. The property of a conductor that restricts its internal flow of electrons is:

    a. Friction

    b. Power

    c. Current

    d. Resistance

4. In physics, _____ is the force that opposes the relative motion of two bodies in contact.

    a. Resistance

    b. Abrasiveness

    c. Friction

    d. Antagonism

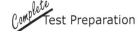
Complete Test Preparation

5. What is the difference, of any, between kinetic energy and potential energy?

a. Kinetic energy is the energy of a body that results from heat while potential energy is the energy possessed by an object that is chilled

b. Kinetic energy is the energy of a body that results from motion while potential energy is the energy possessed by an object by virtue of its position or state, e.g., as in a compressed spring.

c. There is no difference between kinetic and potential energy; all energy is the same.

d. Potential energy is the energy of a body that results from motion while kinetic energy is the energy possessed by an object by virtue of its position or state, e.g., as in a compressed spring.

6. What are considered the four fundamental forces of nature?

a. Gravity, electromagnetic force, weak nuclear force, and strong nuclear force

b. Gravity, electromagnetic force, negative nuclear force, and positive nuclear force

c. Polarity, electromagnetic force, weak nuclear force, and strong nuclear force

d. Gravity, chemical magnetic force, weak nuclear force, and strong nuclear force

7. Starting with the weakest, arrange the fundamental forces of nature in order of strength.

a. Gravity, Weak Nuclear Force, Electromagnetic Force, Strong Nuclear Force

b. Weak Nuclear Force, Gravity, Electromagnetic Force, Strong Nuclear Force

c. Strong Nuclear Force, Weak Nuclear Force, Electromagnetic Force, Gravity

d. Gravity, Strong Nuclear Force, Weak Nuclear Force, Electromagnetic Force

8. What is the difference between Strong Nuclear Force and Weak Nuclear Force?

a. The Strong Nuclear Force is an attractive force that binds protons and neutrons and maintains the structure of the nucleus, and the Weak Nuclear Force is responsible for the radioactive beta decay and other subatomic reactions.

b. The Strong Nuclear Force is responsible for the radioactive beta decay and other subatomic reactions, and the Weak Nuclear Force is an attractive force that binds protons and neutrons and maintains the structure of the nucleus.

c. The Weak Nuclear Force is feeble and the Strong Nuclear Force is robust.

d. The Strong Nuclear Force is a negative force that releases protons and neutrons and threatens the structure of the nucleus, and the Weak Nuclear Force is an attractive force that binds protons and neutrons and maintains the structure of the nucleus.

 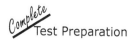

9. The Law of Conservation of Mass states that:

a. No detectable gain but, depending on the substances used, some loss can occur in chemical reactions.

b. No detectable gain or loss occurs in chemical reactions.

c. No detectable loss but some gain occurs in chemical reactions.

d. Depending on the substances used, substantial gain or loss can occur in chemical reactions.

10. What is the difference, if any, between convection and heat radiation?

a. Thermal radiation is the transfer of heat from one place to another by the movement of fluids; convection is electromagnetic radiation emitted from all matter due to its possessing thermal energy.

b. Convection is the transfer of heat from one place to another by the movement of fluids; thermal radiation is nuclear energy emitted from all matter due to its possessing thermal energy.

c. Convection is the transfer of heat from one place to another by the movement of fluids; thermal radiation is electromagnetic radiation emitted from all matter due to its possessing thermal energy.

d. Convection is the transfer of heat from one place to another by the movement of fluids; thermal radiation is the barely detectable light emitted from all matter due to its possessing thermal energy.

11. In _____ cells, the cell cycle is the cycle of events involving cell division, including _____, _____, and _____.

a. Prokaryotic, meiosis, cytokinesis, and interphase

b. Eukaryotic, meiosis, cytokinesis, and interphase

c. Eukaryotic, mitosis, kinematisis, and interphase

d. Eukaryotic, mitosis, cytokinesis, and interphase

12. Which, if any, of the following statements about prokaryotic cells is false?

a. Prokaryotic cells include such organisms as E. coli and Streptococcus.

b. Prokaryotic cells lack internal membranes and organelles.

c. Prokaryotic cells break down food using cellular respiration and fermentation.

d. All of these statements are true.

 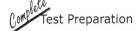

13. _____ **is a nucleic acid that carries the genetic information in the cell and is capable of self-replication.**

    a. RNA

    b. Triglyceride

    c. DNA

    d. DAR

14. The complementary bases found in DNA are _____ and _____ or _____ and _____.

    a. Adenine and thymine or cytosine and guanine

    b. Cytosine and thymine or adenine and guanine

    c. Adenine and cytosine or thymine and guanine

    d. None of the above

15. A/an _____ is the basic structural unit of nucleic acids (DNA or RNA); their sequence determines individual hereditary characteristics.

    a. Gene

    b. Nucleotide

    c. Phosphate

    d. Nitrogen base

16. _____ is a _____ that plays an important role in the creation of new _____.

    a. Deoxyribonucleic acid (DNA) is a chain of nucleotides that plays an important role in the creation of new proteins.

    b. Ribonucleic acid (RNA) is a chain of nucleotides that plays an important role in the creation of new proteins.

    c. Ribonucleic acid (RNA) is a cluster of enzymes that plays an important role in the creation of new proteins.

    d. Ribonucleic acid (RNA) is a chain of nucleotides that plays an important role in the creation of new genes.

17. Which, if any, of the following statements are false?

    a. A mutation is a permanent change in the DNA sequence of a gene.

    b. Mutations in a gene's DNA sequence can alter the amino acid sequence of the protein encoded by the gene.

    c. Mutations in DNA sequences usually occur spontaneously.

    d. Mutations in DNA sequences are caused by exposure to environmental agents

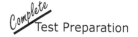

such as sunshine.

18. _____ reactions occur in every cell and use _____ to convert glucose to energy; _____organisms such as many bacteria can release energy without the use of _____.

a. Aerobic reactions occur in every cell and use oxygen to convert glucose to energy; anaerobic organisms such as many bacteria can release energy without the use of oxygen.

b. Anaerobic reactions occur in every cell and use oxygen to convert glucose to energy; aerobic organisms such as many bacteria can release energy without the use of oxygen.

c. Aerobic reactions occur in every cell and use exercise to convert glucose to energy; anaerobic organisms such as many bacteria can release energy without the use of exercise.

d. Analogic reactions occur in every cell and use oxygen to convert glucose to energy; anaerobic organisms such as many bacteria can release energy without the use of oxygen.

19. _____ are a collection of similar cells that group together to perform a specialized function.

a. Ephithelia

b. Organs

c. Systems

d. Tissues

20. _____ tissue serves as membranes lining organs and helping to keep the body's organs separate, in place and protected; an example is the outer layer of the skin.

a. Epithelial

b. Connective

c. Nerve

d. Protein

21. Tissue that adds support and structure to the body and frequently contains fibrous strands of collagen is _____ tissue.

a. Epithelial

b. Muscle

c. Nerve

d. Connective

22. _____ tissue is a specialized tissue that can contract and contains the specialized proteins actin and myosin that slide past one another and allow movement.

    a. Epithelial

    b. Muscle

    c. Nerve

    d. Connective

23. _____ tissue contains two types of cells: neurons and glial cells and has the ability to generate and conduct electrical signals in the body.

    a. Nerve

    b. Connective

    c. Epithelial

    d. Muscle

24. A/an _____ is a group of tissues that perform a specific function or group of functions.

    a. System

    b. Tissue

    c. Group

    d. Organ

25. Among animals, examples of _____ are the heart, lungs, brain, eye, stomach, and bones; plant _____ include the roots, stems, leaves, flowers, seeds and fruits.

    a. Systems

    b. Organs

    c. Tissues

    d. Phylum

26. Our bodies have ____ different _____, including _____, _____, and _____.

    a. Our bodies have 5 different systems, including circulatory, digestive, and lymphatic.

    b. Our bodies have 11 different systems, including circulatory, digestive, and heart.

    c. Our bodies have 11 different systems, including circulatory, digestive, and lymphatic.

    d. Our bodies have 12 different systems, including circulatory, bowel, and lymphatic.

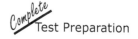

27. The _____ system absorbs excess fluid, preventing tissues from swelling, defends the body against microorganisms and harmful foreign particles, and facilitates the absorption of fat.

    a. Vascular

    b. Digestive

    c. Circulatory

    d. Lymphatic

28. The _____ system consists of _____, _____, and _____ that transport _____ to and from all tissues

    a. The vascular system consists of arteries, veins, and capillaries that transport oxygen to and from all tissues.

    b. The lymphatic system consists of arteries, veins, and capillaries that transport oxygen to and from all tissues.

    c. The vascular system consists of arteries, stratums, and capillaries that transport oxygen to and from all tissues.

    d. The vascular system consists of arteries, veins, and ducts that transport oxygen to and from all tissues.

29. What are the differences, if any, between arteries, veins, and capillaries?

    a. Veins carry oxygenated blood away from the heart, arteries return oxygen-depleted blood to the heart, and capillaries are thin-walled blood vessels in which gas/ nutrient/ waste exchange occurs.

    b. Capillaries carry oxygenated blood away from the heart, veins return oxygen-depleted blood to the heart, and capillaries are thin-walled blood vessels in which gas/ nutrient/ waste exchange occurs.

    c. There are no differences; all perform the same function in different parts of the body.

    d. Arteries carry oxygenated blood away from the heart, veins return oxygen-depleted blood to the heart, and capillaries are thin-walled blood vessels in which gas/ nutrient/ waste exchange occurs.

30. The _____ is the primary organ of the digestive tract, and may be subdivided into three segments, the _____, the _____, and the _____.

    a. The stomach is the primary organ of the digestive tract, and may be subdivided into three segments, the duodenum, the jejunum, and the ileum.

    b. The small intestine is the primary organ of the digestive tract, and may be subdivided into three segments, the duodenum, the jejunum, and the ileum.

    c. The large intestine is the primary organ of the digestive tract, and may be subdivided into three segments, the duodenum, the jejunum, and the ileum.

    d. The small intestine is the primary organ of the digestive tract, and may be subdivided into three segments, the duodenum, the jejunum, and the ilex.

31. The _____system defends our bodies against infections and disease through three types of response systems: the _____ response, the _____ response, and the _____ response.

    a. The vascular system defends our bodies against infections and disease through three types of response systems: the anatomic response, the inflammatory response, and the immune response.

    b. The immune system defends our bodies against infections and disease through three types of response systems: the anatomic response, the inflammatory response, and the immune response.

    c. The immune system defends our bodies against infections and disease through three types of response systems: the automatic response, the flammatory response, and the immune response.

    d. The epithelial system defends our bodies against infections and disease through three types of response systems: the anatomic response, the inflammatory response, and the immune response.

32. The _____ system is composed of all of the bones, cartilage, muscles, joints, tendons and ligaments in a person's body.

    a. Musculoskeletal

    b. Muscular

    c. Skeletal

    d. Connective

33. The _____ is a muscular tube lined by a special layer of cells, called _____; its primary purpose is to break food down into _____, which can be absorbed into the body to provide energy.

    a. The epithelium tract is a muscular tube lined by a special layer of cells, called gastric; its primary purpose is to break food down into nutrients, which can be absorbed into the body to provide energy.

    b. The gastrointestinal tract is a muscular tube lined by a special layer of cells, called ileum; its primary purpose is to break food down into oxygen, which can be absorbed into the body to provide energy.

    c. The gastrointestinal tract is a muscular tube lined by a special layer of cells, called epithelium; its primary purpose is to break food down into nutrients, which can be absorbed into the body to provide energy.

    d. The esophageal tract is a muscular tube lined by a special layer of cells, called epithelium; its primary purpose is to break food down into nutrients, which can be absorbed into the body to provide energy.

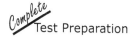

34. The _____ states that, in a chemical change, _____ can be neither _____ nor _____, but only changed from _____.

a. The Law of the Preservation of Matter states that, in a chemical change, energy can be neither created nor destroyed, but only changed from one form to another.

b. The Law of the Conservation of Energy states that, in a chemical change, energy can be neither created nor destroyed, but only changed from one atomic number to another.

c. The Law of the Conservation of Energy states that, in a chemical change, energy can be neither created nor destroyed, but only changed from one form to another.

d. The Law of the Conservation of Energy states that, in a chemical change, energy can be neither duplicated nor destroyed, but only changed from one form to another.

35. A _____ is a process that transforms one set of chemical substances to another; the substances used are known as _____ and those formed are _____.

a. A chemical change is a process that transforms one set of chemical substances to another; the substances used are known as products and those formed are reactants.

b. A biological change is a process that transforms one set of chemical substances to another; the substances used are known as reactants and those formed are products.

c. A chemical change is a process that transforms one set of chemical substances to another; the substances used are known as reactants and those formed are products.

d. A chemical variation is a process that transforms one set of chemical substances to another; the substances used are known as reactants and those formed are products.

36. _____ is the series of chemical reactions resulting in the _____ of organic compounds, and _____ is the series of chemical reactions that _____ larger molecules.

a. Anabolism is the series of chemical reactions resulting in the synthesis of inorganic compounds, and catabolism is a series of chemical reactions that break down larger molecules.

b. Anabolism is the series of chemical reactions resulting in the synthesis of organic compounds, and catabolism is a series of chemical reactions that combine larger molecules.

c. Catabolism is the series of chemical reactions resulting in the synthesis of organic compounds, and anabolism is a series of chemical reactions that break down larger molecules.

d. Anabolism is the series of chemical reactions resulting in the synthesis of organic compounds, and catabolism is a series of chemical reactions that break down larger molecules.

37. A(n) _____ is a chemical involved in, but not changed by, a chemical reaction by which chemical bonds are _____ and reactions _____.

   a. A propellant is a chemical involved in, but not changed by, a chemical reaction by which chemical bonds are weakened and reactions accelerated.

   b. A reagent is a chemical involved in, but not changed by, a chemical reaction by which chemical bonds are strengthened and reactions accelerated.

   c. A catalyst is a chemical involved in, but not changed by, a chemical reaction by which chemical bonds are weakened and reactions slowed.

   d. A catalyst is a chemical involved in, but not changed by, a chemical reaction by which chemical bonds are weakened and reactions accelerated.

38. _____ is the most abundant element in the Earth's crust and appears on the Atomic Table as the letter ____.

   a. Nitrogen, N

   b. Oxygen, O

   c. Silicon, Si

   d. Sodium, Na

39. _____ states that when two elements combine with each other to form more than one compound, the weights of one element that combine with a fixed weight of the other are in a ratio of small whole numbers.

   a. The Law of Multiple Proportions

   b. The Law of Definite Proportions

   c. The Law of the Conservation of Energy

   d. The Law of Averages

40. _____ stats that every chemical compound contains fixed and constant proportions (by weight) of its constituent elements.

   a. The Law of Multiple Proportions

   b. The Law of the Preservation of Matter

   c. The Law of the Conservation of Energy

   d. The Law of Definite Proportions

Complete Test Preparation

41. _____ states that, in a given _____, _____ can have the _____.

a. The Law of Definite Proportions states that, in a given atom, no two electrons can have the same set of four quantum numbers.

b. The Pauli Exclusion Principle states that, in a given atom, no four electrons can have the same set of two quantum numbers.

c. The Pauli Exclusion Principle states that, in a given molecule, no two electrons can have a different set of four quantum numbers.

d. The Pauli Exclusion Principle states that, in a given atom, no two electrons can have the same set of four quantum numbers.

42. According to the tenets of Dalton's atomic theory, which of the following is true:

a. All matter is made up of tiny, interconnected particles called atoms.

b. All atoms of an element are alike in weight, and this weight is specific to the kind of atom.

c. Atoms can be subdivided, created, or destroyed.

d. In chemical reactions, atoms are not combined, separated, or rearranged.

43. Atoms of _____ _____ combine in _____ _____ ratios to form chemical _____.

a. Atoms of different elements combine in simple whole-number ratios to form chemical compounds.

b. Atoms of different components combine in simple fractional ratios to form chemical compounds.

c. Atoms of the same element combine in simple whole-number ratios to form chemical compounds.

d. Atoms of different elements combine in simple whole-number ratios to form chemical mixtures.

44. Which of the following statements about the periodic table of the elements are true?

a. On the periodic table, the elements are arranged according to their atomic mass.

b. The way in which the elements are arranged allows for predictions about their behavior.

c. The vertical columns of the table are called rows.

d. The horizontal rows of the table are called groups.

45. _____ _____ is the minimum amount of energy required to remove an electron from an atom or ion in the gas phase.

    a. Ionization energy

    b. Valence energy

    c. Atomic energy

    d. Ionic energy

46. A(an) _____ _____ is one half the distance between nuclei of atoms of the same element, when the atoms are bound by a single covalent bond or are in a metallic crystal.

    a. Ionic radius

    b. Metallic radius

    c. Covalent radius

    d. Atomic radius

47. What are the differences, if any, between anions and cations?

    a. An anion is a negatively charged ion, and a cation is a positively charged ion.

    b. Anions are typically formed by nonmetals, and metals usually form cations.

    c. A & B

    d. None of the Above

48. The radius of atoms obtained from _____ bond lengths is called the _____ radius; the radius from interatomic distances in metallic crystals is called the _____ radius.

    a. The radius of atoms obtained from valent bond lengths is called the valent radius; the radius from interatomic distances in metallic crystals is called the metallic radius.

    b. The radius of atoms obtained from covalent bond lengths is called the covalent radius; the radius from interatomic distances in nonmetallic crystals is called the nonmetallic radius.

    c. The radius of atoms obtained from covalent bond lengths is called the covalent radius; the radius from interatomic distances in metallic crystals is called the metallic radius.

    d. The radius of atoms obtained from covalent bond lengths is called the covalent radius; the radius from interatomic distances in ionic crystals is called the ionic radius.

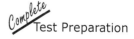

49. A(an) _____ _____ is a regular variation in element properties with _____ atomic number that is ultimately due to _____ variations in atomic structure.

   a. A episodic trend is a regular variation in element properties with increasing atomic number that is ultimately due to regular variations in atomic structure.

   b. A periodic trend is a regular variation in element properties with decreasing atomic number that is ultimately due to regular variations in atomic structure.

   c. A periodic trend is a regular variation in element properties with increasing atomic number that is ultimately due to irregular variations in atomic structure.

   d. A periodic trend is a regular variation in element properties with increasing atomic number that is ultimately due to regular variations in atomic structure.

50. Which of the following statements about nonmetals are false?

   a. A nonmetal is a substance that conducts heat and electricity poorly

   b. The majority of the known chemical elements are nonmetals

   c. A nonmetal is brittle or waxy or gaseous

   d. All of the above are true

Anatomy and Physiology

1. Fluid balance might be negatively impacted when the_____ fail.

   a. Kidneys

   b. Ears

   c. Nose

   d. Legs

2. Fluid balance is important, because _____ comprises about 60-70% of a person's weight.

   a. Calcium

   b. Water

   c. Iron

   d. Bone

3. As a person moves from adolescence to later adulthood, his metabolism

   a. Begins to get higher

   b. Begins to get lower

   c. Stabilizes

   d. Fluctuates wildly

4. "Met" refers to

    a. Mitosis

    b. The person's heart rate

    c. The person's blood pressure

    d. The person's metabolic rate

5. Fluid balance is important, because the human body loses water every day through urination, perspiration, feces, and

    a. Breathing

    b. Resting

    c. Meditating

    d. Outbursts of temper

6. The smallest unit of life in our bodies is the

    a. Atom

    b. Molecule

    c. Proton

    d. Cell

7. One of the functions of the cell membrane is to

    a. Divide into other cells

    b. Control what moves into and out of the cell

    c. Fight infection

    d. Trap bacteria

8. The process of a larger cell dividing into two or more smaller cells is

    a. Cell division

    b. Cell multiplication

    c. Mitosis

    d. Metabolism

9. Prophase, metaphase, anaphase, and telophase are all phases of

    a. Cell division

    b. Infection

    c. Mitosis

    d. Adrenaline

10. Mitosis is a scientific term that, in layman's terms, just means

    a. Cellular disease.

    b. Nuclear cell division (division of the cell nucleus).

    c. Infection.

    d. Atomic fusion.

11. The stage of mitosis in which the chromatin condenses and becomes a chromosome is

    a. Prophase

    b. Metaphase

    c. Anaphase

    d. Telophase

12. The stage of mitosis in which the chromosomes begin to align is _____.

    a. Prophase

    b. Metaphase

    c. Anaphase

    d. Telophase

13. The stage of mitosis in which the paired chromosomes separate, each going to an opposite pole of the cell, is _____.

    a. Metaphase

    b. Prophase

    c. Anaphase

    d. None of the Above

14. The stage of mitosis in which the two chromosomes are cordoned into new nuclei within the daughter cells is _____.

    a. Metaphase

    b. Prophase

    c. Anaphase

    d. Telophase

 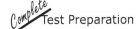

15. Squamous, cuboidal and columnar are three kinds of what kind of cell tissue?
_____

    a. Epidermis

    b. Epithelial tissue

    c. Nerve tissue

    d. Muscle tissue

16. An important function of epithelial tissue is _____.

    a. Strengthen the muscles.

    b. Acting as a protective barrier for the human body.

    c. Protect the nerves.

    d. nonexistent; it has been found to have no known function.

17. An important function of connective tissue is _____.

    a. Acting as a protective barrier for the human body.

    b. Protect the muscles.

    c. Storage of energy.

    d. Strengthen the nerves.

18. Muscle tissue has the ability to _____**, bringing out movement and the ability to work.**

    a. Divide and conquer.

    b. Replicate at will.

    c. Relax and contract.

    d. Sleep.

19. Nervous tissue is specialized to

    a. Do work.

    b. Protect the body.

    c. Teach the person to relax.

    d. React to stimuli.

20. Cells known as _____ make up nerve tissue.

    a. Neurons.

    b. Protons

    c. Molecules

    d. Atoms

21. The _____ system protects the person's body from damage.

    a. Circulatory

    b. Musculoskeletal

    c. Integumentary

    d. Digestive

22. The integumentary system comprises the _____ and its various appendages.

    a. Skeleton

    b. Brain

    c. Skin

    d. Heart

23. An example of appendages contained within the integumentary system are _____.

    a. Lungs

    b. Hair and nails

    c. Nostrils

    d. Ears

24. In addition to protecting the body, an example of a benefit of the integumentary system is its function of _____.

    a. Circulating blood.

    b. Digesting food.

    c. Processing information.

    d. Regulating temperature.

25. How many layers of skin are contained within the human integumentary system (skin)?

    a. One

    b. Two

    c. Three

    d. Four

Practice Test 1 - Answer Key

Section 1 – Reading Comprehension

1. B
We can infer from this passage that sickness from an infectious disease can be easily transmitted from one person to another.

From the passage, "Infectious pathologies are also called communicable diseases or transmissible diseases, due to their potential of transmission from one person or species to another by a replicating agent (as opposed to a toxin)."

2. A
Two other names for infectious pathologies are communicable diseases and transmissible diseases.

From the passage, "Infectious pathologies are also called communicable diseases or transmissible diseases, due to their potential of transmission from one person or species to another by a replicating agent (as opposed to a toxin)."

3. C
Infectivity describes the ability of an organism to enter, survive and multiply in the host. This is taken directly from the passage, and is a definition type question.

Definition type questions can be answered quickly and easily by scanning the passage for the word you are asked to define.

"Infectivity" is an unusual word, so it is quick and easy to scan the passage looking for this word.

4. B
We know an infection is not synonymous with an infectious disease because an infection may not cause important clinical symptoms or impair host function.

5. C
We can infer from the passage that, a virus is too small to be seen with the naked eye. Clearly, if they are too small to be seen with a microscope, then they are too small to be seen with the naked eye.

6. D
Viruses infect all types of organisms. This is taken directly from the passage, "Viruses infect all types of organisms, from animals and plants to bacteria and single-celled organisms."

7. C
The passage does not say exactly how many parts prions and viroids consist of. It does say, "Unlike prions and viroids, viruses consist of two or three parts ..." so we can infer they consist of either less than two or more than three parts.

8. B
A common virus spread by coughing and sneezing is Influenza.

9. C

The cumulus stage of a thunderstorm is the beginning of the thunderstorm.

This is taken directly from the passage, "The first stage of a thunderstorm is the cumulus, or developing stage."

10. D

The passage lists four ways that air is heated. One of the ways is, heat created by water vapor condensing into liquid.

11. A

The sequence of events can be taken from these sentences:

As the moisture carried by the [1] air currents rises, it rapidly cools into liquid drops of water, which appear as cumulus clouds. As the water vapor condenses into liquid, it [2] releases heat, which warms the air. This in turn causes the air to become less dense than the surrounding dry air and [3] rise further.

12. C

The purpose of this text is to explain when meteorologists consider a thunderstorm severe.

The main idea is the first sentence, "The United States National Weather Service classifies thunderstorms as severe when they reach a predetermined level." After the first sentence, the passage explains and elaborates on this idea. Everything is this passage is related to this idea, and there are no other major ideas in this passage that are central to the whole passage.

13. A

From this passage, we can infer that different areas and countries have different criteria for determining a severe storm.

From the passage we can see that most of the US has a criteria of, winds over 50 knots (58 mph or 93 km/h), and hail ¾ inch (2 cm). For the Central US, hail must be 1 inch (2.5 cm) in diameter. In Canada, winds must be 90 km/h or greater, hail 2 centimeters in diameter or greater, and rainfall more than 50 millimeters in 1 hour, or 75 millimeters in 3 hours.

Option D is incorrect because the Canadian system is the same for hail, 2 centimeters in diameter.

14. C

With hail above the minimum size of 2.5 cm. diameter, the Central Region of the United States National Weather Service would issue a severe thunderstorm warning.

15. D

Clouds in space are made of different materials attracted by gravity. Clouds on Earth are made of water droplets or ice crystals.

Choice D is the best answer. Notice also that Choice D is the most specific.

16. C

The main idea is the first sentence of the passage; a cloud is a visible mass of droplets or frozen crystals floating in the atmosphere above the surface of the Earth or other planetary body.

The main idea is very often the first sentence of the paragraph.

17. C

Nephology, which is the study of cloud physics.

18. C

This question asks about the process, and gives options that can be confirmed or eliminated easily.

From the passage, "Dense, deep clouds reflect most light, so they appear white, at least from the top. Cloud droplets scatter light very efficiently, so the further into a cloud light travels, the weaker it gets. This accounts for the gray or dark appearance at the base of large clouds."

We can eliminate choice A, since water droplets inside the cloud do not reflect light is false.

We can eliminate choice B, since, water droplets outside the cloud reflect light, it appears dark, is false.

Choice C is correct.

19. A

The correct order of ingredients is brown sugar, baking soda and chocolate chips.

20. B

Sturdy: strong, solid in structure or person. In context, Stir in chocolate chips by hand with a *sturdy* wooden spoon.

21. A

Disperse: to scatter in different directions or break up. In context, Stir until the chocolate chips and nuts are evenly *dispersed.*

22. B

You can stop stirring the nuts when they are evenly distributed. From the passage, "Stir until the chocolate chips and nuts are evenly dispersed."

23. A

Larvae spend most of their time in search of food and their food is leaves.

24. B

From the passage, the ants provide some degree of protection

25. C

The association is mutual so both benefit.

26. A

Navy SEALS are the maritime component of the United States Special Operations Command (USSOCOM).

27. C

Working underwater separates SEALs from other military units. This is taken directly from the passage.

28. D

SEALs also belong to the Navy and the Coast Guard.

29. A

The CIA also participated. From the passage, the raid was conducted by a "team of 40 *CIA-led* Navy SEALS."

30. C

From the passage, "The Navy SEALs were part of the Naval Special Warfare Development Group, previously called "Team 6". "

31. B

This question is taken directly from the passage.

32. A

The Egyptians believed gods loved gardens.

33. B

Cypresses and palms were the most popular trees in Assyrian Gardens.

34. B

Vegetable gardens came before ornamental gardens.

The earliest forms of gardens emerged from the people's need to grow herbs and vegetables. It was only later that rich individuals created gardens for the purely decorative purpose.

35. A

The ancient Roman gardens are known by their statues and sculptures ...

36. D

After the fall of Rome, gardening was only for medicinal purposes, AND gardening declined in the Middle Ages, so we can infer gardening declined after the fall of Rome.

37. C

From the passage, "After the fall of Rome gardening was only done with the purpose of growing medicinal herbs and decorating church altars," so Choice C.

38. B

From the passage, "Mosaics and glazed tiles used to decorate elaborate fountains are specific to Islamic gardens."

 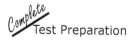

39. B

From the passage, "Often called "rainforests of the sea", coral reefs form some of the most diverse ecosystems on Earth."

40. A

Read the passage carefully – "The polyps are like tiny sea anemones, to which they are closely related."

41. C

This question is designed to confuse by giving variation of the same information. Read the passage carefully for the correct answer.

42. D

This question is designed to confuse by giving variation of the same information. Read the passage carefully for the correct answer.

43. B

Designed to confuse by offering variations of the same information. Read the passage carefully for the correct time sequence.

44. A

From the passage, "As communities established themselves on the shelves, the reefs grew upwards, pacing the rising sea levels. Reefs that rose too slowly became drowned reefs, covered by so much water that there was insufficient light." Here, "pacing" is the key word, so Choice A, "at the same rate... "

From this we can infer that coral reefs grew at the same rate (pacing) as the rising water level.

45. A

Reefs that grew too slowly died from a lack of light. From the passage, "Reefs that rose too slowly became drowned reefs, covered by so much water there was insufficient light."

Section II – Math Answer Key

1. A
1/3 X 3/4 = 3/12 = 1/4

2. D
75/1500 = 15/300 = 3/60 = 1/20

3. D
3.14 + 2.73 = 5.87 and 5.87 + 23.7 = 29.57

4. B
Spent 15% - 100% - 15% = 85%

5. C
To convert a decimal to a fraction, take the places of decimal as your denominator, in this case 2, so in 0.27, '7' is in the 100th place, so the fraction is 27/100 and 0.33 becomes 33/100.

Next estimate the answer quickly to eliminate obvious wrong choices. 27/100 is about 1/4 and 33/100 is 1/3. 1/3 is slightly larger than 1/4, and 1/4 + 1/4 is 1/2, so the answer will be slightly larger than 1/2.

Looking at the choices, Choice A can be eliminated since 3/6 = 1/2. Choice D, 2/7 is less than 1/2 and can also be eliminated. so the answer is going to be Choice B or Choice C.

Do the calculation, 0.27 + 0.33 = 0.60 and 0.60 = 60/100 = 3/5, Choice C is correct.

6. D
3.13 + 7.87 = 11 and 11 X 5 = 55

7. B
2/4 X 3/4 = 6/16, and lowest terms = 3/8

8. D
2/3-2/5 = 10-6 /15 = 4/15

9. C
2/7 + 2/3 = 6+14 /21 (21 is the common denominator) = 20/21

10. B
2/3 x 60 = 40 and 1.5 x 75 = 15, 40 + 15 = 55

11. C
This is an easy question, and shows how you can solve some questions without doing the calculations. The question is, 8 is what percent of 40. Take easy percentages for an approximate answer and see what you get.

10% is easy to calculate because you can drop the zero, or move the decimal point. 10% of 40 = 4, and 8 = 2 X 4, so, 8 must be 2 X 10% = 20%.

Here are the calculations which confirm the quick approximation.
8/40 = X/100 = 8 * 100 / 40X = 800/40 = X = 20

12. D
This is the same type of question which illustrates another method to quickly solve without doing the calculations. The question is, 9 is what percent of 36?

Ask, what is the relationship between 9 and 36? 9 X 4 = 36 so they are related by a fac-

 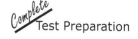

tor of 4. If 9 is related to 36 by a factor of 4, then what is related to 100 (to get a percent) by a factor of 4?

To visualize:

9 X 4 = 36
Z X 4 = 100

So the answer is 25. 9 has the same relation to 36 as 25 has to 100.

Here are the calculations which confirm the quick approximation.
9/36 = X/100 = 9 * 100 / 36X = 900/36 = 25

13. C
3/10 * 90 = 3 * 90/10 = 27

14. B
4/100 * 36 = .4 * 36/100 = .144

15. A
5 mg/10/mg X 1 tab/1 = .5 tablets

16. B
Step 1: Set up the formula to calculate the dose to be given in mg as per weight of the child:-
Dose ordered X Weight in Kg = Dose to be given
Step 2: 20 mg X 12 kg = 240 mg
240 mg/80 mg X 1 tab/1 = 240/80 = 3 tablets

17. A
Set up the formula to calculate the dose to be given in mg as per weight of the child:-
Dose ordered X Weight in Kg = Dose to be given
Step 2: 20 mg X 20 kg = 400 mg (Convert 44 lb to Kg, 1 lb = 0.4536 kg, hence 44 lb = 19.95 kg approx. 20 kg)
400 mg/80 mg X 1 tab/1 = 400/80 = 5 tablets

18. B
3000 units/5000 units X 1 ml/1 = 3000/5000 = 0.6 ml

19. C
60 mg/80 mg X 1 ml/1 = 60/80 = 0.75 ml

20. A
Dose ordered X Weight in Kg = Dose to be given
16 mg X 15 kg = 240 mg
240 mg/80 mg X 1 tab/1 = 240/80 = 3 tablets

21. C
(Convert 1 g = 1000 mg)

1000 mg/1000 mg X 1 tsp/1 = 1000/1000 = 1 tsp

22. D
10 units/200 units X 1 ml/1 = 10/200 = 0.05 ml

23. B
$(4)(3)^3 = (4)(27) = 108$

24. A
1000g = 1kg., 0.007 = 1000 x 0.007 = 7g.

25. C
4 quarts = 1 gallon, 16 quarts = 16/4 = 4 gallons

26. C
1 teaspoon = 4.93 milliliters (U.S.), 2 tp = 4.93 x 2 = 9.86 ml.

27. D
1,000 meters = 1 kilometer, 200 m = 200/1,000 = 0.2 km.

28. B
12 inches = 1 ft., 72 inches = 72/12 = 6 feet

29. C
1 yard = 3 feet, 3 yards = 3 feet x 3 = 9 feet

30. B
0.45 kg = 1 pound, 1 kg. = 1/0.45 and 45 kg = 1/0.45 x 45 = 45 = 99.208, or 100 pounds

31. C
1 g = 1,000 mg. 0.63 g = 0.63 x 1,000 = 630 mg.

32. D
To solve for x,
5x – 7x + 3 = -1
5x – 7x = -1 -3
-2x = -4
x = -4/ -2
x = 2

33. C
To solve for x, first simplify the equation
5x + 2x + 14 = 14x – 7
7x + 14 = 4x -7
7x – 14x + 14 = -7
7x – 14x = -7 – 14
-7x = -21
x = -21/-7

x=3
34. A
5z + 5 = 3z +6 + 11
5z -3z + 5 =6 + 11
5z – 3z = 6 + 11 -5
2z = 17 – 5
2z = 12
z= 12/2
z= 6

35. C
5z + 5 = 3z +6 + 11
5z -3z + 5 =6 + 11
5z – 3z = 6 + 11 -5
2z = 17 – 5
2z = 12
z= 12/2
z= 6

36. D
Price increased by \$5 (\$25-\$20). The percent increase is
5/20 x 100 = 5 x 5=25%

37. C
Price decreased by \$5 (\$25-\$20). The percent increase = 5/25 x 100 = 5 x 4 =20%

38. D
30/100 x 150 = 3 x 15 = 45 (increase in number of correct answers). So the number of correct answers in second test = 150 + 45 = 195

39. B
Let total number of players= X
Let the number of players with long hair=Y and the number of players with short hair=Z
Then X = 4+Z
Y= 12% of X
Z= X - 4
12.5% of X = 4
Converting from decimal to fraction gives 12.5%=125/10 x 1/100=125/1000, therefore 12.5% of =125/1000X=4
Solve for X by multiplying both sides by 1000/125, X=4 x 1000/125=32
Z = x – 4
Z = 32 – 4
z or number of short haired players = 28

40. D
2 glasses are broken for 43 customers so 1 glass breaks for every 43/2 customers served, therefore 10 glasses implies 43/2 x 10=215

41. D

 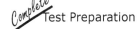

As the lawn is square, the length of one side will be = $\sqrt{62500}$ = 250 meters. Therefore, the perimeters will be: 250 × 4 = 1000 meters
The total cost will be 1000 × 5.5 = $5500

42. D

The price of all the single items is same and there are 13 total items. So the total cost will be 13 × 1.3 = $16.9. After 3.5 percent tax this amount will become 16.9 × 1.035 = $17.5.

43. C

Area of the square = 12 × 12 = 144 cm²
Let x be the width, then 2x be the length of rectangle, so its area will be $2x^2$ and perimeter will be 2(2x+x)=6x
According to the condition
$2x^2$ = 144
X = 8.48 cm
The perimeter will be
Perimeter=6×8.48
=50.88
=51 cm.

44. B

There are 50 balls in the basket now. Let x be the number of yellow balls to be added to make 65%. So the equation becomes

X + 15 /X + 50 = 65/100
X = 50

45. D

Let x be number of rows, and number of trees in a row. So equation becomes
X^2 = 65536
X = 256

46. B

First calculate the number of stores to distribute 5 kg portions: 550 - (20 x 15) - (10 x 12) = 130. Then 130/5 = 26 shops. His distribution is then: 15 x 6.4 = $96, 12 x 3.4 = $40.8, 26 x 1.8 × 26 = $46.8, Total = $183.6. Then subtract the distribution costs: Total number of stores = 15 + 12 + 26 = 53, 53 x 3 = $159 distribution costs. Then calculate profit: $183.6 - 159 = $24.60

47. D

Each tree will require a 10-meter diametric space around its stem. So 65 trees can be planted along 650-meter side. Similarly, 65 along the other side. However, along the 780 meter side, the first tree will be after 10 meters at both edges, so 76 trees can be planted long that side.

Total number of trees then will be 65×2+76×2=282

48. A

 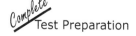

As one tree requires 10-meter diametric space, or, a 10-meter space on all four sides will be left. Therefore, the dimensions left are 630×760=478,800 m².

49. B
X/2 – 250 = 3X/7
X = $3500

50. A
The probability that the 1ˢᵗ ball drawn is red = 4/11
The probability that the 2ⁿᵈ ball drawn is green = 5/10
The combined probability will then be 4/11 X 5/10 = 20/110 = 2/11

Section III English Answer Key

1. A
The third conditional is used for talking about an unreal situation (a situation that did not happen) in the past. For example, "If I had studied harder, [if clause] I would have passed the exam" [main clause]. This has the same meaning as, "I failed the exam, because I didn't study hard enough."

2. D
The third conditional is used for talking about an unreal situation (a situation that did not happen) in the past. For example, "If I had studied harder, [if clause] I would have passed the exam" [main clause]. This has the same meaning as, "I failed the exam, because I didn't study hard enough."

3. B
In double negative sentences, one of the negatives is replaced with "any."

4. C
In double negative sentences, one of the negatives is replaced with "any."

5. D
The present perfect tense cannot be used with specific time expressions such as yesterday, one year ago, last week, when I was a child, at that moment, that day, one day, etc. The present perfect tense is used with unspecific expressions such as ever, never, once, many times, several times, before, so far, already, yet, etc.

6. C
The present perfect tense cannot be used with specific time expressions such as yesterday, one year ago, last week, when I was a child, at that moment, that day, one day, etc. The present perfect tense is used with unspecific expressions such as ever, never, once, many times, several times, before, so far, already, yet, etc.

7. A
"Went" is used in the simple past tense. "Gone" is used in the past perfect tense.

 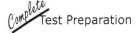

8. B

"Went" is used in the simple past tense. "Gone" is used in the past perfect tense.

9. D

"It's" is a contraction for it is or it has. "Its" is a possessive pronoun.

10. C

"It's" is a contraction for it is or it has. "Its" is a possessive pronoun.

11. B

The sentence refers to a person, so "who" is the only correct option.

12. A

The sentence requires the past perfect "has always been known." Furthermore, this is the only grammatically correct choice.

13. C

The superlative, "hottest," is used when expressing a temperature greater than that of anything to which it is being compared.

14. D

When comparing two items, use "the taller." When comparing more than two items, use "the tallest."

15. B

The past perfect form is used to describe an event that occurred in the past and prior to another event. Here there are two things that happened, both of them in the past, and something the person wanted to do.

Event 1: Kiss came to town
Event 2: All the tickets sold out
What I wanted to do: Buy a ticket

The events are arranged:

When KISS came to town, all of the tickets had been sold out before I could buy one.

16. A

The subject is "rules" so the present tense plural form, "are," is used to agree with "realize."

17. C

The simple past tense, "had," is correct because it refers to completed action in the past.

18. D

The simple past tense, "sank," is correct because it refers to completed action in the past.

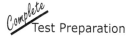

19. A

"Who" is correct because the question uses an active construction. "To whom was first place given?" is passive construction.

20. D

"Which" is correct, because the files are objects and not people.

21. C

The simple present tense, "rises," is correct.

22. A

"Lie" does not require a direct object, while "lay" does. The old woman might lie on the couch, which has no direct object, or she might lay the book down, which has the direct object, "the book."

23. D

The simple present tense, "falls," is correct because it is repeated action.

24. A

The present progressive, "building models," is correct in this sentence; it is required to match the other present progressive verbs.

25. A

"Affect" is a verb, while "effect" is a noun.

26. D

"Than" is used for comparison. "Then" is used to indicate a point in time.

27. C

"There" indicates a state of existence. "Their" is used for third person plural possession. "They're" is the contracted form of "they are."

28. A

"There" indicates a state of existence. "Their" is used for third person plural possession. "They're" is the contraction of "they are."

29. C

"Your" is the possessive form of "you." "You're" is the contraction of "you are."

30. C

"Your" is the possessive form of "you." "You're" is the contraction of "you are."

31. A

Disease is a singular noun.

32. C

Both "dog" and "cat" in this sentence are singular nouns and require the article "a."

33. A

The word "principal" is a synonym for primary or major. "Principle" means a fundamental truth.

34. D

The article "a" come before a noun that begins with a consonant, while "an" comes before a noun that begins with a vowel.

35. A

"Except" means to exclude something. "Accept" means to receive something, or to agree to an idea.

36. A

"Advise" is a verb that means to offer advice, which is a noun.

37. C

"Adapt" means to change or accommodate. "Adopt" means to accept, embrace, or to assume responsibility or ownership for something or someone.

38. D

"Among" is used with more than two items, while "between" is limited to two items.

39. D

"At" refers to a specific time or location, while "about" is approximate.

40. B

"Beside" means next to, and "besides" means in addition to.

41. A

"Can" is used when describing ability or capability. "May" is a request or the granting of permission.

42. B

"Continuous" means a time period without interruption, or ongoing. "Continual" is used for actions that are frequent and repetitive, or that continue almost without interruption.

43. A

"Emigrate" means to leave one's country, usually in order to immigrate to another country to live.

44. A

"Farther" is reserved for physical distance, and "further" is used for figurative distance, or to mean "in addition."

45. B

"Former" refers to the first of two things; "latter" to the second of two things.

 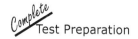

46. D
"Healthy" describes people or animals that are in good health. "Healthful" is generally used in formal speech or writing, and refers to things that are good for health.

47. C
"Lie" does not require a direct object, while "lay" does. In this sentence, "lay" is followed by the direct object, "the books."

48. C
"Lie" does not require a direct object, while "lay" does. In this sentence, "lay" is followed by the direct object, "the books."

49. C
This is the correct choice.

50. B
"Learn" means to receive and integrate knowledge or an experience. "Teach" means to impart knowledge to another.

Section III Part II – Vocabulary

1. C
Edify VERB to instruct or improve morally or intellectually.

2. B
Egress NOUN an exit or way out.

3. A
Confidential ADJECTIVE kept secret within a certain circle of persons; not intended to be known publicly.

4. C
Felony NOUN serious criminal offence that is punishable by death or imprisonment above a year.

5. B
Foment VERB to encourage or incite troublesome acts.

6. A
Funereal ADJECTIVE dignified, solemn that is appropriate for a funeral.

7. B
Geniality NOUN warmth and kindness of disposition.

8. C
Genteel ADJECTIVE polite and well mannered.

 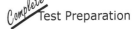

9. D
Goad VERB to encourage, stimulate or incite and provoke.

10. B
Heinous ADJECTIVE shocking, terrible or wicked.

11. A
Harbinger NOUN a person of thing that tells or announces the coming of someone or something.

12. D
Homologous ADJECTIVE similar or identical.

13. B
Ignoble ADJECTIVE common, not honorable or noble.

14. A
Immaterial ADJECTIVE irrelevant not having substance or matter.

15. A
Impeccable ADJECTIVE perfect, no faults or errors.

16. D
Juxtapose VERB place side by side for contrast or comparison.

17. D
Junta NOUN ruling council of a military government.

18. C
Laggard NOUN someone who takes more time than necessary.

19. B
Languid ADJECTIVE lacking enthusiasm, strength or energy.

20. D
Magnate NOUN a person of influence, rank or distinction.

21. C
Malady NOUN a lingering disease or ailment of the human body.

22. B
Nimble ADJECTIVE quick and light in movement.

23. B
Racket NOUN a loud noise.

24. C
Nuptial NOUN of or pertaining to wedding and marriage.

25. A
Ostensible ADJECTIVE meant for open display; apparent.

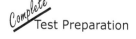

26. C
Octavo NOUN a sheet of paper 7 to 10 inches high and 4.5 to 6 inches wide, the size varying with the large original sheet used to create it. Made by folding the original sheet three times to produce eight leaves.

27. A
Pallid ADJECTIVE appearing weak, pale, or wan.

28. C
Panorama NOUN a picture or series of pictures representing a continuous scene.

29. B
Paradox NOUN a self contradictory statement that can only be true if false and vice versa.

30. A
Querulous ADJECTIVE often complaining; suggesting a complaint in expression; fretful, whining.

31. D
Mollify VERB to ease a burden; make less painful; to comfort; soothe.

32. C
Redundant ADJECTIVE repetitive or needlessly wordy.

33. C
Bicker VERB to quarrel in a tiresome, insulting manner.

34. C
Sombre ADJECTIVE dark; gloomy.

35. A
Maverick NOUN showing independence in thoughts or actions.

36. D
Tenuous ADJECTIVE thin in substance or consistency.

37. A
Pandemonium NOUN chaos; tumultuous or lawless violence.

38. A
Perpetual ADJECTIVE continuing uninterrupted.

39. B
Denigrate VERB to treat as worthless; belittle, degrade or disparage.

40. D
Mundane ADJECTIVE ordinary; not new.

 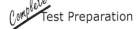

41. B
Importune VERB to harass with persistent requests.

42. D
Volatile ADJECTIVE explosive.

43. B
Plaintive ADJECTIVE sorrowful, mournful or melancholic.

44. A
Nexus NOUN a form of connection.

45. D
Conjoin VERB to join together; to unite; to combine.

46. B
Petrify VERB to harden organic matter by permeating with water and depositing dissolved minerals.

47. B
Inherent ADJECTIVE naturally a part or consequence of something.

48. C
Torpid ADJECTIVE lazy, lethargic or apathetic.

49. A
Gregarious ADJECTIVE Describing one who enjoys being in crowds and socializing.

50. C
Alloy VERB to mix or combine; often used of metals.[17]

Section IV – Science Answer Key

1. C
Electric potential is a fundamental interaction between the magnetic field and the presence and motion of an electric charge. Electric potential is the capacity of an electric field to do work on an electric charge, typically measured in volts, while electromagnetism is a fundamental interaction between the magnetic field and the presence and motion of an electric charge

2. D
An ohm (Ω) is a unit of electrical voltage is not true.
Note: An ohm is a unit of electrical resistance.

3. D
The property of a conductor that restricts its internal flow of electrons is **resistance**.

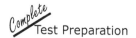

4. C
In physics, friction is the force that opposes the relative motion of two bodies in contact.

5. B
Kinetic energy is the energy of a body that results from motion while potential energy is the energy possessed by an object by virtue of its position or state, e.g., as in a compressed spring.

6. A
The four fundamental forces of nature are gravity, electromagnetic force, weak nuclear force, and strong nuclear force.
Note: Electromagnetic force is more commonly known as electricity.

7. A
Starting with the weakest, the fundamental forces of nature in order of strength are, Gravity, Weak nuclear force, Electromagnetic force, Strong nuclear force.
Note: Although gravitational force is the weakest of the four, it acts over great distances. Electromagnetic force is of order 1039 times stronger than gravity.[18]

8. A
The Strong Nuclear Force is an attractive force that binds protons and neutrons and maintains the structure of the nucleus, and the Weak Nuclear Force is responsible for the radioactive beta decay and other subatomic reactions.
Note: The Weak Nuclear Force is so named because it is only effective for short distances. Nevertheless, it is through the Weak Nuclear Force that the sun provides us with energy by allowing one element to change into another element.[18]

9. B
No detectable gain or loss occurs in chemical reactions.
Note: No detectable gain or loss in mass occurs in chemical reactions. However, the state of a substance may change in a chemical reaction. For example, substances involving in a chemical reaction can change from solid states to gaseous states but the total mass will not change.[5]

10. C
Convection is the transfer of heat from one place to another by the movement of fluids; thermal radiation is electromagnetic radiation emitted from all matter due to its possessing thermal energy.

Note: In physics, the term "fluid" means any substance that deforms under shear stress; it includes liquids, gases, plasmas, and some plastic solids. Sunlight is solar electromagnetic radiation generated by the hot plasma of the Sun, and this thermal radiation heats the Earth.[19]

11. D
In **Eukaryotic** cells, the cell cycle is the cycle of events involving cell division, including **mitosis, cytokinesis,** and **interphase**.

 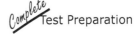

12. D
All of these statements are true.

13. C
DNA is a nucleic acid that carries the genetic information in the cell and is capable of self-replication.

14. A
The complementary bases found in DNA are **adenine** and **thymine** or **cytosine** and **guanine**.

15. B
A **nucleotide** is the basic structural unit of nucleic acids (DNA or RNA); their sequence determines individual hereditary characteristics.

16. B
Ribonucleic acid (RNA) is a **chain of nucleotides** that plays an important role in the creation of new **proteins**.

17. C
Mutations in DNA sequences usually occur spontaneously is false.

Note: Mutations result when the DNA polymerase makes a mistake, which happens about once every 100,000,000 bases. Actually, the number of mistakes that remain incorporated into the DNA is even lower than this because cells contain special DNA repair proteins that fix many of the mistakes in the DNA that are caused by mutagens. The repair proteins see which nucleotides are paired incorrectly, and then change the wrong base to the right one.[20]

18. A
Aerobic reactions occur in every cell and use **oxygen** to convert glucose to energy; **anaerobic** organisms such as many bacteria can release energy without the use of **oxygen**.

Note: The anaerobic process occurs in the cytoplasm and is only moderately efficient. The aerobic cycle takes place in the mitochondria and results in the greatest release of energy.[21]

19. D
Tissues are a collection of similar cells that group together to perform a specialized function.

20. A
Epithelial tissue serves as membranes lining organs and helping to keep the body's organs separate, in place and protected; an example is the outer layer of the skin.

21. D
Tissue that adds support and structure to the body and frequently contains fibrous strands of collagen is **connective** tissue.

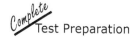

Note: Some examples of connective tissue include the inner layers of skin, tendons, ligaments, cartilage, bone and fat tissue. In addition to these more recognizable forms of connective tissue, blood is also considered a form of connective tissue.[22]

22. B
Muscle tissue is a specialized tissue that can contract and contains the specialized proteins actin and myosin that slide past one another and allow movement.

23. A
N**erve** tissue contains two types of cells: neurons and glial cells and has the ability to generate and conduct electrical signals in the body.

24. D
An organ is a group of tissues that perform a specific function or group of functions.

25. B
Among animals, examples of **organs** are the heart, lungs, brain, eye, stomach, and bones; plant **organs** include the roots, stems, leaves, flowers, seeds and fruits.

26. C
Our bodies have **11** different **systems**, including **circulatory, digestive**, and **lymphatic**.
Note: Other systems include the endocrine, immune, muscular, nervous, reproductive, respiratory, skeletal, and urinary systems.[23]

27. D
The Lymphatic system absorbs excess fluid, preventing tissues from swelling, defends the   body against microorganisms and harmful foreign particles, and facilitates the absorption of fat.

28. A
The **vascular** system consists of **arteries, veins**, and **capillaries** that transport oxygen to and from all tissues.

Note: The cardiovascular system refers to the heart (cardio) and blood vessels (vascular). The circulatory system is a more general term encompassing the blood, blood vessels, heart, lymph, and lymph vessels.[23]

29. D
Arteries carry oxygenated blood away from the heart, veins return oxygen-depleted blood to the heart, and capillaries are thin-walled blood vessels in which gas/ nutrient/ waste exchange occurs.

Note: An easy way to remember the difference between an artery and a vein is that Arteries carry Away from the heart.

30. B
The small **intestine** is the primary organ of the digestive tract, and may be subdivided into three segments, the **duodenum**, the **jejunum**, and the **ileum**.

31. B

The **immune** system defends our bodies against infections and disease through three types of response systems: the **anatomic** response, the **inflammatory** response, and the **immune** response.

32. A

The **musculoskeletal** system is composed of all of the bones, cartilage, muscles, joints, tendons and ligaments in a person's body.

33. C

The **gastrointestinal** tract is a muscular tube lined by a special layer of cells, called **epithelium**; its primary purpose is to break food down into **nutrients**, which can be absorbed into the body to provide energy.

34. C

The **Law of the Conservation of Energy** states that, in a chemical change, **energy** can be neither **created** nor **destroyed**, but only changed from **one form to another**.

35. C

A **chemical change** is a process that transforms one set of chemical substances to another; the substances used are known as **reactants** and those formed are products.

36. D

Anabolism is the series of chemical reactions resulting in the **synthesis** of organic compounds, and **catabolism** is a series of chemical reactions that **break down** larger molecules.

37. D

A **catalyst** is a chemical involved in, but not changed by, a chemical reaction by which chemical bonds are **weakened** and reactions **accelerated**.

Note: Enzymes function as organic catalysts and allow many chemical reactions to occur within the homeostatic constraints of a living system. Enzymes can act rapidly, as in the case of carbonic anhydrase (enzymes typically end in the -ase suffix), which causes the chemicals to react 107 times faster than without the enzyme present.

38. B

Oxygen is the most abundant element in the Earth's crust and appears on the Atomic Table as the letter '**O**'.

39. A

The Law of Multiple Proportions states that when two elements combine with each other to form more than one compound, the weights of one element that combine with a fixed weight of the other are in a ratio of small whole numbers.

40. D

The Law of Definite Proportions states that every chemical compound contains fixed and constant proportions (by weight) of its constituent elements.
Note: Although many experimenters had long assumed the truth of the principle in gen-

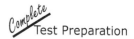

eral, the French chemist Joseph-Louis Proust first accumulated conclusive evidence for it in a series of researches on the composition of many substances, especially the oxides of iron (1797).[25]

41. C
The Pauli Exclusion Principle states that, in a given **molecule, no two electrons can** have **a different set of four quantum numbers**.

42. B
According to the tenets of Dalton's atomic theory, **All atoms of an element are alike in weight, and this weight is specific to the kind of atom.**

43. A
Atoms of **different elements** combine in **simple whole-number** ratios to form chemical **compounds**.

44. B
The following statement about the periodic table is true, **the way in which the elements are arranged allows predictions to made about their behavior.**

45. A
Ionization energy is the minimum amount of energy required to remove an electron from an atom or ion in the gas phase.

46. D
An **atomic radius** is one-half the distance between nuclei of atoms of the same element, when the atoms are bound by a single covalent bond or are in a metallic crystal.

47. A & B are correct.
An anion is a negatively charged ion, and a cation is a positively charged ion.
Anions are typically formed by nonmetals, and metals usually form cations.

48. C
The radius of atoms obtained from **covalent** bond lengths is called the **covalent** radius; the radius from interatomic distances in metallic crystals is called the **metallic** radius.

49. D
A **periodic trend** is a regular variation in element properties with **increasing** atomic number that is ultimately due to **regular** variations in atomic structure.

50. D
All of these statements are true.

 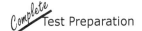

Anatomy and Physiology

1. A
Kidneys are responsible for regulating fluid balance.

2. B
Fluid balance is important, because water comprises about 60-70% of a person's weight.

3. B
Metabolism slows with aging.

4. D
"Met" refers to **the person's metabolic rate.**

5. A
Fluid balance is important, because the human body loses water every day through urination, perspiration, feces, and **breathing**.

6. D
The smallest unit of life in our bodies is the **cell**.

7. B
The cell membrane or plasma membrane is a biological membrane that separates the interior of all cells from the outside environment. The cell membrane is selectively permeable to ions and organic molecules and controls the movement of substances in and out of cells.[26]

8. A
Cell division is the process by which a parent cell divides into two or more daughter cells. Cell division is usually a small segment of a larger cell cycle.

9. C
Mitosis is the process by which a eukaryotic cell separates the chromosomes in its cell nucleus into two identical sets in two separate nuclei. The process of mitosis is fast and highly complex. The sequence of events is divided into stages corresponding to the completion of one set of activities and the start of the next. These stages are interphase, prophase, prometaphase, metaphase, anaphase and telophase.[27]

10. B
Mitosis is the process by which a eukaryotic cell separates the chromosomes in its cell nucleus into two identical sets in two separate nuclei.[27]

11. A
Prophase, is a stage of mitosis in which the chromatin condenses (it becomes shorter and fatter) into a highly ordered structure called a chromosome in which the chromatin becomes visible.[28]

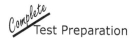

12. B
Metaphase is a stage of mitosis in the eukaryotic cell cycle in which condensed & highly coiled chromosomes, carrying genetic information, align in the middle of the cell before being separated into each of the two daughter cells. Preceded by events in prometaphase and followed by anaphase, microtubules formed in prophase have already found and attached themselves to kinetochores in metaphase[29]

13. D
Anaphase, from the ancient Greek ἀνά (up) and φάσις (stage), is the stage of mitosis or meiosis when chromosomes move to opposite poles of the cell.
Anaphase begins with the regulated triggering of the metaphase-to-anaphase transition. Metaphase ends with the destruction of cyclin, which is required for the function of metaphase cyclin-dependent kinases (M-Cdks). Anaphase is initiated with the cleavage of securin, a protein that inhibits the protease known as separase. Separase then cleaves cohesin, a protein responsible for holding sister chromatids together.[30]

14. D
Telophase is a stage in both meiosis and mitosis in a eukaryotic cell. During telophase, the effects of prophase and prometaphase events are reversed. Two daughter nuclei form in the cell. The nuclear envelopes of the daughter cells are formed from the fragments of the nuclear envelope of the parent cell. As the nuclear envelope forms around each pair of chromatids, the nucleoli reappear.[31]

15. B
Epithelium is one of the four basic types of animal tissue, along with connective tissue, muscle tissue and nervous tissue. Epithelial tissues line the cavities and surfaces of structures throughout the body, and form many glands. Functions of epithelial cells include secretion, selective absorption, protection, transcellular transport and detection of sensation.
Simple epithelial tissues are generally classified by the shape of their cells. The four major classes of simple epithelium are: (1) simple squamous; (2) simple cuboidal; (3) simple columnar; (4) pseudostratified.[32]

16. B
Epithelial tissue **acts as a protective barrier for the human body.**

17. C
The functions of connective tissue are, Storage of energy, Protection of organs, Providing structural framework for the body and Connection of body tissues.

18. C
Muscle tissue has the ability to **relax and contract**, bringing out movement and the ability to work.

19. D
Nervous tissue is specialized to **react to stimuli**.

 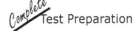

20. A

Neurons make up nerve tissue.

21. C

The integumentary system is the organ system that protects the body from damage, comprising the skin and its appendages, including hair, scales, feathers, and nails.

22. C

The integumentary system comprises the **skin** and its various appendages, including hair, scales, feathers, and nails.

23. B

The appendages of the integumentary system are hair, scales, feathers, and nails.

24. D

The integumentary system has a variety of functions; it may serve to waterproof, cushion, and protect the deeper tissues, excrete wastes, and **regulate temperature**, and is the attachment site for sensory receptors to detect pain, sensation, pressure, and temperature.

25. C

The human skin (integumentary) is composed of a minimum of 3 major layers of tissue, the Epidermis, the Dermis and Hypodermis.

Practice Test Questions Set 2

Section I – Reading Comprehension

Questions: 45
Time: 45 Minutes

Section II – Math

Questions: 50
Time: 50 Minutes

Section III – Part I - English Grammar

Questions: 50
Time: 50 Minutes

Section III – Part II – Vocabulary

Questions: 50
Time: 50 Minutes

Section IV – Science – Part I – Chemistry & Biology

Questions: 50
Time: 50 Minutes

Section IV – Science – Part II – Anatomy & Physiology

Questions: 25
Time: 25 Minutes

The practice test portion presents questions that are representative of the type of question you should expect to find on the HESI. However, they are not intended to match exactly what is on the HESI.

For the best results, take this Practice Test as if it were the real exam. Set aside time when you will not be disturbed, and a location that is quiet and free of distractions. Read the instructions carefully, read each question carefully, and answer to the best of your ability.

Use the bubble answer sheets provided. When you have completed the Practice Test, check your answer against the Answer Key and read the explanation provided.

NOTE: The Science, Anatomy and Physiology and English sections are optional. Check with your school for exam details.

Section I – Reading Comprehension Answer Sheet

1. Ⓐ Ⓑ Ⓒ Ⓓ   18. Ⓐ Ⓑ Ⓒ Ⓓ   35. Ⓐ Ⓑ Ⓒ Ⓓ

2. Ⓐ Ⓑ Ⓒ Ⓓ   19. Ⓐ Ⓑ Ⓒ Ⓓ   36. Ⓐ Ⓑ Ⓒ Ⓓ

3. Ⓐ Ⓑ Ⓒ Ⓓ   20. Ⓐ Ⓑ Ⓒ Ⓓ   37. Ⓐ Ⓑ Ⓒ Ⓓ

4. Ⓐ Ⓑ Ⓒ Ⓓ   21. Ⓐ Ⓑ Ⓒ Ⓓ   38. Ⓐ Ⓑ Ⓒ Ⓓ

5. Ⓐ Ⓑ Ⓒ Ⓓ   22. Ⓐ Ⓑ Ⓒ Ⓓ   39. Ⓐ Ⓑ Ⓒ Ⓓ

6. Ⓐ Ⓑ Ⓒ Ⓓ   23. Ⓐ Ⓑ Ⓒ Ⓓ   40. Ⓐ Ⓑ Ⓒ Ⓓ

7. Ⓐ Ⓑ Ⓒ Ⓓ   24. Ⓐ Ⓑ Ⓒ Ⓓ   41. Ⓐ Ⓑ Ⓒ Ⓓ

8. Ⓐ Ⓑ Ⓒ Ⓓ   25. Ⓐ Ⓑ Ⓒ Ⓓ   42. Ⓐ Ⓑ Ⓒ Ⓓ

9. Ⓐ Ⓑ Ⓒ Ⓓ   26. Ⓐ Ⓑ Ⓒ Ⓓ   43. Ⓐ Ⓑ Ⓒ Ⓓ

10. Ⓐ Ⓑ Ⓒ Ⓓ   27. Ⓐ Ⓑ Ⓒ Ⓓ   44. Ⓐ Ⓑ Ⓒ Ⓓ

11. Ⓐ Ⓑ Ⓒ Ⓓ   28. Ⓐ Ⓑ Ⓒ Ⓓ   45. Ⓐ Ⓑ Ⓒ Ⓓ

12. Ⓐ Ⓑ Ⓒ Ⓓ   29. Ⓐ Ⓑ Ⓒ Ⓓ   46. Ⓐ Ⓑ Ⓒ Ⓓ

13. Ⓐ Ⓑ Ⓒ Ⓓ   30. Ⓐ Ⓑ Ⓒ Ⓓ   47. Ⓐ Ⓑ Ⓒ Ⓓ

14. Ⓐ Ⓑ Ⓒ Ⓓ   31. Ⓐ Ⓑ Ⓒ Ⓓ   48. Ⓐ Ⓑ Ⓒ Ⓓ

15. Ⓐ Ⓑ Ⓒ Ⓓ   32. Ⓐ Ⓑ Ⓒ Ⓓ   49. Ⓐ Ⓑ Ⓒ Ⓓ

16. Ⓐ Ⓑ Ⓒ Ⓓ   33. Ⓐ Ⓑ Ⓒ Ⓓ   50. Ⓐ Ⓑ Ⓒ Ⓓ

17. Ⓐ Ⓑ Ⓒ Ⓓ   34. Ⓐ Ⓑ Ⓒ Ⓓ

Section II – Math – Answer Sheet

1. Ⓐ Ⓑ Ⓒ Ⓓ	21. Ⓐ Ⓑ Ⓒ Ⓓ	41. Ⓐ Ⓑ Ⓒ Ⓓ
2. Ⓐ Ⓑ Ⓒ Ⓓ	22. Ⓐ Ⓑ Ⓒ Ⓓ	42. Ⓐ Ⓑ Ⓒ Ⓓ
3. Ⓐ Ⓑ Ⓒ Ⓓ	23. Ⓐ Ⓑ Ⓒ Ⓓ	43. Ⓐ Ⓑ Ⓒ Ⓓ
4. Ⓐ Ⓑ Ⓒ Ⓓ	24. Ⓐ Ⓑ Ⓒ Ⓓ	44. Ⓐ Ⓑ Ⓒ Ⓓ
5. Ⓐ Ⓑ Ⓒ Ⓓ	25. Ⓐ Ⓑ Ⓒ Ⓓ	45. Ⓐ Ⓑ Ⓒ Ⓓ
6. Ⓐ Ⓑ Ⓒ Ⓓ	26. Ⓐ Ⓑ Ⓒ Ⓓ	46. Ⓐ Ⓑ Ⓒ Ⓓ
7. Ⓐ Ⓑ Ⓒ Ⓓ	27. Ⓐ Ⓑ Ⓒ Ⓓ	47. Ⓐ Ⓑ Ⓒ Ⓓ
8. Ⓐ Ⓑ Ⓒ Ⓓ	28. Ⓐ Ⓑ Ⓒ Ⓓ	48. Ⓐ Ⓑ Ⓒ Ⓓ
9. Ⓐ Ⓑ Ⓒ Ⓓ	29. Ⓐ Ⓑ Ⓒ Ⓓ	49. Ⓐ Ⓑ Ⓒ Ⓓ
10. Ⓐ Ⓑ Ⓒ Ⓓ	30. Ⓐ Ⓑ Ⓒ Ⓓ	50. Ⓐ Ⓑ Ⓒ Ⓓ
11. Ⓐ Ⓑ Ⓒ Ⓓ	31. Ⓐ Ⓑ Ⓒ Ⓓ	51. Ⓐ Ⓑ Ⓒ Ⓓ
12. Ⓐ Ⓑ Ⓒ Ⓓ	32. Ⓐ Ⓑ Ⓒ Ⓓ	52. Ⓐ Ⓑ Ⓒ Ⓓ
13. Ⓐ Ⓑ Ⓒ Ⓓ	33. Ⓐ Ⓑ Ⓒ Ⓓ	53. Ⓐ Ⓑ Ⓒ Ⓓ
14. Ⓐ Ⓑ Ⓒ Ⓓ	34. Ⓐ Ⓑ Ⓒ Ⓓ	54. Ⓐ Ⓑ Ⓒ Ⓓ
15. Ⓐ Ⓑ Ⓒ Ⓓ	35. Ⓐ Ⓑ Ⓒ Ⓓ	55. Ⓐ Ⓑ Ⓒ Ⓓ
16. Ⓐ Ⓑ Ⓒ Ⓓ	36. Ⓐ Ⓑ Ⓒ Ⓓ	56. Ⓐ Ⓑ Ⓒ Ⓓ
17. Ⓐ Ⓑ Ⓒ Ⓓ	37. Ⓐ Ⓑ Ⓒ Ⓓ	57. Ⓐ Ⓑ Ⓒ Ⓓ
18. Ⓐ Ⓑ Ⓒ Ⓓ	38. Ⓐ Ⓑ Ⓒ Ⓓ	58. Ⓐ Ⓑ Ⓒ Ⓓ
19. Ⓐ Ⓑ Ⓒ Ⓓ	39. Ⓐ Ⓑ Ⓒ Ⓓ	59. Ⓐ Ⓑ Ⓒ Ⓓ
20. Ⓐ Ⓑ Ⓒ Ⓓ	40. Ⓐ Ⓑ Ⓒ Ⓓ	60. Ⓐ Ⓑ Ⓒ Ⓓ

Section III – Answer Sheet English Grammar

1. Ⓐ Ⓑ Ⓒ Ⓓ   18. Ⓐ Ⓑ Ⓒ Ⓓ   35. Ⓐ Ⓑ Ⓒ Ⓓ
2. Ⓐ Ⓑ Ⓒ Ⓓ   19. Ⓐ Ⓑ Ⓒ Ⓓ   36. Ⓐ Ⓑ Ⓒ Ⓓ
3. Ⓐ Ⓑ Ⓒ Ⓓ   20. Ⓐ Ⓑ Ⓒ Ⓓ   37. Ⓐ Ⓑ Ⓒ Ⓓ
4. Ⓐ Ⓑ Ⓒ Ⓓ   21. Ⓐ Ⓑ Ⓒ Ⓓ   38. Ⓐ Ⓑ Ⓒ Ⓓ
5. Ⓐ Ⓑ Ⓒ Ⓓ   22. Ⓐ Ⓑ Ⓒ Ⓓ   39. Ⓐ Ⓑ Ⓒ Ⓓ
6. Ⓐ Ⓑ Ⓒ Ⓓ   23. Ⓐ Ⓑ Ⓒ Ⓓ   40. Ⓐ Ⓑ Ⓒ Ⓓ
7. Ⓐ Ⓑ Ⓒ Ⓓ   24. Ⓐ Ⓑ Ⓒ Ⓓ   41. Ⓐ Ⓑ Ⓒ Ⓓ
8. Ⓐ Ⓑ Ⓒ Ⓓ   25. Ⓐ Ⓑ Ⓒ Ⓓ   42. Ⓐ Ⓑ Ⓒ Ⓓ
9. Ⓐ Ⓑ Ⓒ Ⓓ   26. Ⓐ Ⓑ Ⓒ Ⓓ   43. Ⓐ Ⓑ Ⓒ Ⓓ
10. Ⓐ Ⓑ Ⓒ Ⓓ   27. Ⓐ Ⓑ Ⓒ Ⓓ   44. Ⓐ Ⓑ Ⓒ Ⓓ
11. Ⓐ Ⓑ Ⓒ Ⓓ   28. Ⓐ Ⓑ Ⓒ Ⓓ   45. Ⓐ Ⓑ Ⓒ Ⓓ
12. Ⓐ Ⓑ Ⓒ Ⓓ   29. Ⓐ Ⓑ Ⓒ Ⓓ   46. Ⓐ Ⓑ Ⓒ Ⓓ
13. Ⓐ Ⓑ Ⓒ Ⓓ   30. Ⓐ Ⓑ Ⓒ Ⓓ   47. Ⓐ Ⓑ Ⓒ Ⓓ
14. Ⓐ Ⓑ Ⓒ Ⓓ   31. Ⓐ Ⓑ Ⓒ Ⓓ   48. Ⓐ Ⓑ Ⓒ Ⓓ
15. Ⓐ Ⓑ Ⓒ Ⓓ   32. Ⓐ Ⓑ Ⓒ Ⓓ   49. Ⓐ Ⓑ Ⓒ Ⓓ
16. Ⓐ Ⓑ Ⓒ Ⓓ   33. Ⓐ Ⓑ Ⓒ Ⓓ   50. Ⓐ Ⓑ Ⓒ Ⓓ
17. Ⓐ Ⓑ Ⓒ Ⓓ   34. Ⓐ Ⓑ Ⓒ Ⓓ

Section III Part II – Vocabulary Answer Sheet

1. (A) (B) (C) (D)   21. (A) (B) (C) (D)   41. (A) (B) (C) (D)

2. (A) (B) (C) (D)   22. (A) (B) (C) (D)   42. (A) (B) (C) (D)

3. (A) (B) (C) (D)   23. (A) (B) (C) (D)   43. (A) (B) (C) (D)

4. (A) (B) (C) (D)   24. (A) (B) (C) (D)   44. (A) (B) (C) (D)

5. (A) (B) (C) (D)   25. (A) (B) (C) (D)   45. (A) (B) (C) (D)

6. (A) (B) (C) (D)   26. (A) (B) (C) (D)   46. (A) (B) (C) (D)

7. (A) (B) (C) (D)   27. (A) (B) (C) (D)   47. (A) (B) (C) (D)

8. (A) (B) (C) (D)   28. (A) (B) (C) (D)   48. (A) (B) (C) (D)

9. (A) (B) (C) (D)   29. (A) (B) (C) (D)   49. (A) (B) (C) (D)

10. (A) (B) (C) (D)   30. (A) (B) (C) (D)   50. (A) (B) (C) (D)

11. (A) (B) (C) (D)   31. (A) (B) (C) (D)   51. (A) (B) (C) (D)

12. (A) (B) (C) (D)   32. (A) (B) (C) (D)   52. (A) (B) (C) (D)

13. (A) (B) (C) (D)   33. (A) (B) (C) (D)   53. (A) (B) (C) (D)

14. (A) (B) (C) (D)   34. (A) (B) (C) (D)   54. (A) (B) (C) (D)

15. (A) (B) (C) (D)   35. (A) (B) (C) (D)   55. (A) (B) (C) (D)

16. (A) (B) (C) (D)   36. (A) (B) (C) (D)   56. (A) (B) (C) (D)

17. (A) (B) (C) (D)   37. (A) (B) (C) (D)   57. (A) (B) (C) (D)

18. (A) (B) (C) (D)   38. (A) (B) (C) (D)   58. (A) (B) (C) (D)

19. (A) (B) (C) (D)   39. (A) (B) (C) (D)   59. (A) (B) (C) (D)

20. (A) (B) (C) (D)   40. (A) (B) (C) (D)   60. (A) (B) (C) (D)

Section IV – Science Part I - Chemistry & Biology

1. (A) (B) (C) (D)
2. (A) (B) (C) (D)
3. (A) (B) (C) (D)
4. (A) (B) (C) (D)
5. (A) (B) (C) (D)
6. (A) (B) (C) (D)
7. (A) (B) (C) (D)
8. (A) (B) (C) (D)
9. (A) (B) (C) (D)
10. (A) (B) (C) (D)
11. (A) (B) (C) (D)
12. (A) (B) (C) (D)
13. (A) (B) (C) (D)
14. (A) (B) (C) (D)
15. (A) (B) (C) (D)
16. (A) (B) (C) (D)
17. (A) (B) (C) (D)

18. (A) (B) (C) (D)
19. (A) (B) (C) (D)
20. (A) (B) (C) (D)
21. (A) (B) (C) (D)
22. (A) (B) (C) (D)
23. (A) (B) (C) (D)
24. (A) (B) (C) (D)
25. (A) (B) (C) (D)
26. (A) (B) (C) (D)
27. (A) (B) (C) (D)
28. (A) (B) (C) (D)
29. (A) (B) (C) (D)
30. (A) (B) (C) (D)
31. (A) (B) (C) (D)
32. (A) (B) (C) (D)
33. (A) (B) (C) (D)
34. (A) (B) (C) (D)

35. (A) (B) (C) (D)
36. (A) (B) (C) (D)
37. (A) (B) (C) (D)
38. (A) (B) (C) (D)
39. (A) (B) (C) (D)
40. (A) (B) (C) (D)
41. (A) (B) (C) (D)
42. (A) (B) (C) (D)
43. (A) (B) (C) (D)
44. (A) (B) (C) (D)
45. (A) (B) (C) (D)
46. (A) (B) (C) (D)
47. (A) (B) (C) (D)
48. (A) (B) (C) (D)
49. (A) (B) (C) (D)
50. (A) (B) (C) (D)

Section IV - Anatomy and Physiology Answer Sheet

1. (A) (B) (C) (D)   18. (A) (B) (C) (D)   35. (A) (B) (C) (D)

2. (A) (B) (C) (D)   19. (A) (B) (C) (D)   36. (A) (B) (C) (D)

3. (A) (B) (C) (D)   20. (A) (B) (C) (D)   37. (A) (B) (C) (D)

4. (A) (B) (C) (D)   21. (A) (B) (C) (D)   38. (A) (B) (C) (D)

5. (A) (B) (C) (D)   22. (A) (B) (C) (D)   39. (A) (B) (C) (D)

6. (A) (B) (C) (D)   23. (A) (B) (C) (D)   40. (A) (B) (C) (D)

7. (A) (B) (C) (D)   24. (A) (B) (C) (D)   41. (A) (B) (C) (D)

8. (A) (B) (C) (D)   25. (A) (B) (C) (D)   42. (A) (B) (C) (D)

9. (A) (B) (C) (D)   26. (A) (B) (C) (D)   43. (A) (B) (C) (D)

10. (A) (B) (C) (D)   27. (A) (B) (C) (D)   44. (A) (B) (C) (D)

11. (A) (B) (C) (D)   28. (A) (B) (C) (D)   45. (A) (B) (C) (D)

12. (A) (B) (C) (D)   29. (A) (B) (C) (D)   46. (A) (B) (C) (D)

13. (A) (B) (C) (D)   30. (A) (B) (C) (D)   47. (A) (B) (C) (D)

14. (A) (B) (C) (D)   31. (A) (B) (C) (D)   48. (A) (B) (C) (D)

15. (A) (B) (C) (D)   32. (A) (B) (C) (D)   49. (A) (B) (C) (D)

16. (A) (B) (C) (D)   33. (A) (B) (C) (D)   50. (A) (B) (C) (D)

17. (A) (B) (C) (D)   34. (A) (B) (C) (D)

Section I - Reading Comprehension

Questions 1-4 refer to the following passage.

Passage 1 - The Respiratory System

The respiratory system's function is to allow oxygen exchange through all parts of the body. The anatomy or structure of the exchange system, and the uses of the exchanged gases, varies depending on the organism. In humans and other mammals, for example, the anatomical features of the respiratory system include airways, lungs, and the respiratory muscles. Molecules of oxygen and carbon dioxide are passively exchanged, by diffusion, between the gaseous external environment and the blood. This exchange process occurs in the alveolar region of the lungs.

Other animals, such as insects, have respiratory systems with very simple anatomical features, and in amphibians even the skin plays a vital role in gas exchange. Plants also have respiratory systems but the direction of gas exchange can be opposite to that of animals.

The respiratory system can also be divided into physiological, or functional, zones. These include the conducting zone (the region for gas transport from the outside atmosphere to just above the alveoli), the transitional zone, and the respiratory zone (the alveolar region where gas exchange occurs). [33]

1. What can we infer from the first paragraph in this passage?

    a. Human and mammal respiratory systems are the same

    b. The lungs are an important part of the respiratory system

    c. The respiratory system varies in different mammals

    d. Oxygen and carbon dioxide are passive exchanged by the respiratory system

2. What is the process by which molecules of oxygen and carbon dioxide are passively exchanged?

    a. Transfusion

    b. Affusion

    c. Diffusion

    d. Respiratory confusion

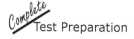

3. What organ plays an important role in gas exchange in amphibians?

    a. The skin

    b. The lungs

    c. The gills

    d. The mouth

4. What are the three physiological zones of the respiratory system?

    a. Conducting, transitional, respiratory zones

    b. Redacting, transitional, circulatory zones

    c. Conducting, circulatory, inhibiting zones

    d. Transitional, inhibiting, conducting zones

Questions 5-8 refer to the following passage.

ABC Electric Warranty

ABC Electric Company warrants that its products are free from defects in material and workmanship. Subject to the conditions and limitations set forth below, ABC Electric will, at its option, either repair or replace any part of its products that prove defective due to improper workmanship or materials.

This limited warranty does not cover any damage to the product from improper installation, accident, abuse, misuse, natural disaster, insufficient or excessive electrical supply, abnormal mechanical or environmental conditions, or any unauthorized disassembly, repair, or modification.

This limited warranty also does not apply to any product on which the original identification information has been altered, or removed, has not been handled or packaged correctly, or has been sold as second-hand.

This limited warranty covers only repair, replacement, refund or credit for defective ABC Electric products, as provided above.

5. I tried to repair my ABC Electric blender, but could not, so can I get it repaired under this warranty?

    a. Yes, the warranty still covers the blender

    b. No, the warranty does not cover the blender

    c. Uncertain. ABC Electric may or may not cover repairs under this warranty

6. My ABC Electric fan is not working. Will ABC Electric provide a new one or repair this one?

    a. ABC Electric will repair my fan

    b. ABC Electric will replace my fan

    c. ABC Electric could either replace or repair my fan can request either a replacement or a repair.

7. My stove was damaged in a flood. Does this warranty cover my stove?

    a. Yes, it is covered.

    b. No, it is not covered.

    c. It may or may not be covered.

    d. ABC Electric will decide if it is covered

8. Which of the following is an example of improper workmanship?

    a. Missing parts

    b. Defective parts

    c. Scratches on the front

    d. None of the above

Questions 9 – 12 refer to the following passage.

Passage 3 – Mythology

The main characters in myths are usually gods or supernatural heroes. As sacred stories, rulers and priests have traditionally endorsed their myths and as a result, myths have a close link with religion and politics. In the society where a myth originates, the natives believe the myth is a true account of the remote past. In fact, many societies have two categories of traditional narrative—(1) "true stories", or myths, and (2) "false stories", or fables.

Myths generally take place during a primordial age, when the world was still young, prior to achieving its current form. These stories explain how the world gained its current form and why the culture developed its customs, institutions, and taboos. Closely related to myth are legend and folktale. Myths, legends, and folktales are different types of traditional stories. Unlike myths, folktales can take place at any time and any place, and the natives do not usually consider them true or sacred. Legends, on the other hand, are similar to myths in that many people have traditionally considered them true. Legends take place in a more recent time, when the world was much as it is today. In addition, legends generally feature humans as their main characters, whereas myths have super-human characters. [34]

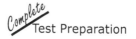

9. We can infer from this passage that

    a. Folktales took place in a time far past, before civilization covered the earth

    b. Humankind uses myth to explain how the world was created

    c. Myths revolve around gods or supernatural beings; the local community usually accepts these stories as not true

    d. The only difference between a myth and a legend is the time setting of the story

10. The main purpose of this passage is

    a. To distinguish between many types of traditional stories, and explain the background of some traditional story categories

    b. To determine whether myths and legends might be true accounts of history

    c. To show the importance of folktales how these traditional stories made life more bearable in harder times

    d. None of the Above

11. How are folktales different from myths?

    a. Folktales and myth are the same

    b. Folktales are not true and generally not sacred and take place anytime

    c. Myths are not true and generally not sacred and take place anytime

    d. Folktales explained the formation of the world and myths do not

12. How are legends and myth similar?

    a. Many people believe legends and myths are true, myths take place in modern day, and legends are about ordinary people

    b. Many people believe legends and myths are true, legends take place in modern day, and legends are about ordinary people

    c. Many people believe legends and myths are true, legends take place in modern day, and myths are about ordinary people

    d. Many people believe legends and myths are not true, legends take place in mod-ern day, and legends are about ordinary people

Questions 13-18 refer to the following passage.

Passage 4 – Myths, Legend and Folklore

Cultural historians draw a distinction between myth, legend and folktale simply as a way to group traditional stories. However, in many cultures, drawing a sharp line between myths and legends is not that simple. Instead of dividing their traditional stories

 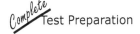

into myths, legends, and folktales, some cultures divide them into two categories. The first category roughly corresponds to folktales, and the second is one that combines myths and legends. Similarly, we can not always separate myths from folktales. One society might consider a story true, making it a myth. Another society may believe the story is fiction, which makes it a folktale. In fact, when a myth loses its status as part of a religious system, it often takes on traits more typical of folktales, with its formerly divine characters now appearing as human heroes, giants, or fairies. Myth, legend, and folktale are only a few of the categories of traditional stories. Other categories include anecdotes and some kinds of jokes. Traditional stories, in turn, are only one category within the much larger category of folklore, which also includes items such as gestures, costumes, and music. [33]

13. The main idea of this passage is that

a. Myths, fables, and folktales are not the same thing, and each describes a specific type of story

b. Traditional stories can be categorized in different ways by different people

c. Cultures use myths for religious purposes, and when this is no longer true, the people forget and discard these myths

d. Myths can never become folk tales, because one is true, and the other is false

14. The terms myth and legend are

a. Categories that are synonymous with true and false

b. Categories that group traditional stories according to certain characteristics

c. Interchangeable, because both terms mean a story that is passed down from generation to generation

d. Meant to distinguish between a story that involves a hero and a cultural message and a story meant only to entertain

15. Traditional story categories not only include myths and legends, but

a. Can also include gestures, since some cultures passed these down before the written and spoken word

b. In addition, folklore refers to stories involving fables and fairy tales

c. These story categories can also include folk music and traditional dress

d. Traditional stories themselves are a part of the larger category of folklore, which may also include costumes, gestures, and music

 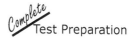

16. This passage shows that

    a. There is a distinct difference between a myth and a legend, although both are folktales

    b. Myths are folktales, but folktales are not myths

    c. Myths, legends, and folktales play an important part in tradition and the past, and are a rich and colorful part of history

    d. Most cultures consider myths to be true

Questions 17-19 refer to the following passage.

Passage 5 – Insects

Humans regard certain insects as pests and attempt to control them with insecticides and many other techniques. Some insects damage crops by feeding on sap, leaves or fruits, a few bite humans and livestock, alive and dead, to feed on blood and some are capable of transmitting diseases to humans, pets and live-stock. Many other insects are considered ecologically beneficial and a few provide direct economic benefit. Silkworms and bees, for example, have been domesticated for the production of silk and honey, respectively. [35]

17. How do humans control insects?

    a. By training them

    b. Using insecticides and other techniques

    c. In many different ways

    d. Humans do not control insects

18. Why do humans control insects?

    a. Because they do not like them

    b. Because they damage crops

    c. Because they damage buildings

    d. Because they damage the soil

19. How do insects damage crops?

    a. By feeding on crops

    b. By transmitting disease

    c. By laying eggs on crops

    d. None of the above

 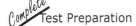

Questions 20-24 refer to the following passage.

Passage 6 – Trees I

Trees are an important part of the natural landscape because they prevent erosion and protect ecosystems in and under their branches. Trees also play an important role in producing oxygen and reducing carbon dioxide in the atmosphere, as well as moderating ground temperatures. Trees are important elements in landscaping and agriculture, both for their visual appeal and for their crops, such as apples, and other fruit. Wood from trees is a building material, and a primary energy source in many developing countries. Trees also play a role in many of the world's mythologies. [36]

20. What are two reasons trees are important in the natural landscape?

    a. They prevent erosion and produce oxygen

    b. They produce fruit and are important elements in landscaping

    c. Trees are not important in the natural landscape

    d. Trees produce carbon dioxide and prevent erosion

21. What kind of ecosystems do trees protect?

    a. Trees do not protect ecosystems

    b. Weather sheltered ecosystems

    c. Ecosystems around the base and under the branches

    d. All of the above

22. Which of the following is true?

    a. Trees provide a primary food source in the developing world

    b. Trees provide a primary building material in the developing world

    c. Trees provide a primary energy source in the developing world

    d. Trees provide a primary oxygen source in the developing world

23. Why are trees important for agriculture?

    a. Because of their crops

    b. Because they shelter ecosystems

    c. Because they are a source of energy

    d. Because of their visual appeal

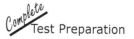

24. What do trees do to the atmosphere?

    a. Trees produce carbon dioxide and reduce oxygen

    b. Trees product oxygen and carbon dioxide

    c. Trees reduce oxygen and carbon dioxide

    d. Trees produce oxygen and reduce carbon dioxide

Questions 25-28 refer to the following passage.

Passage 7 – Trees II

With an estimated 100,000 species, trees represent 25 percent of all living plant species. The majority of tree species grow in tropical regions of the world and many of these areas have not been surveyed by botanists, making species diversity poorly understood. The earliest trees were tree ferns and horsetails, which grew in forests in the Carboniferous period. Tree ferns still survive, but the only surviving horsetails are no longer in tree form. Later, in the Triassic period, conifers and ginkgos, appeared, followed by flowering plants after that in the Cretaceous period. [35]

25. Do botanists understand the number of tree species?

    a. Yes botanists know exactly how many tree species there are

    b. No, the species diversity is not well understood

    c. Yes, botanists are sure

    d. No, botanists have no idea

26. Where do most trees species grow?

    a. Most tree species grow in tropical regions.

    b. There is no one area where most tree species grow.

    c. Tree species grow in 25% of the world.

    d. There are 100,000 tree species.

27. What tree(s) survived from the Carboniferous period?

    a. 25% of all trees.

    b. Horsetails.

    c. Conifers.

    d. Tree Ferns.

 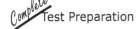

28. Choose the correct list below, ranked from oldest to youngest trees.

   a. Flowering plants, conifers and ginkgos, tree ferns and horsetails.

   b. Tree ferns and horsetails, conifers and ginkgos, flowering plants.

   c. Tree ferns and horsetails, flowering plants, conifers and ginkgos.

   d. Conifers and ginkgos, tree ferns and horsetails, flowering plants.

Questions 29 - 30 refer to the following passage.

Lowest Price Guarantee

Get it for less. Guaranteed!

ABC Electric will beat any advertised price by 10% of the difference.

   1) If you find a lower advertised price, we will beat it by 10% of the difference.

   2) If you find a lower advertised price within 30 days* of your purchase we will beat it by 10% of the difference.

   3) If our own price is reduced within 30 days* of your purchase, bring in your receipt and we will refund the difference.

*14 days for computers, monitors, printers, laptops, tablets, cellular & wireless devices, home security products, projectors, camcorders, digital cameras, radar detectors, portable DVD players, DJ and pro-audio equipment, and air conditioners.

29. I bought a radar detector 15 days ago and saw an ad for the same model only cheaper. Can I get 10% of the difference refunded?

   a. Yes. Since it is less than 30 days, you can get 10% of the difference refunded.

   b. No. Since it is more than 14 days, you cannot get 10% of the difference re-funded.

   c. It depends on the cashier.

   d. Yes. You can get the difference refunded.

30. I bought a flat-screen TV for $500 10 days ago and found an advertisement for the same TV, at another store, on sale for $400. How much will ABC refund under this guarantee?

   a. $100

   b. $110

   c. $10

   d. $400

 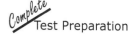

Questions 31-33 refer to the following passage.

Passage 9 - Insects

Insects have segmented bodies supported by an exoskeleton, a hard outer covering made mostly of chitin. The segments of the body are organized into three distinctive connected units, a head, a thorax, and an abdomen. The head supports a pair of antennae, a pair of compound eyes, and three sets of appendages that form the mouthparts.

The thorax has six segmented legs and, if present in the species, two or four wings. The abdomen consists of eleven segments, though in a few species these segments may be fused together or very small.

Overall, there are 24 segments. The abdomen also contains most of the digestive, respiratory, excretory and reproductive internal structures. There is considerable variation and many adaptations in the body parts of insects especially wings, legs, antenna and mouthparts. [36]

31. How many units do insects have?

    a. Insects are divided into 24 units.

    b. Insects are divided into 3 units.

    c. Insects are divided into segments not units.

    d. It depends on the species.

32. Which of the following is true?

    a. All insects have 2 wings.

    b. All insects have 4 wings.

    c. Some insects have 2 wings.

    d. Some insects have 2 or 4 wings.

33. What is true of insect's abdomen?

    a. It contains some of the organs.

    b. It is too small for any organs.

    c. It contains all of the organs.

    d. None of the above.

Questions 34-37 refer to the following passage.

Passage 10 - The Circulatory System

The circulatory system is an organ system that passes nutrients (such as amino acids and electrolytes), gases, hormones, and blood cells to and from cells in the body to help fight diseases and help stabilize body temperature and pH levels.

The circulatory system may be seen strictly as a blood distribution network, but some consider the circulatory system as composed of the cardiovascular system, which distributes blood, and the lymphatic system, which distributes lymph. While humans, as well as other vertebrates, have a closed cardiovascular system (meaning that the blood never leaves the network of arteries, veins and capillaries), some invertebrate groups have an open cardiovascular system. The most primitive animal phyla lack circulatory systems. The lymphatic system, on the other hand, is an open system.

Two types of fluids move through the circulatory system: blood and lymph. The blood, heart, and blood vessels form the cardiovascular system. The lymph, lymph nodes, and lymph vessels form the lymphatic system. The cardiovascular system and the lymphatic system collectively make up the circulatory system.

The main components of the human cardiovascular system are the heart and the blood vessels. It includes: the pulmonary circulation, a "loop" through the lungs where blood is oxygenated; and the systemic circulation, a "loop" through the rest of the body to provide oxygenated blood. An average adult contains five to six quarts (roughly 4.7 to 5.7 liters) of blood, which consists of plasma, red blood cells, white blood cells, and platelets. Also, the digestive system works with the circulatory system to provide the nutrients the system needs to keep the heart pumping. [37]

34. What can we infer from the first paragraph?

    a. An important purpose of the circulatory system is that of fighting diseases.

    b. The most important function of the circulatory system is to give the person energy.

    c. The least important function of the circulatory system is that of growing skin cells.

    d. The entire purpose of the circulatory system is not known.

35. Do humans have an open or closed circulatory system?

    a. Open

    b. Closed

    c. Usually open, though sometimes closed

    d. Usually closed, though sometimes open

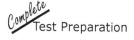

36. In addition to blood, what two components form the cardiovascular system?

    a. The heart and the lungs

    b. The lungs and the veins

    c. The heart and the blood vessels

    d. The blood vessels and the nerves

37. Which system, along with the circulatory system, helps provide nutrients to keep the human heart pumping?

    a. The skeletal system

    b. The digestive system

    c. The immune system

    d. The nervous system

Questions 38-41 refer to the following passage.

Passage 11 - Blood

Blood is a specialized bodily fluid that delivers nutrients and oxygen to the body's cells and transports waste products away.

In vertebrates, blood consists of blood cells suspended in a liquid called blood plasma. Plasma, which comprises 55% of blood fluid, is mostly water (90% by volume), and contains dissolved proteins, glucose, mineral ions, hormones, carbon dioxide, platelets and the blood cells themselves.

Blood cells are mainly red blood cells (also called RBCs or erythrocytes) and white blood cells, including leukocytes and platelets. Red blood cells are the most abundant cells, and contain an iron-containing protein called hemoglobin that transports oxygen through the body.

The pumping action of the heart circulates blood around the body through blood vessels. In animals with lungs, arterial blood carries oxygen from inhaled air to the tissues of the body, and venous blood carries carbon dioxide, a waste product of metabolism produced by cells, from the tissues to the lungs to be exhaled. [38]

38. What can we infer from the first paragraph in this passage?

    a. Blood is responsible for transporting oxygen to the cells.

    b. Blood is only red when it reaches the outside of the body.

    c. Each person has about six pints of blood.

    d. Blood's true function was only learned in the last century.

39. What liquid are blood cells suspended?

  a. Plasma

  b. Water

  c. Liquid nitrogen

  d. A mixture consisting largely of human milk

40. Which of these is not contained in blood plasma?

  a. Hormones

  b. Mineral ions

  c. Calcium

  d. Glucose

41. Which body part exhales carbon dioxide after venous blood has carried it from body tissues?

  a. The lungs

  b. The skin cells

  c. The bowels

  d. The sweat glands

Questions 42-45 refer to the following passage.

Passage 12 - The Human Skeleton

The human skeleton consists of both fused and individual bones supported and supplemented by ligaments, tendons, muscles and cartilage. It serves as a scaffold which supports organs, anchors muscles, and protects organs such as the brain, lungs and heart. The biggest bone in the body is the femur in the upper leg, and the smallest is the stapes bone in the middle ear. In an adult, the skeleton comprises around 14% of the total body weight, and half of this weight is water.

Fused bones include the pelvis and the cranium. Not all bones are interconnected directly: There are three bones in each middle ear called the ossicles that articulate only with each other. The thyoid bone, which is located in the neck, and serves as the point of attachment for the tongue, does not articulate with any other bones in the body, being supported by muscles and ligaments.

There are 206 bones in the adult human skeleton, which varies between individuals and with age - newborn babies have over 270 bones, some of which fuse together. These bones are organized into a longitudinal axis, the axial skeleton, to which the appendicular skeleton is attached. [39]

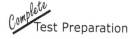

42. What is the main idea of this passage?

a. The human skeleton is an important and complicated system of the body.

b. There are 206 bones in the typical human body.

c. In a child, the skeleton represents 14% of the body weight.

d. Bones become more fragile as we age.

43. How many bones are located in the human middle ear?

a. 3

b. 2

c. 1

d. 0

44. Which of the following is not true about the number of bones in the human skeleton?

a. The typical skeleton has 206 bones.

b. The number of bones stays the same throughout one's lifetime.

c. Newborn babies have about 270 bones.

d. As a baby grows older, some of its bones fuse together.

45. What is the appendicular skeleton attached to?

a. The exoskeleton.

b. The radial skeleton.

c. The rotating skeleton.

d. The axial skeleton.

Section II – Math

1. 8327 – 1278 =

    a. 7149

    b. 7209

    c. 6059

    d. 7049

2. 294 X 21 =

    a. 6017

    b. 6174

    c. 6728

    d. 5679

3. 1278 + 4920 =

    a. 6298

    b. 6108

    c. 6198

    d. 6098

4. 285 * 12 =

    a. 3420

    b. 3402

    c. 3024

    d. 2322

5. 4120 – 3216 =

    a. 903

    b. 804

    c. 904

    d. 1904

6. 2417 + 1004 =

    a. 3401

    b. 4321

    c. 3402

    d. 3421

7. 1440 ÷ 12 =

    a. 122

    b. 120

    c. 110

    d. 132

8. 2713 – 1308 =

    a. 1450

    b. 1445

    c. 1405

    d. 1455

9. It is known that $x^2+4x=5$. Then x can be

    a. 0

    b. -5

    c. 1

    d. Either (b) or (c)

10. (a+b)2 = 4ab. What is necessarily correct?

    a. a > b

    b. a < b

    c. a = b

    d. None of the Above

11. The sum of the digits of a 2-digit number is 12. If we switch the digits, the number we get will be greater than the initial one by 36. Find the initial number.

    a. 39

    b. 48

    c. 57

    d. 75

12. Two friends traveled to a nearby city. In the second day they travelled 75 miles more than the first day, and in the third day, they travelled a third of the distance covered in the second day. How many miles did they cover in the first day, if the total travelled was 170 miles?

    a. 30 miles

    b. 35 miles

    c. 105 miles

    d. 135 miles

13. Kate's father is 32 years older than Kate is. In 5 years, he will be five times older. How old is Kate?

    a. 2

    b. 3

    c. 5

    d. 6

14. If Lynn can type a page in p minutes, what portion of the page can she do in 5 minutes?

    a. $5/p$

    b. $p - 5$

    c. $p + 5$

    d. $p/5$

15. If Sally can paint a house in 4 hours, and John can paint the same house in 6 hours, how long will it take for both of them to paint the house together?

    a. 2 hours and 24 minutes

    b. 3 hours and 12 minutes

    c. 3 hours and 44 minutes

    d. 4 hours and 10 minutes

16. Employees of a discount appliance store receive an additional 20% off the lowest price on any item. If an employee purchases a dishwasher during a 15% off sale, how much will he pay if the dishwasher originally cost $450?

    a. $280.90

    b. $287

    c. $292.50

    d. $306

17. The sale price of a car is $12,590, which is 20% off the original price. What is the original price?

    a. $14,310.40

    b. $14,990.90

    c. $15,108.00

    d. $15,737.50

18. A goat eats 214 kg. of hay in 60 days, while a cow eats the same amount in 15 days. How long will it take them to eat this hay together?

    a. 37.5

    b. 75

    c. 12

    d. 15

19. Express 25% as a fraction.

    a. 1/4

    b. 7/40

    c. 6/25

    d. 8/28

20. Express 125% as a decimal.

    a. .125

    b. 12.5

    c. 1.25

    d. 125

21. Solve for x: 30 is 40% of x

    a. 60

    b. 90

    c. 85

    d. 75

22. 12 ½% of x is equal to 50. Solve for x.

    a. 300

    b. 400

    c. 450

    d. 350

23. Express 24/56 as a reduced common fraction.

    a. 4/9

    b. 4/11

    c. 3/7

    d. 3/8

24. Express 87% as a decimal.

    a. .087

    b. 8.7

    c. .87

    d. 87

25. 60 is 75% of x. Solve for x.

    a. 80

    b. 90

    c. 75

    d. 70

26. 60% of x is 12. Solve for x.

    a. 18

    b. 15

    c. 25

    d. 20

27. Express 71/1000 as a decimal.

    a. .71

    b. .0071

    c. .071

    d. 7.1

28. 4.7 + .9 + .01 =

   a. 5.5
   b. 6.51
   c. 5.61
   d. 5.7

29. .33 × .59 =

   a. .1947
   b. 1.947
   c. .0197
   d. .1817

30. .84 ÷ .7 =

   a. .12
   b. 12
   c. .012
   d. 1.2

31. What number is in the ten thousandths place in 1.7389?

   a. 1
   b. 8
   c. 9
   d. 3

32. .87 - .48 =

   a. .39
   b. .49
   c. .41
   d. .37

33. The physician ordered 100 mg Ibuprofen/kg of body weight; on hand is 230 mg/ tablet. The child weighs 50 lb. How many tablets will you give?

   a. 10 tablets
   b. 5 tablets
   c. 1 tablet
   d. 12 tablets

34. The physician ordered 1,000 units of heparin; 5,000 U/mL is on hand. How many milliliters will you give?

    a. 0.002 ml

    b. 0.2 ml

    c. 0.02 ml

    d. 2 ml

35. Simplify 4^3

    a. 20

    b. 32

    c. 64

    d. 108

36. The physician ordered 5 mL of Capacitate; 15 mL/tsp is on hand. How many teaspoons will you give?

    a. 0.05 tsp

    b. 0.03 tsp

    c. 0.5 tsp

    d. 0.3 tsp

37. The physician orders 70 mg morphine sulphate; 1 g/mL is on hand. How many mL will you give?

    a. 0.05 ml

    b. 0.07 ml

    c. 0.04 ml

    d. 0.007 ml

38. The physician ordered 200 mg amoxicillin. The pharmacy stocks amoxicillin 400 mg per tsp. How many teaspoons will you give?

    a. 0.55 tsp

    b. 0.25 tsp

    c. 0.5 tsp

    d. 0.05 tsp

39. The physician ordered 600 mg ibuprofen po; the office stocks amoxicillin 200 mg per tablet. How many tablets will you give?

    a. 3.5 tablets

    b. 2 tablets

    c. 5 tablets

    d. 3 tablets

40. The manager of a weaving factory estimates that if 10 machines run on 100% efficiency for 8 hours, they will produce 1450 meters of cloth. However, due to some technical problems, 4 machines run of 95% efficiency and the remaining 6 at 90% efficiency. How many meters of cloth can these machines will produce in 8 hours?

    a. 1334 meters

    b. 1310 meters

    c. 1300 meters

    d. 1285 meters

41. Convert 60 feet to inches.

    a. 700 inches

    b. 600 inches

    c. 720 inches

    d. 1,800 inches

42. Convert 25 centimeters to millimeters.

    a. 250 millimeters

    b. 7.5 millimeters

    c. 5 millimeters

    d. 2.5 millimeters

43. Convert 100 millimeters to centimeters.

    a. 10 centimeters

    b. 1,000 centimeters

    c. 1100 centimeters

    d. 50 centimeters

44. Convert 3 gallons to quarts.

    a. 15 quarts

    b. 6 quarts

    c. 12 quarts

    d. 32 quarts

45. 2000 mm. =

    a. 2 m

    b. 200 m

    c. 0.002 m

    d. 0.02 m

46. 0.05 ml. =

    a. 50 liters

    b. 0.00005 liters

    c. 5 liters

    d. 0.0005 liters

47. 30 mg is the same mass as:

    a. 0.0003 kg.

    b. 0.03 grams

    c. 300 decigrams

    d. 0.3 grams

48. 0.101 mm. =

    a. .0101 cm

    b. 1.01 cm

    c. 0.00101 cm

    d. 10.10 cm

49. Smith and Simon are playing a card game. Smith will win if a card drawn from a deck of 52 is either 7 or a diamond, and Simon will win if the drawn card is an even number. Which statement is more likely to be correct?

    a. Smith will win more games.

    b. Simon will win more games.

    c. They have same winning probability.

    d. A decision cannot be made from the provided data.

50. How much water can be stored in a cylindrical container 5 meters in diameter and 12 meters high?

    a. 223.65m³

    b. 235.65m³

    c. 240.65m³

    d. 252.65m³

Section III – English Grammar

1. Elaine promised to bring the camera _____ at the mall yesterday.

    a. by me
    b. with me
    c. at me
    d. to me

2. Last night, he _____ the sleeping bag down beside my mattress.

    a. lay
    b. laid
    c. lain
    d. has laid

3. I would have bought the shirt for you if _____.

    a. I had known you liked it.
    b. I have known you liked it.
    c. I would know you liked it.
    d. I know you liked it.

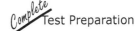

4. Many believers still hope _____ proof of the existence of ghosts.

    a. two find

    b. to find

    c. to found

    d. to have been found

Fill in the blank.

5. All of the people at the school, including the teachers and _____ were glad when summer break came.

    a. students:

    b. students,

    c. students;

    d. students

6. To _____, Anne was on time for her math class.

    a. everybody's surprise

    b. every body's surprise

    c. everybodys surprise

    d. everybodys' surprise

7. If he _____ the textbook like he was supposed to, he would have known what was on the test.

    a. will have read

    b. shouldn't have read

    c. would have read

    d. had read

8. Following the tornado, telephone poles _____ all over the street.

    a. laid

    b. lied

    c. were lying

    d. were laying

9. In Edgar Allen Poe's _____ Edgar Allen Poe describes a man with a guilty conscience.

    a. short story, "The Tell-Tale Heart,"

    b. short story The Tell-Tale Heart,

    c. short story, The Tell-Tale Heart

    d. short story. "the Tell-Tale Heart,"

10. Billboards are considered an important part of advertising for big business, _____ by their critics.

    a. but, an eyesore;

    b. but, " an eyesore,"

    c. but an eyesore

    d. but-an eyesore-

11. I can never remember how to use those two common words, "sell," meaning to trade a product for money, or _____ meaning an event where products are traded for less money than usual.

    a. sale-

    b. "sale,"

    c. "sale

    d. "to sale,"

12. The class just finished reading _____ a short story by Carl Stephenson about a plantation owner's battle with army ants.

    a. "Leinengen versus the Ants",

    b. Leinengen versus the Ants,

    c. "Leinengen versus the Ants,"

    d. Leinengen versus the Ants

13. After the car was fixed, it _____ again.

    a. ran good

    b. ran well

    c. would have run well

    d. ran more well

14. "Where does the sun go during the _____ asked little Kathy.

   a. night,"

   b. night"?,

   c. night,?"

   d. night?"

15. When I was a child, my mother taught me to say thank you, holding the door open for other, and cover my mouth when yawning or coughing.

   a. When I was a child, my mother teaching me to say thank you, to hold the door open for others, and cover my mouth when yawning or coughing.

   b. When I was a child, my mother taught me say thank you, to hold the door open for others, and to covering my mouth when yawning or coughing.

   c. When I was a child, my mother taught me saying thank you, holding the door open for others, and to cover my mouth when yawning or coughing.

   d. When I was a child, my mother taught me to say thank you, hold the door open for others, and cover my mouth when yawning or coughing.

16. Mother is talking to a man that wants to hire her to be a receptionist.

   a. Mother is talking to a man who wants to hire her to be a receptionist.

   b. Mother is talked to a man who wants to hire her to be a receptionist.

   c. Mother is talking to a man who wants to her. To be a receptionist.

   d. Mother is talking to a man hiring her who to be a receptionist.

17. Those comic books, which was for sale at the magazine shop, are now quite valuable.

   a. Those comics books which were for sale, at the magazine shop are now quite valuable.

   b. Those comic books, which were for sale at the magazine, shop, are now quite valuable.

   c. Those comic books, which were for sale at the magazine shop, are now, quite valuable

   d. Those comic books, which were for sale at the magazine shop, are now quite valuable.

18. If you want to sell your car, it's important being honest with the buyer.

    a. If you want to sell your car, being honest with the buyer is important.

    b. If you want to sell your car, to be honest with the buyer is important.

    c. If you wanting to sell your car, being honest with the buyer are important.

    d. If you want to selling your car, to be honest with the buyer is important.

19. Although today the boy was nice to my brother, they usually was quite mean to him.

    a. Although today the boy was nice to my brother, they were usually quite mean to him.

    b. Although today the boy was nice to my brother, he was usually quite mean to him.

    c. Although today the boy were nice to my brother, he is usually quite mean to him.

    d. Although today the boy was nice to my brother, he were usually quite mean to him.

Combine the Sentences into one Simpler Sentence with the Same Meaning.

20. The customers were impatient for the store to open. The customers rushed inside as soon as the doors were open.

    a. Although the customers were impatient for the store to open, the doors were opened as soon as the customers rushed inside.

    b. Although the doors were opened before customers rushed inside, the customers were impatient for the store to open.

    c. The customers, who were impatient for the store to open, rushed inside as soon as the doors were open.

    d. Although the doors were opened by impatient customers, they rushed inside before the store was open.

21. I should enter my dog in a dog pageant. Everyone says that my dog, whose name is Skipper, is the most beautiful one they've ever seen."

    a. Because my dog's name is Skipper, my dog was entered in the pageant and everyone said he was the mot beautiful dog that they've ever seen.

    b. I should enter my dog in a dog pageant, since everyone says that Skipper is the most beautiful dog they've ever seen.

    c. Before I entered my dog in the dog pageant, Skipper said that he was the most beautiful dog that he'd ever seen.

    d. Skipper entered my dog in the dog pageant because he was the most beautiful one that anyone had ever seen.

Complete Test Preparation

22. The doctor was not looking forward to meeting Mrs. Lucas. The doctor would have to tell Mrs. Lucas that she has cancer. The doctor hated giving bad news to patients.

a. The doctor hated giving bad news, and so he was not looking forward to meeting Mrs. Lucas because he would have to tell her that she has cancer.

b. The doctor has cancer and was not looking forward to meeting Mrs. Lucas and telling her this bad news.

c. Before the doctor met Mrs. Lucas, he had to give his the patients the bad news that Mrs. Lucas has cancer.

d. The doctor was not looking forward to giving the bad news to his patients that he had to tell Mrs. Lucas that his patients have cancer.

23. Mom hates shopping. We were out of bread, milk and eggs. Mom went to the supermarket.

a. Because we were out of bread, milk and eggs, Mom hated shopping at the supermarket.

b. Although she hates shopping, Mom went to the supermarket since we were out of bread, milk and eggs.

c. Although we were out of bread, milk and eggs, Mom still hated shopping at the supermarket and went there anyway.

d. Because Mom hated shopping at the supermarket, she went to there to buy her bread, milk and eggs.

24. I hate needles. I want to give blood. I can't give blood.

a. Although I hate needles, I can't give blood even even if I wanted to.

b. Because I hate needles, I can't give blood, although I want to.

c. Whenever I hate needles, I give blood although I can't give blood.

d. Whenever I can't give blood, I give blood anyway, although I hate needles.

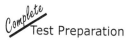

Section III – Vocabulary

Vocabulary

1. NOUN Use of too many words.

   a. Verbiage

   b. Outspoken

   c. Inveigh

   d. Precarious

2. NOUN An aide or assistant.

   a. Attache

   b. Influx

   c. Mien

   d. Knoll

3. VERB To cause or inflict especially related to harm or injury.

   a. Wreak

   b. Mandible

   c. Tremulous

   d. Juxtapose

4. ADJECTIVE Foolish, without understanding.

   a. Coinage

   b. Witless

   c. Distinctive

   d. Nullify

5. ADJECTIVE Strong fear of strangers.

   a. Xenophobia

   b. Agoraphobia

   c. Frightful

   d. Genteel

6. NOUN Highest point, highest state or peak.

    a. Towering

    b. Flickers

    c. Zenith

    d. Grouse

7. NOUN Light wind or gentle breeze.

    a. Sea-breeze

    b. Scuttle

    c. Zephyr

    d. Freight

8. NOUN Self evident or clear obvious truth.

    a. Truism

    b. Catharsis

    c. Libertine

    d. Tractable

9. ADJECTIVE Beyond what is obvious or evident.

    a. Ulterior

    b. Sybarite

    c. Torsion

    d. Trenchant

10. ADJECTIVE Tasteless or bland.

    a. Obstinate

    b. Morose

    c. Inculpate

    d. Vapid

11. NOUN homeless child or stray.

    a. Elegy

    b. Waif

    c. Martyr

    d. Palaver

12. VERB Complaint or criticism.

    a. Obsequies

    b. Whine

    c. Opprobrious

    d. Panacea

13. NOUN Subordinate of lesser rank or authority.

    a. Palliate

    b. Plebeian

    c. Underling

    d. Expiate

14. NOUN A young animal that is between 1 and 2 years.

    a. Yearling

    b. Rogue

    c. Gnostic

    d. Billet

15. NOUN Lush green vegetation.

    a. Coquette

    b. Verdure

    c. Ennui

    d. Lugubrious

16. NOUN A person who is very passionate and fanatic about his specific objectives or beliefs.

    a. Plebeian

    b. Zealot

    c. Progenitor

    d. Iconoclast

17. NOUN Dizziness.

    a. Indolence

    b. Percipient

    c. Vertigo

    d. Tenacious

18. ADJECTIVE Obvious or easy to notice.

   a. Important

   b. Conspicuous

   c. Beautiful

   d. Convincing

19. NOUN Disposition to do good.

   a. Happiness

   b. Courage

   c. Kindness

   d. Benevolence

20. ADJECTIVE Full of energy; exuberant; noisy.

   a. Boisterous

   b. Soft

   c. Gentle

   d. Warm

21. VERB To fondle.

   a. Hold

   b. Caress

   c. Facilitate

   d. Neuter

22. ADJECTIVE Outstanding in importance.

   a. Momentous

   b. Spurious

   c. Extraordinary

   d. Secede

23. NOUN An opponent or enemy.

   a. Antagonist

   b. Protagonist

   c. Sophist

   d. Pugilist

24. NOUN A keepsake; an object kept as a reminder of a place or event.

   a. Monument

   b. Memento

   c. Recurrence

   d. Catharsis

25. ADJECTIVE Producing harm in a stealthy, often gradual, manner.

   a. Adulterate

   b. Acquiesce

   c. Insidious

   d. Deceitful

26. Choose the best definition of obfuscate.

   a. Deliberately make noisy

   b. Deliberately make difficult

   c. Deliberately make quiet

   d. Talk about for a long time

27. Choose the best definition of plethora.

   a. Too many

   b. Too few

   c. A lot

   d. A few

28. Choose the best definition of laceration.

   a. A stripe

   b. A mark

   c. A scratch

   d. A cut

29. Choose the best definition of enshroud.

   a. Hold up

   b. Cover

   c. Wear

   d. Take away

30. Choose the best definition of hasten.

    a. To hurry

    b. To climb

    c. To fasten

    d. To worry

31. Choose the best definition of pliable.

    a. Rigid

    b. Fixable

    c. Bendable

    d. None of the Above

32. Choose the best definition of blithe.

    a. Skinny

    b. Tall

    c. Carefree

    d. Lithe

33. Choose the best definition of rescind.

    a. To take back

    b. To give away

    c. To enforce

    d. To straighten

34. Choose the best definition of headstrong.

    a. Does not listen

    b. Stubborn

    c. Willing

    d. To disbelieve

35. Choose the best definition of oblique.

    a. Direct

    b. Indirect

    c. Sharp

    d. Straight

36. Choose the best definition of temper.

    a. To make worse

    b. To aggravate

    c. To soften

    d. None of the Above

37. Choose the best definition of cryptic.

    a. Building in a graveyard

    b. Difficult to understand

    c. Printed in code

    d. None of the above

38. Choose the best definition of curtail.

    a. To cut short

    b. To arrive early

    c. To lengthen

    d. To give back

39. Choose the best definition of heed.

    a. To ignore

    b. To listen

    c. To advise

    d. To pay

40. Choose the best definition of oblivious.

    a. Far Away

    b. Believable

    c. Unbelievable

    d. Totally unaware

41. Choose the best definition of podium.

    a. Speaker

    b. Raised platform

    c. Brief lecture

    d. None of the above

42. Choose the best definition of boorish.

   a. Bad tempered

   b. Bad mannered

   c. Bad looking

   d. Bad smelling

43. Choose the best definition of heresy.

   a. Against the orthodox opinion

   b. Same as the orthodox opinion

   c. An unusual opinion

   d. To have no opinion

44. Choose the best definition of respite.

   a. A drink

   b. Intermission

   c. A rest stop on highways

   d. An interval

45. Choose the best definition of regicide.

   a. To endow or furnish with requisite ability

   b. Killing a king

   c. Disposed to seize by violence or by unlawful or greedy methods

   d. To refresh after labor

46. Choose the best definition of salient.

   a. To make light by fermentation, as dough

   b. Not stringent or energetic

   c. Negligible

   d. Worthy of note or relevant

47. Choose the best definition of sedentary.

   a. Yellowing of the skin

   b. Not moving or sitting in one a place

   c. To wander from place to place

   d. Perplexity

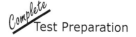

48. Choose the best definition of sedulous.

a. The support on or against which a lever rests

b. Dedicated and diligent

c. To oppose with an equal force

d. The branch of medical science that relates to improving health

49. Choose the best definition of tincture.

a. Alcoholic drink with plant extract used for medicine

b. An artificial trance-sleep

c. A special medicinal drink made by mixing water with plant extracts

d. The point of puncture

50. Choose the best definition of truism.

a. A comparison which directs the mind to the representative object itself

b. Self evident or clear obvious truth

c. A statement that is true but that can hardly be proved

d. False statements

Section IV – Science – Biology and Chemistry

1. Which, if any, of the following statements about the respiratory system are true?

a. The respiratory system consists of all the organs involved in breathing.

b. Organs included in the respiratory system are the nose, pharynx, larynx, trachea, bronchi and lungs.

c. The respiratory system conveys oxygen into our bodies and removes carbon dioxide from our bodies.

d. All of the Above.

 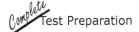

2. The _____ system maintains the body's balance through the release of _____ directly into the bloodstream.

a. The gastrointestinal system maintains the body's balance through the release of hormones directly into the bloodstream.

b. The endocrine system maintains the body's balance through the release of oxygen directly into the bloodstream.

c. The digestive system maintains the body's balance through the release of hormones directly into the bloodstream.

d. The endocrine system maintains the body's balance through the release of hormones directly into the bloodstream.

3. Among others, the endocrine system includes:

a. The pituitary gland

b. The thyroid gland

c. The adrenal glands

d. All of the Above.

4. _____ are contractile organs that cause movement when stimulated; the three types are _____, _____, and _____.

a. Muscles are expansion organs that cause movement when stimulated; the three types are smooth, cardiac, and skeletal.

b. Muscles are contractile organs that cause movement when stimulated; the three types are smooth, cardiac, and skeletal.

c. Muscles are contractile organs that cause movement when stimulated; the three types are semipermeable, cardiac, and skeletal.

d. Muscles are contractile organs that cause movement when stimulated; the three types are respiratory, cardiac, and skeletal.

5. Which of the following is not a function of the skeletal system?

a. Providing the shape and form of our bodies

b. Supporting and protecting the body

c. Producing Blood

d. Storing vitamins

6. What is the number of bones included in the human skeletal system?

a. 412

b. 103

c. Over 300

d. 206

7. _____ are connected to ____ by _____, and _____ are connected to each other by _____.

   a. Muscles are connected to bones by tendons, and bones are connected to each other by ligaments.

   b. Tendons are connected to bones by ligaments, and bones are connected to each other by tendons.

   c. Muscles are connected to bones by ligaments, and bones are connected to each other by tendons.

   d. Ligaments are connected to bones by tendons, and bones are connected to each other by bands.

8. The _____ consists of all the organs involved in the formation and release of urine and includes the kidneys, ureters, bladder and urethra.

   a. The digestive system consists of all the organs involved in the formation and release of urine and includes the kidneys, ureters, bladder and urethra.

   b. The reproductive system consists of all the organs involved in the formation and release of urine and includes the kidneys, ureters, bladder and urethra.

   c. The renal system consists of all the organs involved in the formation and release of urine and includes the kidneys, ureters, bladder and urethra.

   d. The kidney system consists of all the organs involved in the formation and release of urine and includes the kidneys, ureters, bladder and urethra.

9. _____ is a classification of organisms into different categories based on their physical characteristics and presumed natural relationship.

   a. Biology

   b. Taxonomy

   c. Grouping

   d. Nomenclature

10. The order of the hierarchy of levels in the biological classification of organisms is:

   a. Kingdom, phylum, class, order, family, genus, and species

   b. Phylum, kingdom, class, order, family, genus, and species

   c. Order, phylum, class, kingdom, family, genus, and species

   d. Kingdom, phylum, order, class, family, genus, and species

11. Which, if any, of the following statements about the biosphere are correct?

    a. The biosphere is the part of the Earth that supports life.

    b. The biosphere encompasses the Earth's entire surface.

    c. A and B are correct.

    d. None of these statements are correct.

12. Tundra, savannas, grasslands, deserts and rainforests are examples of _____.

    a. Biomasses

    b. Biospheres

    c. Biodiversity

    d. Biomes

13. The mixture of gases surrounding a planet is its _____.

    a. Atmosphere

    b. Stratosphere

    c. Biosphere

    d. Troposphere

14. In order, from lower to upper, the layers of the atmosphere are:

    a. Exosphere, thermosphere, mesosphere, stratosphere, troposphere

    b. Troposphere, stratosphere, mesosphere, thermosphere, exosphere

    c. Mesosphere, troposphere, stratosphere, , thermosphere, exosphere

    d. Thermosphere, troposphere, stratosphere, mesosphere, , exosphere

15. The force per unit area exerted against a surface by the weight of air above that surface in the Earth's atmosphere is the _____ _____.

    a. Gravitational force

    b. Atmospheric pressure

    c. Barometric density

    d. Aneroid pressure

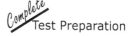
Complete Test Preparation

16. Which, if any, of the following statements are true?

a. Water boils at approximately 100 °C (212 °F) at standard atmospheric pressure.

b. The boiling point is the temperature at which the vapor pressure is higher than the atmospheric pressure around the water.

c. Water boils at a lower temperature in areas of lower pressure.

d. A and C are true.

17. ___ _____ _____ is the effect of the Earth's rotation on the atmosphere and on all objects on the Earth's surface.

a. The Coriolis effect

b. The Corona effect

c. The Archimedes effect

d. The tidal effect

18. Binding membrane of an animal cell is called,

a. Biological membrane

b. Cell coat

c. Unit membrane

d. Plasma membrane

19. The segment of a DNA molecule that determines the amino acid sequence of protein is known as ____?

a. Operator gene

b. Structural gene

c. Regulator gene

d. Modifier gene

20. Cells that line the inner or outer surfaces of organs or body cavities are often linked together by intimate physical connections. These connections are referred to as____

a. Separate desmosomes

b. Ronofilaments

c. Tight junctions

d. Fascia adherenes

21. Which one of the following best describes the function of a cell membrane?

a. It controls the substances entering and leaving the cell.

b. It keeps the cell in shape.

c. It controls the substances entering the cell.

d. It supports the cell structures

22. Which of the following arrangement is seen in the plasma membrane?

a. Lipids with embedded proteins

b. An outer lipid layer and an inner lipid layer

c. Proteins embedded in lipid bilayer

d. Altering protein and lipid layers

23. Genes control heredity in man and other organisms. This gene is ____

a. A segment of DNA

b. A bead like structure on the chromosomes

c. A protein molecule

d. A segment of RNA

24. A(an) _____ _____ is a description of a _____ _____ that gives the chemical formulas of the reactants and the_____ of the reaction, with coefficients introduced so that the number of each type of atom and the total charge is _____ by the reaction.

a. A balanced comparison is a description of a biological reaction that gives the chemical formulas of the reactants and the consequences of the reaction, with co-efficients introduced so that the number of each type of atom and the total charge is unchanged by the reaction.

b. A reactant chemical equation is a description of a chemical reaction that gives the chemical formulas of the reactants and the products of the reaction, with coefficients introduced so that the number of each type of atom and the total charge is unchanged by the reaction.

c. A balanced equation is a description of a chemical reaction that gives the chemical formulas of the reactants and the products of the reaction, with coefficients introduced so that the number of each type of atom and the total charge is changed by the reaction.

d. A balanced equation is a description of a chemical reaction that gives the chemical formulas of the reactants and the products of the reaction, with coefficients introduced so that the number of each type of atom and the total charge is unchanged by the reaction.

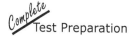

Complete Test Preparation

25. _____ bonds involve a complete sharing of electrons and occurs most commonly between atoms that have partially filled outer shells or energy levels.

    a. Covalent

    b. Ionic

    c. Hydrogen

    d. Proportional

26. The reaction of elements with low electronegativity(almost empty outer shells) with elements with high electronegativity (mostly full outer shells) gives rise to _____ bonds.

    a. Hydrogen

    b. Covalent

    c. Ionic

    d. Nuclear

27. _____ bonds involve electrons that are not equally shared, and may be deemed as an intermediate between the extremes represented by _____ and _____ bonds.

    a. Ionic bonds involve electrons that are not equally shared, and may be deemed as an intermediate between the extremes represented by covalent and polar bonds.

    b. Covalent bonds involve electrons that are not equally shared, and may be deemed as an intermediate between the extremes represented by polar and ionic bonds.

    c. Chemical bonds involve electrons that are not equally shared, and may be deemed as an intermediate between the extremes represented by covalent and ionic bonds.

    d. Polar bonds involve electrons that are not equally shared, and may be deemed as an intermediate between the extremes represented by covalent and ionic bonds.

28. _____ _____ involve an especially strong dipole-dipole force between molecules, and are responsible for the unique properties of water and pin DNA into its characteristic shape.

    a. Oxygen links

    b. Hydrogen bonds

    c. Nitrogen bonds

    d. Dipolar bonds

29. _____ predicts that the solubility (C) of a gas or volatile substance in a liquid is proportional to the partial pressure (P) of the substance over the liquid (P = k C).

     a. Boyle's law

     b. Gay-Lussac's Law

     c. Henry's law

     d. Charles' law

30. _____ states that the pressure of an ideal gas is inversely proportional to its volume, if the temperature and amount of gas are held constant.

     a. Henry's law

     b. Dalton's law

     c. Brown's law

     d. Boyle's law

31. Which of the following statements, if any, are correct?

     a. pH is a measure of effective concentration of hydrogen ions in a solution, and is approximately related to the molarity of H+ by pH = - log [H+]

     b. pH is a measure of effective concentration of oxygen ions in a solution, and is approximately related to the molarity of O+ by pH = - log [O+]

     c. pH is a measure of effective concentration of hydrogen atoms in a solution, and is approximately related to the polarity of H+ by pH = - log [H+]

     d. Acidity is a measure of effective concentration of hydrogen ions in a solution, and is approximately related to the molarity of H+ by pH = - log [H+]

32. Four factors that affect rates of reaction are:

     a. Barometric pressure, particle size, concentration, and the presence of a facilitator

     b. Temperature, particle size, concentration, and the presence of a catalyst

     c. Temperature, container material, elevation, and the presence of instability

     d. Volatility, particle size, concentration, and the presence of a catalyst

 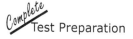

33. One factor that affects rates of reaction is concentration. Which of these statements about concentration is/are correct?

a. A higher concentration of reactants causes more effective collisions per unit time, leading to an increased reaction rate.

b. A lower concentration of reactants causes more effective collisions per unit time, leading to an increased reaction rate.

c. A higher concentration of reactants causes more effective collisions per unit time, leading to a decreased reaction rate.

d. A higher concentration of reactants causes less effective collisions per unit time, leading to an increased reaction rate.

34. _____ is expressed by the equation: $P_{tot} = P_a + P_b$, whereby P is pressure, P_{tot} is total pressure, P_a and P_b are component pressures.

a. Henry's law

b. Dalton's law

c. Boyle's law

d. Gay-Lussac's law

35. A/an _____ is an element with both metallic and non-metallic properties. Examples are silicon, arsenic, and germanium.

a. Metalloid

b. Conglomerate

c. Semi-metal

d. Amalgamate

36. Which, if any, of these statements about solubility are correct?

a. The solubility of a substance is its concentration in a saturated solution.

b. Substances with solubilities much less than 1 g/100 mL of solvent are usually considered insoluble.

c. A saturated solution is one which does not dissolve any more solute.

d. All of these statements are correct.

37. Which, if any, of the following statements are false?

a. In an endothermic process, solubility increases with the increase in temperature and decreases if the temperature decreases.

b. In an exothermic process, solubility decreases with an increase in temperature.

c. All of the Above.

d. None of the Above.

38. _____ is the spontaneous, random movement of small particles suspended in liquid, caused by the unbalanced impacts of molecules on the particle.

    a. Brownian motion

    b. Grey's kinesis

    c. Boyle's wave

    d. None of the above

39. _____ is defined as the number of cycles of a wave that move past a fixed observation point per second.

    a. Wave

    b. Wavelength

    c. Frequency

    d. Wavefunction

40. _____ is defined as the distance between adjacent peaks (or adjacent troughs) on a wave.

    a. Frequency

    b. Wavenumber

    c. Wave oscillation

    d. Wavelength

41. _____ is a mathematical function that gives the amplitude of a wave as a function of position (and sometimes, as a function of time and/or electron spin).

    a. Wavelength

    b. Frequency

    c. Wavenumber

    d. Wavefunction

42. In the periodic table the elements are arranged in

    a. Order of increasing atomic number

    b. Alphabetical order

    c. Order of increasing metallic properties

    d. Order of increasing neutron content

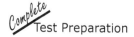

43. A molecule of water contains hydrogen and oxygen in a 1:8 ratio by mass. This is a statement of _____ .

    a. The law of multiple proportions

    b. The law of conservation of mass

    c. The law of conservation of energy

    d. The law of constant composition

44. Different isotopes of a particular element contain the same number of _____ .

    a. Protons

    b. Neutrons

    c. Protons and neutrons

    d. Protons, neutrons and electrons

45. The s block and p block elements are collectively known as _____ ?

    a. Transition elements

    b. Active elements

    c. Representative elements

    d. Inactive elements

46. Who was the English scientist who made accurate observations on how pressure and volume are related?

    a. Charles

    b. Combine

    c. Boyle

    d. Gay-Lussac

47. When pressure on a gas is reduced to half what happens to its volume?

    a. The volume stays the same

    b. The volume decreases

    c. The volume rises then falls

    d. The volume increases

48. What is the standard temperature in Kelvin?

    a. 25 Kelvin

    b. 273 Kelvin

    c. 0 kelvin

    d. 373 Kelvin

49. Real gases approach ideal behavior under which of the following conditions?

    a. At high pressure and high temperature

    b. At low pressure and high temperature

    c. Near the boiling point of water

    d. Real gases can never exhibit ideal behavior

50. The temperature and volume of a gas are directly related. This is a statement of:

    a. Combined Gas Law

    b. Boyle's Law

    c. Charles' Law

    d. The Ideal Gas Law

Anatomy and Physiology

1. The names of the three layers of skin are,

    a. Proton, neuron, nucleus.

    b. Epidural, Mitochondria, chromosome

    c. Inner, outer, local

    d. Epidermis, dermis and sub dermis.

2. Which sub-layer of skin gives it flexibility?

    a. The dermis

    b. Epidermis

    c. Subdermis

    d. Dermatology

3. An example of a minor ailment of the integumentary system is,

   a. Skin cancer

   b. Acne

   c. Common cold

   d. Flu

4. An example of a serious ailment of the integumentary system is

   a. Acne

   b. Skin cancer

   c. Heart disease

   d. High blood pressure

5. Which body system is comprised mostly of bones?

   a. Respiratory

   b. Endocrine

   c. Musculoskeletal

   d. Integumentary

6. Joints are an example of what within the musculoskeletal system?

   a. Bone tissue

   b. Connective tissue

   c. Muscles

   d. Nerves

7. One of the primary purposes of the musculoskeletal system is

   a. Providing stability to the body.

   b. Distributing blood.

   c. Providing infection-control.

   d. Eliminating waste.

8. Another primary purpose of the musculoskeletal system is

   a. Moving oxygen.

   b. Cleansing the blood stream.

   c. Relaxing the mind.

   d. Providing form for the body

9. What makes it sometimes difficult to diagnose an ailment within the musculo-skeletal system?

     a. Bones resist X-rays.

     b. There are no diseases associated with the musculoskeletal system.

     c. Its close proximity to other organs within the body.

     d. Its distant proximity away from other organs within the body.

10. What is cartilage?

     a. A flexible, connective tissue that keeps bones from rubbing against each other.

     b. The material that comprises the brain.

     c. A part of human blood responsible for fighting infection.

     d. Another name for the femur.

11. What is osteoporosis?

     a. A brain disorder that moves to the leg bones.

     b. A condition in which nerves become fragile.

     c. An ailment in which muscles deteriorate.

     d. An ailment in which bones become fragile because of loss of tissue

12. Marfan syndrome is an example of an ailment that, rather than affecting the bones themselves, afflicts

     a. The muscles.

     b. The nerves.

     c. The heart.

     d. The connective tissue.

13. Which system can be thought of as the blood distribution system?

     a. Digestive system.

     b. Musculoskeletal system.

     c. Endocrine system.

     d. Circulatory system

14. _____ are examples of nutrients passed along via the circulatory system.

   a. Citric acids
   b. Amino acids
   c. Proteins
   d. Nuclei

15. Other than blood, what else moves through the circulatory system?

   a. Traces of bone
   b. Sweat
   c. Lymph
   d. Mercury

16. What are the main components of the circulatory system?

   a. The heart, veins and blood vessels.
   b. The heart, brain, and ears.
   c. The nose, throat and ears.
   d. The lungs, stomach, and kidneys.

17. Which disease of the circulatory system is one of the most frequent causes of death in North America?

   a. The cold
   b. Pneumonia
   c. Arthritis
   d. Heart disease

18. One disease of the circulatory system which is often mistakenly thought to be a heart attack is

   a. Cardiac arrest
   b. High blood pressure
   c. Angina
   d. Acid reflux

 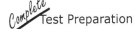

19. What is a more common name for the circulatory system disease known as hypertension?

    a. Anemia

    b. High blood pressure

    c. Angina

    d. Cardiac arrest

20. A condition in which the heart beats too fast, too slow, or with an irregular beat is called

    a. Hypertension

    b. Angina

    c. Cardiac arrest

    d. Arrythmia

21. What is the respiratory system?

    a. The system that brings oxygen into the body and expels carbon dioxide from the body.

    b. The system that sends blood to and from the heart.

    c. The system that processes food that enters the body.

    d. The system that expels urine from the body.

22. Which of the following is an example of an important component of the respiratory system?

    a. The cornea

    b. The lungs

    c. The kidneys

    d. The stomach

23. The exchange of oxygen for carbon dioxide takes place in the alveolar area of

    a. The throat

    b. The ears

    c. The appendix

    d. The lungs

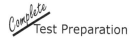

24. The part of the body that initiates inhalation is

   a. The lungs
   b. The diaphragm
   c. The larynx
   d. The kidneys

25. Exhalation generally uses the

   a. Abdominal muscles
   b. Chest muscles.
   c. The esophagus.
   d. The nasal passageway.

Practice Test Questions Set II Answer Key

1. B

We can infer an important part of the respiratory system are the lungs. From the passage, "Molecules of oxygen and carbon dioxide are passively exchanged, by diffusion, between the gaseous external environment and the blood. This exchange process occurs in the alveolar region of the lungs."

Therefore, one of the primary functions for the respiratory system is the exchange of oxygen and carbon dioxide, and this process occurs in the lungs. We can therefore infer that the lungs are an important part of the respiratory system.

2. C

The process by which molecules of oxygen and carbon dioxide are passively exchanged is diffusion.

This is a definition type question. Scan the passage for references to "oxygen," "carbon dioxide," or "exchanged."

3. A

The organ that plays an important role in gas exchange in amphibians is the skin.

Scan the passage for references to "amphibians," and find the answer.

4. A

The three physiological zones of the respiratory system are Conducting, transitional, respiratory zones.

5. B

This warranty does not cover a product that you have tried to fix yourself. From paragraph two, "This limited warranty does not cover ... any unauthorized disassembly, repair, or modification. "

6. C

ABC Electric could either replace or repair the fan, provided the other conditions are met. ABC Electric has the option to repair or replace.

7. B

The warranty does not cover a stove damaged in a flood. From the passage, "This limited warranty does not cover any damage to the product from improper installation, accident, abuse, misuse, natural disaster, insufficient or excessive electrical supply, abnormal mechanical or environmental conditions."

A flood is an "abnormal environmental condition," and a natural disaster, so it is not covered.

8. A

A missing part is an example of defective workmanship. This is an error made in the manufacturing process. A defective part is not considered workmanship.

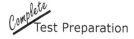

9. B

The first paragraph tells us that myths are a true account of the remote past.

The second paragraph tells us that, "myths generally take place during a primordial age, when the world was still young, prior to achieving its current form."

Putting these two together, we can infer that humankind used myth to explain how the world was created.

10. A

This passage is about different types of stories. First, the passage explains myths, and then compares other types of stories to myths.

11. B

From the passage, "Unlike myths, folktales can take place at any time and any place, and the natives do not usually consider them true or sacred."

12. B

This question gives options with choices for the three different characteristics of myth and legend. The options are,

- True or not true

- Takes place in modern day

- About ordinary people

For this type of question, where two things are compared for different characteristics, you can easily eliminate wrong answers using only one of the choices. Take myths: myths are believed to be true, do not take place in modern day, and are not about ordinary people.

Make a list as follows,

True or not true - True

Takes place in modern day - No

About ordinary people - No

Now check the options quickly. Option A is wrong (myths do not take place in modern day). Option B looks good. Put a check beside it. Option C is incorrect (myths are about ordinary people), and Option D is incorrect (myths are not true), so the answer must be Option B.

13. B

This passage describes the different categories for traditional stories. The other options are facts from the passage, not the main idea of the passage. The main idea of a passage will always be the most general statement. For example, Option A, Myths, fables, and folktales are not the same thing, and each describes a specific type of story. This is a true statement from the passage, but not the main idea of the passage, since the passage also talks about how some cultures may classify a story as a myth and others as a

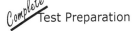

folktale.

The statement, from Option B, Traditional stories can be categorized in different ways by different people, is a more general statement that describes the passage.

14. B
Option B is the best choice, categories that group traditional stories according to certain characteristics.

Options A and C are false and can be eliminated right away. Option D is designed to confuse. Option D may be true, but it is not mentioned in the passage.

15. D
The best answer is D, traditional stories themselves are a part of the larger category of folklore, which may also include costumes, gestures, and music.

All of the other options are false. Traditional stories are part of the larger category of Folklore, which includes other things, not the other way around.

16. A
There is a distinct difference between a myth and a legend, although both are folktales.

17. B
The techniques for controlling insects are taken directly from the first sentence.

18. B
The inference is humans control pests because they damage crops.

19. A
Feeding on crops is the best choice, even though A and C are also correct.

20. A
Choice A is a re-wording of text from the passage.

21. C
This is taken directly from the passage.

22. C
Although trees are used as a building material, this is not their primary use. Trees are a primary energy source.

23. A
This is taken directly from the passage.

24. D
This question is designed to confuse by presenting different options for the two chemicals, oxygen and carbon dioxide. One is produced, and one is reduced. Read the passage carefully to see which is reduced and which is produced.

25. B
The inference is botanists have not surveyed all of the tropical areas so they do not know the number of species.

 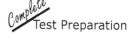

26. A

This is taken directly from the passage.

27. D

Tree-ferns survived the Carboniferous period. This is a fact-based question about the Carboniferous period. "Carboniferous" is an unusual word, so the fastest way to answer this question is to scan the pas-sage for the word "Carboniferous" and find the answer.

28. B

Here is the passage with the oldest to youngest trees.

The earliest trees were [1] tree ferns and horsetails, which grew in forests in the Carboniferous period. Tree ferns still survive, but the only surviving horsetails are no longer in tree form. Later, in the Triassic period, [2] conifers and ginkgos, appeared, [3] followed by flowering plants after that in the Cretaceous period.

29. B

The time limit for radar detectors is 14 days. Since you made the purchase 15 days ago, you do not qualify for the guarantee.

30. B

Since you made the purchase 10 days ago, you are covered by the guarantee. Since it is an advertised price at a different store, ABC Electric will "beat" the price by 10% of the difference, which is,

500 – 400 = 100 – difference in price

100 X 10% = \$10 – 10% of the difference

The advertised lower price is \$400. ABC will beat this price by 10% so they will refund \$100 + 10 = \$110.

31. B

From the first paragraph, "The segments of the body are organized into three distinctive connected units, a head, a thorax, and an abdomen."

This question tries to confuse 'segments' and 'units.'

32. D

This question tries to confuse. Read the passage carefully to find reference to the number of wings. "...if present in the species, two or four wings."

From this, we can conclude some insects have no wings, (if present ...) some have 2 wings and some have 4 wings.

33. A

The question asks about the abdomen and choices refer to organs in the abdomen. The passage says, "The abdomen also contains most of the digestive, respiratory, ... "

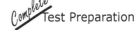

The choices are,

> a. It contains some of the organs.
> b. It is too small for any organs.
> c. It contains all of the organs.
> d. None of the above.

Choice A is true, but we need to see if there is better choice before answering. Choice B is not true. Choice C is not true since the relevant sentence says 'most' not 'all.' Choice D can be eliminated since Choice A is true.

Given there is not better choice, Choice A is the best choice answer.

34. A
We can infer that an important purpose of the circulatory system is that of fighting diseases.

35. A
Humans have an open circulatory system.

36. C
In addition to blood, the heart and the blood vessels form the cardiovascular system.

37. B
The digestive system, along with the circulatory system, helps provide nutrients to keep the human heart pumping.

38. A
We can infer that blood is responsible for transporting oxygen to the cells.

39. A
Human blood cells suspended in Plasma.

40. C
Calcium is not contained in blood plasma.

From the passage, "[Blood Plasma] contains dissolved proteins, glucose, mineral ions, hormones, carbon dioxide, platelets and the blood cells themselves."

41. A
The lungs exhale the carbon dioxide after venous blood has been carried from body tissues.

42. A
The main idea of this passage is that the human skeleton is an important and complicated system of the body.

We can infer the skeleton is important because it protects important organs like brain,

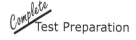

lungs and heart. We know the skeleton is complicated because it consists of a number of parts, (ligaments, tendons, muscles and cartilage) and 206 bones.

This general statement best describes the passage. The other choices are details mentioned in the passage.

43. A
There are three bones are located in the human middle ear. This is a fact-based question taken directly from the passage.

44. B
The number of bones stays the same throughout one's lifetime is not true. From the passage, "There are 206 bones in the adult human skeleton, which varies between individuals and with age."

45. D
The appendicular skeleton attached to the axial skeleton.   This is a fact-based question.

Section II – Math

1. D
8327 – 1278 = 7049

2. B
294 X 21 = 6174

3. C
1278 + 4920 = 6198

4. A
285 * 12 = 3420

5. C
4120 – 3216 = 904

6. D
2417 + 1004 = 3421

7. B
1440 ÷ 12 = 120

8. C
2713 – 1308 = 1405

9. D

$x^2 + 4x = 5$, $x^2 + 4x - 5 = 0$, $x^2 + 5x - x - 5 = 0$, factorize $x(x+5) - 1(x+5) = o$, $(x+5)(x-1)=0$. $x + 5 = 0$ or $x - 1 = 0$, $x = 0 - 5$ or $x = 0 + 1$, $x = -5$ or $x = 1$, either b or c.

10. C

Open parenthesis: $2a + 2b = 4ab$, divide both sides by $2 = a+b=2ab$ or $a+b=ab + ab$, therefore $a=ab$ and $b=ab$, therefore $a=b$.

11. B

Let the XY represent the initial number, $X + Y = 12$, $YX=XY+ 36$, Only b = 48 satisfies both equations above from the given options.

12. A

13. B

Let the father's age=Y, and Kate's age=X, therefore $Y=32+X$, in 5yrs $y=5x$, substituting for Y will be $5x = 32+X$, $5x - x = 32$, $4X=32$, $X= 32/8$, $x = 8$, Kate will be 8 in 5 yrs time, so Kate's present age = 8 - 5 = 3.

14. D

15. A

Let X represent the house, Sally paints X in 4hrs or ¼ X per 1hr or 60 minutes, John paints X in 6 hours or at 1/6X per 1hr or 60mins. Working together, they will paint 1/4x + 1/6x in 1hr or 60minutes = 10/24x = 5/12x every 60 minutes, to paint x = 60 minutes x 12/5 = 144 minutes or 2 hrs and 24 minutes.

16. D

The cost of the dishwasher = $450, 15% discount = 15/100 x 450 = $67.5,
The new price = 450 – 67.5 = $382.5, 20% discount on lowest price = 20/100 x 382.5 = $76.5,
so the final price = $306.

17. D

Original price = x,
80/100 = 12590/X,
80X = 1259000,
X = 15737.50.

18. C

Total hay = 214 kg,
The goat eats at a rate of 214/60days = 3.6kg per day.
The Cow eats at a rate of 214/15 = 14.3kg per day,
Together they eat 3.6 + 14.3 = 17.9 per day.
At a rate of 17.9kg per day, they will consume 214kg in 214/17.9 = 11.96 or 12 days approx.

19. A

25% = 25/100 = 1/4

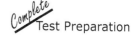

20. C
125/100 = 1.25

21. D
40/100 = 30/X = 40X = 30*100 = 3000/40 = 75

22. B
12.5/100 = 50/X = 12.5X = 50 * 100 = 5000/12.5 = 400

23. C
24/56 = 3/7 (divide numerator and denominator by 8)

24. C
Converting percent to decimal – divide percent by 100 and remove the % sign. 87% = 87/100 = .87

25. A
60 has the same relation to X as 75 to 100 – so
60/X = 75/100
6000 = 75X
X = 80

26. D
60 has the same relationship to 100 as 12 does to X – so
60/100 = 12/X
1200 = 60X
X = 20

27. C
Converting a fraction into a decimal – divide the numerator by the denominator – so 71/1000 = .071. Dividing by 1000 moves the decimal point 3 places.

28. C
4.7 + .9 + .01 = 5.61

29. A
.33 × .59 = .1947

30. D
.84 ÷ .7 = 1.2

31. C
9 is in the ten thousandths place in 1.7389.

32. A
.87 - .48 = .39

33. A
Step 1: Set up the formula to calculate the dose to be given in mg as per weight of the

child:-
Dose ordered X Weight in Kg = Dose to be given
Step 2: 100 mg X 23 kg = 2300 mg
(Convert 50 lb to Kg, 1 lb = 0.4536 kg, hence 50 lb = 50 X 0.4536 = 22.68 kg approx. 23 kg)
2300 mg/230 mg X 1 tablet/1 = 2300/230 = 10 tablets

34. B
1000 units/5000 units X 1 ml/1 = 1000/5000 = 0.2 ml

35. C
4 x 4 x 4 = 64

36. D
5 ml/15 ml kX 1 tsp/1 = 5/15 = 0.3 tsp

37. B
70 mg/1000 mg X 1 ml/1 = 70/1000 – 0.07 ml
(Convert 1 g = 1000 mg)

38. C
200 mg/400 mg X 1 tsp/1 = 200/400 = 0.5 tsp

39. D
600 mg/ 200 mg X 1 tablet/1 = 600/200 = 3 tablets

40. A
At 100% efficiency 1 machine produces 1450/10 = 145 m of cloth.
At 95% efficiency, 4 machines produce 4 X 0.95 X 145 = 551 m of cloth.
At 90% efficiency, 6 machines produce 6 X 0.90 X 145 = 783 m of cloth.

Total cloth produced = 551 + 783 = 1334 m

41. C
1 foot = 12 inches, 60 feet = 60 x 12 = 720 inches.

42. A
1 centimeter = 10 millimeter, 25 centimeter = 25 X 10 = 250.

43. A
1 millimeter = 10 centimeter, 100 millimeter = 100/10 = 10 centimeters.

44. C
1 gallon = 4 quarts, 3 gallons = 3 x 4 = 12 quarts.

45. A
There are 1000 mm in a meter.

46. B

There are 1000 ml in a liter. 0.05/1000 = 0.00005 liters.

47. D

There are 1000 mg in a gram. 30/1000 = 0.03 grams.

48. A

There are 10 mm in a cm. 0.101/10 = .0101

49. B

There are 52 cards in total. Smith has 16 cards in which he can win. Therefore, his probability of winning in a single game will be 16/52. Simon has 20 winning cards so his probability of winning in single draw is 20/52.

50. B

The formula of the volume of cylinder is = π r²h
Where π is 3.142, r is radius of the cross sectional area, and h is the height.
So the volume will be = $3.142 \times 2.5^2 \times 12 = 235.65m^3$.

51. C

The area of a 7 centimeter pizza is $\prod(3.5)^2 = 38.48$ cm²
The weight of 1 cm² of pizza will be 750/38.48 = 1949 grams
The area of 8.2 cm diameter pizza is $\prod(4.1)^2 = 52.81$ cm²
The difference in area is 52.81 – 38.48 = 14.33 cm²
The difference in weight will be 19.49 X 14.33 = 279.29 grams.

Section IV – English Grammar

1. D

The preposition "to" is correct. "To" here means give.

2. A

"Lie" means to recline, and does not take an object. "lay" means to place and does take an object.

3. A

Past unreal conditional. Takes the form,
[If ... Past Perfect ..., ... would have + past participle ...]

4. B

This sentence is in the present tense, so "to find" is correct.

5. B

The comma separates a phrase.

6. A

Possessive pronouns ending in s take an apostrophe before the 's': one's; everyone's;

Pass the HESI!

somebody's, nobody else's, etc.

7. D

When talking about something that didn't happen in the past, use the past perfect (if I had done).

8. C

"Lie" means to recline, and does not take an object. "Lay" means to place and does take an object. Peter lay the books on the table (the books are the direct object), or the telephone poles were lying on the road (no direct object).

9. A

Titles of short stories are enclosed in quotation marks.

10. C

No additional punctuation is required here.

11. B

Here the word "sale" is used as a "word" and not as a word in the sentence, so quotation marks are used.

12. C

Titles of short stories are enclosed in quotation marks, and commas always go inside quotation marks.

13. B

"Ran well" is correct. "Ran good" is never correct.

14. D

Commas and periods always go inside quotation marks. Question marks that are part of a quote also go inside quotation marks; however, if the writer quotes a statement as part of a larger question, the question mark is placed after the quotation mark.

15. D

The sentence starts with a phrase, which is separated by a comma and then lists the things the speaker's mother taught, to say thank you, etc. Each of the items in the list are separated by a comma.

16. A

When referring to a person, use "who" instead of "that."

17. A

The comma separates a phrase starting with 'which.'

18. A

"Being honest," present tense is the best choice. "The buyer" is singular so use "is."

19. C

The subject in the first phrase, "the boy," has to agree with the subject in the second phrase, "he is."

20. C
These two sentences can be combined into one sentence with 2 clauses separated by a comma.

21. B
These two sentences can be combined and the phrase, 'whose name is Skipper,' deleted.

22. A
These three sentences can be combined using 'although,' and 'even if.'

23. B
These two sentences can be combined into one sentence with two clauses separated by a comma.

24. A
These three sentences can be combined using 'although,' and 'since.'

Section V - Vocabulary

1. A
Verbiage NOUN speech with too many words.

2. A
Attache NOUN an aide or assistant.

3. A
Wreak VERB to cause or inflict especially related to harm or injury.

4. B
Witless ADJECTIVE foolish, without understanding.

5. A
Xenophobia NOUN a strong fear of strangers.

6. C
Zenith NOUN highest point, highest state or peak.

7. C
Zephyr NOUN light wind or gentle breeze.

8. A
Truism NOUN self evident or clear obvious truth.

9. A
Ulterior ADJECTIVE beyond what is obvious or evident.

10. D
Vapid ADJECTIVE tasteless or bland.

11. B
Waif NOUN homeless child or stray.

12. B
Whine VERB Complaint or criticism.

13. C
Underling NOUN subordinate of lesser rank or authority.

14. A
Yearling NOUN a young animal that is between 1 and 2 years.

15. B
Verdure NOUN lush green vegetation.

16. B
Zealot NOUN a person who is very passionate and fanatic about his specific objectives or beliefs.

17. C
Vertigo NOUN dizziness.

18. B
Conspicuous ADJECTIVE obvious or easy to notice.

19. D
Benevolence NOUN disposition to do good.

20. A
Boisterous ADJECTIVE full of energy; exuberant; noisy.

21. B
Fondle VERB to touch or stroke.

22. A
Momentous ADJECTIVE outstanding in importance.

23. A
Antagonist NOUN an opponent or enemy.

24. B
Memento NOUN a keepsake; an object kept as a reminder of a place or event.

25. C
Insidious ADJECTIVE producing harm in a stealthy, often gradual, manner.

26. B
Obfuscate VERB to deliberately make more confusing in order to conceal the truth.

27. A
Plethora NOUN an excessive amount or number; an abundance.

28. D
Laceration NOUN an irregular open wound caused by a blunt impact to soft tissue.

29. B
Enshroud VERB to cover with (or as if with) a shroud.

30. A
Hasten VERB to move in a quick fashion.

31. C
Pliable ADJECTIVE soft, flexible, easily bent; formed, shaped or molded.

32. C
Carefree ADJECTIVE indifferent, careless, showing a lack of concern.

33. A
Rescind VERB to repeal, annul, or declare void; to take (something such as a rule or contract) out of effect.

34. B
Headstrong ADJECTIVE determined to do as one pleases, and not as others want.

35. B
Oblique ADJECTIVE not straightforward; indirect; obscure; hence, disingenuous; underhand; perverse; sinister.

36. C
Temper VERB to moderate or control.

37. B
Cryptic ADJECTIVE mystified or of an obscure nature.

38. A
Curtail VERB to shorten or abridge the duration of something; to truncate.

39. B
Heed VERB to mind; to regard with care; to take notice of; to attend to; to observe.

40. D
Oblivious ADJECTIVE lacking awareness; unmindful.

41. B
Podium NOUN a platform on which to stand, as when conducting an orchestra or preaching at a pulpit.

42. B
Boorish ADJECTIVE behaving as a boor; rough in manners; rude; uncultured.

43. A
Heresy NOUN a controversial or unorthodox opinion held by a member of a group, as in politics, philosophy or science.

44. B
Respite NOUN a brief interval of rest or relief.

45. B
Regicide VERB to kill a king.

46. D
Salient ADJECTIVE worthy of note or relevant.

47. B
Sedentary ADJECTIVE not moving or sitting in one place.

48. B
Sedulous ADJECTIVE dedicated and diligent.

49. A
Tincture NOUN alcoholic drink with plant extract used for medicine.

50. B
Truism NOUN self-evident or clear obvious truth. [17]

Section IV – Science – Biology and Chemistry

1. D
All of the statements are true.

  a. The respiratory system consists of all the organs involved in breathing.

  b. Organs included in the respiratory system are the nose, pharynx, larynx, trachea, bronchi and lungs.

  c. The respiratory system conveys oxygen into our bodies and removes carbon dioxide from our bodies.

2. D
The **endocrine** system maintains the body's balance through the release of **hormones** directly into the bloodstream.

3. D
All of the above.   The endocrine system includes:

  a. The pituitary gland

  b. The thyroid gland

  c. The adrenal glands

4. B
Muscles are contractile organs that cause movement when stimulated; the three types are **smooth**, **cardiac**, and **skeletal**.

5. D
Storing vitamins **is not a function of the skeletal system.**

6. D
There are 206 bones in the skeletal system.

7. A
Muscles are connected to **bones** by **tendons**, and **ligaments connect bones to each other**.

Note: Muscles that cause movement of a joint are connected to two different bones and contract to pull them together. An example would be the contraction of the biceps and a relaxation of the triceps. This produces a bend at the elbow. The contraction of the triceps and relaxation of the biceps produces the effect of straightening the arm.[24]

8. C
The **renal system** consists of all the organs involved in the formation and release of urine and includes the kidneys, ureters, bladder and urethra.

9. B
Taxonomy is a classification of organisms into different categories based on their physical characteristics and presumed natural relationship.

10. A
The order of the hierarchy of levels in the biological classification of organisms is: **Kingdom, phylum, class, order, family, genus, and species.**

Note: A useful mnemonic device to remember this order is:
"Kids Prefer Cheese Over Fried Green Spinach."

11. A and B are correct.
a. The biosphere is the part of the Earth that supports life.
c. The biosphere is limited to the waters of the Earth, a fraction of its crust and the lower regions of the atmosphere.

12. D
Tundra, savannas, grasslands, deserts and rainforests are examples of biomes.

13. A
The mixture of gases surrounding a planet is its **atmosphere**.

14. B
In order, from lower to upper, the layers of the atmosphere are:
troposphere, stratosphere, mesosphere, thermosphere, exosphere.

15. B

The force per unit area exerted against a surface by the weight of air above that surface in the Earth's atmosphere is the **atmospheric pressure**.

16. D A and C are correct.

a. Water boils at approximately 100 °C (212 °F) at standard atmospheric pressure.
c. Water boils at a lower temperature in areas of lower pressure.

17. A

The Coriolis effect is the effect of the Earth's rotation on the atmosphere and on all objects on the Earth's surface.

Note: In the northern hemisphere, the Coriolis effect causes moving objects and currents to be deflected to the right, while in the southern hemisphere, it causes deflection to the left.

18. D

The plasma membrane surrounds the cell and functions as an interface between the living interior of the cell and the nonliving exterior.[40]

19. B

DNA is a nucleic acid that contains the genetic instructions used in the development and functioning of all known living organisms (with the exception of RNA viruses). The DNA segments that carry this genetic information are called genes but other DNA sequences have structural purposes or are involved in regulating the use of this genetic information. Along with RNA and proteins DNA is one of the three major macromolecules that are essential for all known forms of life.[41]

20. C

Tight junctions or zonula occludens are the closely associated areas of two cells whose membranes join forming a virtually impermeable barrier to fluid. It is a type of junctional complex present only in vertebrates. The corresponding junctions that occur in invertebrates are septate junctions.[42]

21. A

The cell membrane is a biological membrane that separates the interior of all cells from the outside environment. The cell membrane is selectively permeable to ions and organic molecules and controls the movement of substances in and out of cells[43]

22. C

The plasma membrane or cell membrane protects the cell from outside forces. It consists of the lipid bilayer with embedded proteins.

23. A

Genes are made from a long molecule called DNA, which is copied and inherited across generations. DNA is made of simple units that line up in a particular order within this large molecule. The order of these units carries genetic information similar to how the order of letters on a page carries information. The language used by DNA is called the genetic code that lets organisms read the information in the genes. This information is

 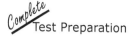

the instructions for constructing and operating a living organism.[41]

24. D
A **balanced equation** is a description of a **chemical reaction** that gives the chemical formulas of the reactants and the **products** of the reaction, with coefficients introduced so that the number of each type of atom and the total charge is **unchanged** by the reaction.

Note: For example, a balanced equation for the reaction of sodium metal ($Na(s)$) with chlorine gas ($Cl_2(g)$) to form table salt ($NaCl(s)$) would be $2 Na(s) + Cl_2(g) = 2 NaCl(s)$, NOT $Na(s) + Cl_2(g) = NaCl(s)$.[44]

25. A
Covalent bonds involve a complete sharing of electrons and occurs most commonly between atoms that have partially filled outer shells or energy levels.
Note: Diamond is strong because it involves a vast network of covalent bonds between the carbon atoms in the diamond. [45]

26. C
The reaction of elements with low electronegativity(almost empty outer shells) with elements with high electronegativity (mostly full outer shells) gives rise to Ionic bonds.

27. D
Polar bonds involve electrons that are not equally shared, and may be deemed as an intermediate between the extremes represented by **covalent** and **ionic** bonds.

28. B
Hydrogen bonds involves an especially strong dipole-dipole force between molecules, and are responsible for the unique properties of water and pin DNA into its characteristic shape.

29. C
Henry's law predicts that the solubility (C) of a gas or volatile substance in a liquid is proportional to the partial pressure (P) of the substance over the liquid (P = k C).

30. D
Boyle's law states that the pressure of an ideal gas is inversely proportional to its volume, if the temperature and amount of gas are held constant.

Note: Doubling gas pressure halves gas volume, if temperature and amount of gas don't change. If the initial pressure and volume are P1 and V1 and the final pressure and volume are P2V2, then P1V1 = P2V2 at fixed temperature and gas amount.[46]

31. A
pH is a measure of effective concentration of hydrogen ions in a solution, and is approximately related to the molarity of H+ by pH = - log [H+]

32. B
Four factors that affect rates of reaction are: **Temperature, particle size, concentra-**

tion, and the presence of a catalyst.

33. A
A higher concentration of reactants causes more effective collisions per unit time, leading to an increased reaction rate.

34. B
Dalton's law is expressed by the equation: $P_{tot} = P_a + P_b$, whereby P is pressure, P_{tot} is total pressure, P_a and P_b are component pressures.

35. A
A **Metalloid** is an element with both metallic and non-metallic properties. Examples are silicon, arsenic, and germanium.

36. D
All of these statements are correct.

37. C
All of the statements are false.

38. A
Brownian motion is the spontaneous, random movement of small particles suspended in liquid, caused by the unbalanced impacts of molecules on the particle.

Note: The discovery of Brownian motion provided strong circumstantial evidence for the existence of molecules.[47]

39. C
Frequency is defined as the number of cycles of a wave that move past a fixed observation point per second.

Note: The SI unit of frequency is the Hertz (Hz).

40. D
Wavelength is defined as the distance between adjacent peaks (or adjacent troughs) on a wave.

Note: Varying the wavelength of light changes its color; varying the wavelength of sound changes its pitch.[48]

41. D
Wavefunction is a mathematical function that gives the amplitude of a wave as a function of position (and sometimes, as a function of time and/or electron spin).
Note: Wavefunctions are used in chemistry to represent the behavior of electrons bound in atoms or molecules.[49]

42. A
The periodic table of the chemical elements (also known as the periodic table or periodic table of the elements) is a tabular display of the 118 known chemical elements

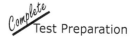

organized by selected properties of their atomic structures. Elements are presented by increasing atomic number, the number of protons in an atom's atomic nucleus. [50]

43. D
In chemistry, the law of definite proportions, sometimes called Proust's Law, states that a chemical compound always contains exactly the same proportion of elements by mass. An equivalent statement is the law of constant composition, which states that all samples of a given chemical compound have the same elemental composition. [51]

44. A
Isotopes are variants of atoms of a particular chemical element that have differing numbers of neutrons.

45. C
In chemistry and atomic physics, main group elements are elements in groups (periodic columns) whose lightest members are represented by helium, lithium, beryllium, boron, carbon, nitrogen, oxygen, and fluorine as arranged in the periodic table of the elements. Main group elements include elements (except hydrogen) in groups 1 and 2 (s-block), and groups 13 to 18 (p-block). [52]

46. A
Jacques Charles was a French chemist famous for his experiments in ballooning. Instead of hot air, he used hydrogen gas to fill balloons that could stay a float longer and travel farther.

47. D
Boyle's law (sometimes referred to as the Boyle-Mariotte law) is one of many gas laws and a special case of the ideal gas law. Boyle's law describes the inversely proportional relationship between the absolute pressure and volume of a gas, if the temperature is kept constant within a closed system. [53]

48. B
Standard temperature = 273 Kelvin

49. A
Real gases approach ideal behavior **at high pressure and high temperature.**

50. C
Charles's Law, or the law of volumes, was found in 1678. It says that, for an ideal gas at constant pressure, the volume is directly proportional to the absolute temperature (in kelvins).[54]

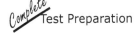

Section VI – Anatomy and Physiology

1. D
The human skin (integumentary) is composed of a minimum of 3 major layers of tissue, the Epidermis, the Dermis and Hypodermis.

2. A
The dermis is the middle layer of skin, composed of dense irregular connective tissues such as collagen with elastin arranged in a diffusely bundled and woven pattern. These layers serve to give elasticity to the integument, allowing stretching and conferring flexibility, while also resisting distortions, wrinkling, and sagging.

3. B
Acne is an example of a minor ailment of the integumentary system.

4. B
Skin cancer is an example of a serious ailment of the integumentary system.

5. C
Musculoskeletal is a body system comprised mostly of the bones.

6. B
Joints are an example of connective tissue within the musculoskeletal system.

7. A
One of the primary purposes of the musculoskeletal system is providing stability to the body.

8. D
Another primary purpose of the musculoskeletal system is providing form for the body.

9. C
It is difficult to diagnose an ailment within the musculoskeletal system because of its close proximity to other organs within the body.

10. A
Cartilage is a flexible connective tissue found in many areas in the bodies of humans and other animals, including the joints between bones, the rib cage, the ear, the nose, the elbow, the knee, the ankle, the bronchial tubes and the intervertebral discs. It is not as hard and rigid as bone but is stiffer and less flexible than muscle.

11. D
Osteoporosis is a disease of bones that leads to an increased risk of fracture. In osteoporosis the bone mineral density (BMD) is reduced, bone micro-architecture is deteriorating, and the amount and variety of proteins in bone is altered. The disease may be classified as primary type 1, primary type 2, or secondary

12. D
Marfan syndrome (also called Marfan's syndrome) is a genetic disorder of the connective

 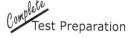

tissue. People with Marfan's tend to be unusually tall, with long limbs and long, thin fingers.

13. D
The circulatory system can be thought of as the blood distribution system.

14. B
The circulatory system is an organ system that passes nutrients (such as amino acids, electrolytes and lymph), gases, hormones, blood cells, etc. to and from cells in the body to help fight diseases and help stabilize body temperature and pH to maintain homeostasis.

15. C
The circulatory system is an organ system that passes nutrients (such as amino acids, electrolytes and lymph), gases, hormones, blood cells, etc. to and from cells in the body to help fight diseases and help stabilize body temperature and pH to maintain homeostasis.[37]

16. A
The main components of the circulatory system are the heart, veins and blood vessels.

17. D
The circulatory system disease that is one of the most frequent causes of death in North America is heart disease.

18. C
Angina is frequently mistaken for a heart attack. Angina pectoris, commonly known as angina, is severe chest pain due to ischemia (a lack of blood, thus a lack of oxygen supply) of the heart muscle, generally due to obstruction or spasm of the coronary arteries (the heart's blood vessels).

19. B
High blood pressure is a more common name for the circulatory system disease known as hypertension. Hypertension (HTN) or high blood pressure is a cardiac chronic medical condition in which the systemic arterial blood pressure is elevated.

20. D
Cardiac dysrhythmia (also known as arrhythmia and irregular heartbeat) is a term for any of a large and heterogeneous group of conditions in which there is abnormal electrical activity in the heart. The heartbeat may be too fast or too slow, and may be regular or irregular.

21. A
The respiratory system is the anatomical system of an organism that introduces respiratory gases to the interior and performs gas exchange. The anatomical features of the respiratory system include airways, lungs, and the respiratory muscles. Molecules of oxygen and carbon dioxide are passively exchanged, by diffusion, between the gaseous external environment and the blood. This exchange process occurs in the alveolar region of the lungs. [33]

22. B

The Lungs are an important component of the respiratory system.

23. D

The exchange of oxygen for carbon dioxide takes place in the alveolar area of the lungs.

24. B

The thoracic diaphragm, or simply the diaphragm, is a sheet of internal skeletal muscle that extends across the bottom of the rib cage. The diaphragm separates the thoracic cavity (heart, lungs & ribs) from the abdominal cavity and performs an important function in respiration.

25. A

Exhalation is often accomplished by the abdominal muscles.

Multiple Choice Secrets How to Answer Reading Comprehension Multiple Choice

H ERE IS A TEST QUESTION:

Which of the following is a helpful tip for taking a multiple-choice test?

a. Answering "B" for all questions.
b. Eliminate all answers that you know cannot be true.
c. Eliminate all answers that seem like they might be true.
d. Cheat off your neighbor.

If you answered B, you are correct. Even if you are not positive about the answer, try to get rid of as many options as possible. Think of it this way: If every item on your test has four possible answers, and if you guess on one of those four answers, you have a one in four chance of getting it right. This means that you should get one question right for every four that you have to guess on.

However, if you can get rid of two answers, then your chances improve to one in two chances. That means you will get a correct answer for every two that you guess.

So much for one of the obvious tips for improving your multiple-choice score. There are many other tips that you may or may not have considered, which will give your grade a boost. Remember, though, that none of these tips is infallible. In fact, some test-writers who know these suggestions deliberately write questions that can confound your system. Most of the time, however, you will do better on the test if you put these tips into practice.

Be prepared with all the materials you will need for the test. Bring several sheets of notebook paper, two or three sharpened pencils, an extra eraser, a high lighter, and three working pens. Why so many? Having extra materials will save you valuable time should a pencil break or a pen stop working. If you are permitted to use other aides such as a calculator, make sure the extra batteries are charged.

By familiarizing yourself with these tips, you increase your chances and who knows; you might just get a lucky break and increase your score by a few points!

TIPS FOR READING THE INSTRUCTIONS.

Pay close attention to the sample questions. Almost all standardized tests offer sample questions, paired with their correct solutions. Go through these to make sure that you understand what they mean and how they arrived at the correct answer. Do not be afraid to ask the test supervisor for help with a sample that confuses you, or instructions that you are unsure of.

Tips for Reading the Question

We could write pages and pages of tips just on reading the test questions. Here are the ones that will help you the most.

- **Think first.** Before you look at the answer, read and think about the question. It is best to try to come up with the correct answer before you look at the options given. This way, when the test-writer tries to trick you with a close answer, you will not fall for it.

- **Make it true or false.** If a question confuses you, then look at each answer option and think of it as a "true" "false" question. Select the one that seems most likely to be "true."

- **Mark the Question.** For some reason, a lot of test-takers are afraid to mark up their test booklet. Unless you are specifically told not to mark in the booklet, you should feel free to use it to your advantage. More on this below.

- **Circle Key Words.** As you are reading the question, underline or circle key words. This helps you to focus on the most critical information needed to solve the problem. For example, if the question said, "Which of these is not a synonym for huge?" You might circle "not," "synonym" and "huge." That clears away the clutter and lets you focus on what is important. More on this below.

- **Always underline these words:** all, none, always, never, most, best, true, false and except.

- **Cross out irrelevant choices.** If you find yourself confused by lengthy questions, cross out anything that you think is irrelevant, obviously wrong, or information that you think is offered to distract you.

- **Do not try to read between the lines.** Usually, questions are written to be

 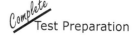

straightforward, with no deep, underlying meaning. The simple answer really is often the correct answer. Do not over-analyze!

GENERAL MULTIPLE CHOICE TIPS.

• **Finding Hints without Cheating** Pssst. There is a way to get hints about a question, even as you are taking the test—and it is completely legal. The key: Use the test itself to find clues about the answer. Here is how to do this. If you find that a question stumps you, read the answers. If you find one that uses the language that your teacher or textbook used, there is a good chance that this is the right answer. That is because on complex topics, teachers and books tend to always use the same or similar language.

Another point: Look out for test questions which are like previous questions. Often, you will find the same information used in more than one question.

• **Before you try eliminating wrong answers, try to solve the problem.** If you know for sure that you have answered the question correctly, then obviously there is no need to eliminate wrong choices. If you cannot solve it, then see how many choices you can eliminate. Now try solving it again and see if one of the remaining answers comes close to your answer. Your chances of getting the answer right have now improved dramatically. Elimination is one of the most powerful strategies and we will discuss in more detail, as well as practice below.

• **Skip if you do not know.** If you simply do not know the answer and do not know how to get the answer, skip it and come back if you have time.

• **Be systematic in your guesses.** For instance, let us say you have six questions that you are able to eliminate some options, and on all of them, you have two possible answers. Pick the same answer for all six of them. If you have gotten down to two options on each of them, then chances are, you will get about three of them right.

• **Rule out answers that seem so general that they do not offer much information.** If an answer said, for example, "Columbus came to the West in the spring," it is probably not the right answer.

• **Use "all of the above" and "none of the above" to your advantage.** For "all of the above," you need not check to make sure that all of them are correct. Just check two of them. If two of the answers are correct, then this probably means they are all correct, and you can select "all." (This, of course, is not always the case, especially if there is also an option for "A and B" or "C and D."). With "all of the above" questions, you only have to find one wrong answer, and then you have eliminated two choices.

• **Let "close" answers be your guide.** The clever test-writer often includes an an-

 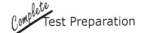

swer that is almost the correct one, in order to throw you off. The clever test-taker, however, can use this to his advantage. If you see two answer options that are strangely similar, then the chances are good that one of those is the correct choice. That means you can rule out the other answers—and thus improve your chances. For instance, if two choices are George Washington and George Washington Carver, among Abraham Lincoln and Thomas Edison, there is a good chance that one of the two Washingtons is right. More on this strategy below.

Watch Out For Trick Questions

Most multiple-choice tests contain a few trick questions. A trick question is one where the test-writer intentionally makes you think that the answer is easier than it really is. Test-writers include trick questions because so many people think that they have mastered the techniques of taking a test that they need not study the material. In only a very few cases will a test have more than a handful of trick questions. Often instructors will include trick questions, where you really have to know your stuff inside-out to answer it correctly. This separates the "A" students from the "B+" students, and the "A" students from the "A+" students.

The best way to beat the trick question is to read the question carefully and break it down into parts. Then break it down into individual words. For instance, if a question asks, "When a plane crashes on the border between the United States and Canada, where are the survivors buried?" if you had looked at each word individually, you would have realized that the last word, "survivors," means that the test writer is talking about burying people who are still alive.

Before You Change That Answer ...

You are probably familiar with the concept by now: your first instinct is usually right. That is why so many people, when giving advice about tests, tell you that unless you are convinced that your first instinct was wrong, do not take a chance. It really is true that in those cases, more people change a right answer to the wrong one than change a wrong answer to a right one.

Let's take that advice a step further, though. Maybe you do not always have to leave your first answer, especially if you think there might be a reasonable chance that your second choice was right. Before you go changing the answer, though, go on and do a few questions and clear your thoughts of the problem question. After you have done a few more, go back and start over from the beginning. Then see if the original answer is still the one that jumps out at you. If so, leave it. If your second thought now jumps out at you, then go ahead and change it. If both are equal in your mind, then leave it with your first hunch.

Answering Step-by-Step.

It might seem rather long and complicated to follow a formula for answering a multiple-choice question. After you have practiced this formula for a while, though, it will come naturally and will not take any time at all. Try to follow these steps below on each question.

Step 1. Cover up the answers while you read the question. See the material in your mind's eye and try to envision what the correct answer is before you expose the answers on the answer sheet.

Step 2. Uncover the responses.

Step 3. Eliminate. Cross out every answer that you know is ridiculous, absurd or that must clearly be wrong. Then work with the answers that remain.

Step 4. Watch for distracters. A distracter is an answer that looks very similar to the correct answer, but is put there to trip you up. If you see two answers that are strikingly similar, the chances are good that one of them is correct. For instance, if you are asked the term for the distance around a square, and two of the responses are "periwinkle" and "perimeter," you can guess that one of these is probably correct, since the words look similar (both start with "peri-"). Guess one of these two and your chances of correcting selecting "perimeter" are 50/50. More on this below.

Step 5. Check! If you see the answer that you saw in your mind, put a light checkmark by it and then see if any of the other choices are better. If not, mark that response as your answer.

Step 6. If all else fails, guess. If you cannot envision the correct response in your head, or figure it out by reading the passage, and if you are left totally clueless as to what the answer should be, guess.

There is a common myth that says choice "C" has a statistically greater chance of being correct. This may be true if your professor is making the test, however, most standardized tests today are generated by computer and the choices are randomized. We do not recommend choosing "C" as a strategy.

That is a quick introduction to multiple-choice to get us warmed up. Next we move on to the strategies and practice test questions section. Each multiple-choice strategy is explained, followed by practice questions using the strategy. Opposite this page is a bubble sheet for answering.

Multiple Choice Answer Sheet

1. (A) (B) (C) (D)	18. (A) (B) (C) (D)	35. (A) (B) (C) (D)
2. (A) (B) (C) (D)	19. (A) (B) (C) (D)	36. (A) (B) (C) (D)
3. (A) (B) (C) (D)	20. (A) (B) (C) (D)	37. (A) (B) (C) (D)
4. (A) (B) (C) (D)	21. (A) (B) (C) (D)	38. (A) (B) (C) (D)
5. (A) (B) (C) (D)	22. (A) (B) (C) (D)	39. (A) (B) (C) (D)
6. (A) (B) (C) (D)	23. (A) (B) (C) (D)	40. (A) (B) (C) (D)
7. (A) (B) (C) (D)	24. (A) (B) (C) (D)	41. (A) (B) (C) (D)
8. (A) (B) (C) (D)	25. (A) (B) (C) (D)	42. (A) (B) (C) (D)
9. (A) (B) (C) (D)	26. (A) (B) (C) (D)	43. (A) (B) (C) (D)
10. (A) (B) (C) (D)	27. (A) (B) (C) (D)	44. (A) (B) (C) (D)
11. (A) (B) (C) (D)	28. (A) (B) (C) (D)	45. (A) (B) (C) (D)
12. (A) (B) (C) (D)	29. (A) (B) (C) (D)	46. (A) (B) (C) (D)
13. (A) (B) (C) (D)	30. (A) (B) (C) (D)	47. (A) (B) (C) (D)
14. (A) (B) (C) (D)	31. (A) (B) (C) (D)	48. (A) (B) (C) (D)
15. (A) (B) (C) (D)	32. (A) (B) (C) (D)	49. (A) (B) (C) (D)
16. (A) (B) (C) (D)	33. (A) (B) (C) (D)	50. (A) (B) (C) (D)
17. (A) (B) (C) (D)	34. (A) (B) (C) (D)	

The following are detailed strategies for answering multiple choice questions with practice questions for each strategy.

Answers appear following this section with a detailed explanation and discussion on each strategy and question, plus tips and analysis.

Strategy 1 - Locate Keywords.

For every question, figure out exactly what the question is asking by locating key words that are in the question.

Directions: Read the passage below and answer the questions using this strategy.

Free range is a method of farming husbandry where the animals are allowed to roam freely instead of being enclosed in a pen. The term is used in two senses that do not overlap completely: as a farmer-centric description of husbandry methods, and as a consumer-centric description of them. Farmers practice free range to achieve free-range or humane certification (and thus capture high prices), to reduce feed costs, to improve the happiness and liveliness of their animals, to produce a higher-quality product, and as a method of raising multiple crops on the same land. [55]

1. The free-range method of farming

    a. Uses a minimum amount of fencing to give animals more room

    b. Can refer to two different things

    c. Is always a very humane method

    d. Only allows for one crop at a time

2. Free range farming is practiced

    a. To obtain free-range certification

    b. To lower the cost of feeding animals

    c. To produce higher quality product

    d. All of the above

3. Free range farming husbandry:

    a. Can mean either farmer described or consumer described methods

    b. Is becoming much more popular in many areas

    c. Has many limits and causes prices to go down

    d. Is only done to make the animals happier and healthier

4. Free range certification is most important to farmers because:

    a. Free-range livestock are less expensive to feed

    b. The price of the product is higher

    c. Both 1 and 2

    d. The animals are kept in smaller enclosures, so more can be produced

Strategy 2 - Watch Negatives.

For every question, no matter what type, look for words that are associated with negatives. These can include always, all, most, never, not, and others that will completely change what is being asked.

Directions: Read the passage below and answer the questions using this strategy.

Male grizzly bears can weight more than 1,000 pounds, but more typically weigh 400 pounds to 770 pounds. The females are on average 38% smaller, at about 250–350 pounds, an example of sexual dimorphism. On average, grizzly bears stand about 1 meter (3.3 ft.) at the shoulder when on all fours and 2 meters (6.6 ft.) on their hind legs, but males often stand 2.44 meters (8 ft.) or more on their hind legs. On average, grizzly bears from the Yukon River area are about 20% smaller than typical grizzlies. [56]

5. Sexual dimorphism does not mean

    a. Male grizzly bears are the same size as the female of the species

    b. All grizzly bears look the same and are the same size

    c. Grizzly bears can be quite large, and weigh more than half a ton

    d. All of the above

6. The size of a full-grown grizzly bear is never

    a. More than 500 pounds

    b. Dependent on what sex the bear is

    c. Determined simply by diet

    d. More than 6 feet tall

7. Grizzly bears from the area of the Yukon River do not

    a. Get as big as most other grizzly bears do

    b. Get the rich and varied food supply needed

    c. Need the same nutrients as other grizzly bears

    d. Get less than 7 feet tall, and weigh close to half of a ton

STRATEGY 3 - READ THE STEM COMPLETELY.

For every question, no matter what type, read the information in the stem and then try to determine the correct answer before you look at the different answers.

Directions: Read the passage below and answer the questions using this strategy.

Formerly, taxonomists listed brown and grizzly bears as separate species. Technically, brown and grizzly bears are classified as the same species, Ursus Arctos. The term "brown bear" is commonly used to refer to the members of this species found in coastal areas where salmon is the primary food source. Brown bears found inland and in northern habitats are often called "grizzlies." Brown bears on Kodiak Island are classified as a distinct subspecies from those on the mainland because they are genetically and physically isolated. The shape of their skulls also differs slightly. [56]

8. Grizzly bears, brown bears, and kodiak bears are all

   a. Arctas Ursinas

   b. Ursus Arctos

   c. Arctos Ursina

   d. Ursula Arctic

9. Kodiak brown bears are classified as a different subspecies because

   a. They are much larger than other brown bears

   b. Their diet is radically different from that of other brown bears

   c. They are not true brown bears but instead a mixture of bear species

   d. Of their genetics and head shape, as well as the physical isolation

10. The term grizzlies, when referring to the brown bear, is used mainly

   a. In eastern areas where the bear grows large

   b. Only in snowy areas where there are low year round temperatures

   c. In the northern and central areas

   d. In areas where the bear has a silver appearance

11. The term brown bear is normally used

   a. When one of the main food sources is salmon

   b. When the bear is small

   c. When the bear is found inland

   d. When the bear has a light brown coat and is very large

Strategy 4 - Read all the choices first.

For every question, no matter what type, make sure to read every option before determining which option is the right one.

Directions: Read the passage below and answer the questions using this strategy.

Jim Martell, a hunter from Idaho, reportedly found and shot a grizzly-polar bear hybrid near Sachs Harbor on Banks Island, Northwest Territories, Canada, on April 16, 2006. Martell had been hunting for polar bears with an official license and a guide, at a cost of $50,000, and killed the animal believing it to be a normal polar bear. Officials took interest in the creature after noticing that it had thick, creamy white fur, typical of polar bears, as well as long claws; a humped back; a shallow face; and brown patches around its eyes, nose, and back, as well as patches on one foot, which are all traits of grizzly bears. If the bear had been adjudicated to be a grizzly, he would have faced a possible CAN$1,000 fine and up to a year in jail. A DNA test conducted by the Wildlife Genetics International in British Columbia confirmed that it was a hybrid, with the mother a polar bear and the father a grizzly. It is the first documented case in the wild, though it was known that this hybrid was biologically possible and other hybrids have been bred in zoos in the past. [57]

12. Which grizzly bear features did the hybrid bear have?

    a. Brown patches in certain areas

    b. Long claws

    c. A shallow face

    d. All of the above

13. The hybrid bear was the result of

    a. A male brown bear and a female grizzly

    b. A female brown bear and a male grizzly bear

    c. A female polar bear and a male grizzly bear

    d. A male polar bear and a female grizzly

14. The hybrid bear tested in this case was

    a. The first case ever known where two different bear species mated successfully

    b. Genetically flawed and prone to many diseases and conditions

    c. A fluke, and a mistake of nature which has never happened before

    d. The first proof of a wild bear hybrid species outside of zoos

 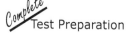

15. Modern science

   a. Has proven that the cubs from two different species will not survive in almost every case

   b. Has known for some time that these hybrid bears were possible

   c. Completely understands how bear hybrids occur and why this happens in nature

   d. Has studied hundreds of bear hybrids in an attempt to learn more

STRATEGY 5 - ELIMINATION.

For every question, no matter what type, eliminating obviously incorrect answers narrows the possible choices. Elimination is probably the most powerful strategy for answering multiple choice.

Directions: Read the passage below and answer the questions using this strategy.

The male peafowl, or peacock, has long been known and valued for its brilliant tail feathers. The bright spots on it are known as "eyes," and inspired the Greek myth that Hera placed the hundred eyes of the slain giant Argus on the tail of her favorite bird. Indian Peafowl are iridescent blue-green or blue in the head, neck and breast. The back, or scapular, feathers are vermiculated in black and white, while the primaries are orange-chestnut. The so-called "tail" of the peacock, also termed the "train," is not the tail quill feathers but highly elongated upper tail feathers. It is mostly bronze-green, with a series of eyes that are best seen when the train is fanned. The actual tail feathers are short and grey-colored and can be seen from behind when a peacock's train is fanned in a courtship display. During the molting season, the males shed their stunning train feathers and reveal the unassuming grey-colored tail which is normally hidden from view beneath the train. The female peacock is duller in comparison. It is mostly brown, with pale under-parts and some green iridescence in the neck, and lacks the long upper tail feathers of the male. [58]

16. The long colorful tail feathers of the peacock

   a. Are only present in the male of the species

   b. Are used by both sexes to warn off predators

   c. Are normally red and blue in color

   d. Are only present for a very short time each year

17. The differences between the male and female peacock are

   a. Size and weight

   b. Coloring and tail feather length

   c. The female does not ever leave the nest

   d. The male sits on and hatches the eggs

18. The term peacock actually refers to

    a. Both sexes from the pheasant family

    b. The eyes on the tail feathers of the bird

    c. The male bird of the peafowl species

    d. The female bird of the peafowl species

19. The gray tail feathers on the male peacock can be seen

    a. When the bird is startled

    b. Only when the bird is searching for food

    c. When the peacock lowers the tail feathers to the ground

    d. During molting

STRATEGY 6 - OPPOSITES.

For every question, no matter what type, look at answers that are opposites. When two answers are opposites, the odds increase that one of them is the correct answer.

Directions: Read the passage below and answer the questions using this strategy.

Smallpox is an infectious disease unique to humans, caused by either of two virus variants, the Variola Major or Variola Minor. The disease is also known by the Latin names Variola or Variola vera, which is a derivative of the Latin varius, meaning spotted.

Smallpox localizes in small blood vessels of the skin and in the mouth and throat. In the skin, this results in a characteristic rash, and later, blisters. Variola Major produces a more serious disease and has an overall mortality rate of 30–35%. Variola Minor causes a milder form of disease (also known as alastrim, cottonpox, milkpox, whitepox, and Cuban itch) which kills about 1% of its victims. Long-term complications of Variola major infection include characteristic scars, commonly on the face, which occur in 65–85% of survivors. Blindness and limb deformities due to arthritis and osteomyelitis are less common complications, seen in about 2–5% of cases. [59]

20. Smallpox

    a. Effects all mammals, including humans

    b. Is caused by a bacteria from contact with dead flesh

    c. Was called the great pox during the fifteenth century

    d. Only affects humans, although other species can carry and transmit the virus

21. Smallpox caused by Variola major has a

    a. Thirty to thirty five percent survival rate

    b. Sixty percent mortality rate

    c. Thirty to thirty five percent mortality rate

    d. Sixty percent survival rate

22. Smallpox caused by Variola minor is

    a. Much more severe, with a greater number of pox and more scarring

    b. Much less severe, with fewer pox and less scarring

    c. Characterized because there are no pox

    d. So minor that no treatment or medical attention is needed

23. Smallpox can be fatal

    a. In between thirty and thirty five percent of those who catch the virus, depending on the type

    b. In between thirty and sixty five percent of those who catch the virus, depending on the type

    c. When no medical treatment is available

    d. Only in developing countries where medical care is poor

STRATEGY 7 - LOOK FOR DIFFERENCES

For every question, no matter what type, look at the two choices that seem to be correct and then examine the differences between the two. Refer to the stem to determine the best answer.

Directions: Read the passage below and answer the questions using this strategy.

Lightning is an atmospheric discharge of electricity accompanied by thunder, which typically occurs during thunderstorms, and sometimes during volcanic eruptions or dust storms. Atmospheric electrical discharges, or bolts of lightning, can travel at speeds of 130,000 mph, and reach temperatures approaching 54,000° F, hot enough to fuse silica sand into glass channels known as fulgurites that are normally hollow and can extend some distance into the ground. There are some 16 million lightning storms in the world every year.

The irrational fear of lightning and thunder is astraphobia.

Lightning can also occur within the ash clouds of volcanic eruptions, or can be caused by violent forest fires which generate sufficient dust to create a static charge.

How lightning initially forms is still a matter of debate: Scientists have studied root causes ranging from atmospheric perturbations (wind, humidity, friction, and atmospheric pressure) to the impact of solar wind and accumulation of charged solar particles. Ice inside a cloud is thought to be a key element in lightning development, and may cause a forcible separation of positive and negative charges within the cloud, thus assisting in the formation of lightning. [11]

24. Astraphobia is

a. Fear of thunder

b. Fear of thunder and lightning

c. Fear of lightning

d. None of the above

25. Lightning occurs

a. Only in thunderstorms

b. In thunderstorms and dust storms

c. In thunderstorms, volcanic eruptions and dust storms

d. In the upper atmosphere

26. Fulgurites are

a. Made of silica

b. Made of glass

c. Made of silica turned in to glass

d. Made of silica and glass

Strategy 8 - Context clues.

Looked at the sentences, and the context to determine the best option. In some cases, the answer to the question may be located right in the passage or question.

Directions: Read the passage below and answer the questions using this strategy.

Venus is one of the four solar terrestrial planets, meaning that, like the Earth, it is a rocky body. In size and mass, it is very similar to the Earth, and is often described as its "sister," or Earth's twin. The diameter of Venus is only 650 km. less than the Earth's, and its mass is 81.5% of the Earth's. However, conditions on the Venusian surface differ radically from those on Earth, due to its dense carbon dioxide atmosphere. The mass of the atmosphere of Venus is 96.5% carbon dioxide, with most of the remaining 3.5% nitrogen.

Venus is the second-closest planet to the Sun, orbiting every 224.7 Earth days. The planet is named after Venus, the Roman goddess of love and beauty. After the Moon, it is the brightest natural object in the night sky, reaching an apparent magnitude of

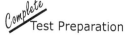

-4.6. Because Venus is an inferior planet from Earth, it never appears to venture far from the Sun: its elongation reaches a maximum of 47.8°. Venus reaches its maximum brightness shortly before sunrise or shortly after sunset, and is often called the Morning Star or the Evening Star. [60]

27. Apparent magnitude is

    a. A measure of darkness

    b. A measure of brightness

    c. The distance from the moon

    d. The distance from the earth

28. The elongation of a planet is

    a. The angular distance from the sun, as seen from earth.

    b. The distance from the sun

    c. The distance form the earth

    d. None of the above

29. Terrestrial planets are

    a. Made of rock

    b. Have people on them

    c. The earth and no others

    d. The same size as Earth

30. How many planets orbit the sun in less than 224.7 days?

    a. 1 planet

    b. Only Venus

    c. 2 planets

    d. 3 planets

STRATEGY 9 - TRY EVERY OPTION.

For definition questions, try out all of the options - one option will fit better than the rest. As you go through the options, use Strategy 5 - Elimination to eliminate obviously incorrect choices as you go.

Directions: Read the passage below and answer the questions using this strategy.

On Earth, common weather phenomena include wind, cloud, rain, snow, fog and dust storms. Less common events include natural disasters such as tornadoes, hurricanes, typhoons and ice storms. Almost all weather phenomena occurs in the troposphere (the lower part of the atmosphere). Weather does occur in the stratosphere and can affect weather lower down in the troposphere, but the exact mechanisms are poorly understood.

Weather occurs primarily due to different temperature and moisture densities. The strong temperature contrast between polar and tropical air gives rise to the jet stream. Weather systems in the mid-latitudes, such as extra tropical cyclones, are caused by instabilities of the jet stream flow. Weather systems in the tropics, such as monsoons or thunderstorms, are caused by different processes.

Because the Earth's axis is tilted relative to its orbital plane, sunlight is incident at different angles at different times of the year. In June the Northern Hemisphere is tilted towards the sun, so at any given Northern Hemisphere latitude, sunlight is more direct than in December. This effect causes seasons. Over thousands to hundreds of thousands of years, changes in Earth's orbital parameters affect the amount and distribution of solar energy received by the Earth and influence long-term climate. [61]

31. The troposphere is

    a. The highest strata of the atmosphere

    b. The lowest strata of the atmosphere

    c. The middle level of the atmosphere

    d. Not part of the atmosphere

32. Monsoons are

    a. Caused by instabilities in the jet stream

    b. Caused by processes other than instabilities in the jet stream

    c. Part of the jet stream

    d. Cause the jet stream

33. Extra-tropical cyclones occur

    a. In the tropics

    b. In temperate zones

    c. In the gulf stream

    d. In mid-latitudes

34. Tilted means:

    a. Slanted

    b. Rotating

    c. Connected to

    d. Bent

STRATEGY 10 - WORK FOR IT.

For questions about supporting details, work is the key. Review the passage to locate the right option. Never forget the choices that you are given are designed to confuse, and they may *seem* reasonable answers to the question. However, if they are not mentioned in the text, they are "red herring" answers.

The best answer is the exact answer mentioned in the text.

Directions: Read the passage below and answer the questions using this strategy.

Ebola is the common term for a group of viruses belonging to genus Ebola virus (EBOV), which is a part of the family Filoviridae, and for the disease that they cause, Ebola hemorrhagic fever. The virus is named after the Ebola River, where the first recognized outbreak of Ebola hemorrhagic fever occurred. The viruses are characterized by long filaments, and have a shape similar to that of the Marburg virus, also in the family Filoviridae, and possessing similar disease symptoms. There are a number of species within the Ebola virus genus, which in turn have a number of specific strains or serotypes. The Zaire virus is the type species, which is also the first discovered and the most lethal. Ebola is transmitted primarily through bodily fluids and to a limited extent through skin. The virus interferes with the endothelial cells lining the interior surface of blood vessels and platelet cells. As the blood vessel walls become damaged and the platelets are unable to coagulate, patients succumb to hypovolemic shock. Ebola first emerged in 1976 in Zaire. It remained largely obscure until 1989 with the outbreak in Reston, Virginia. [59]

35. The Ebola virus received this name because of

    a. The doctor who first discovered the virus

    b. The cure that is used to treat those infected

    c. The river where the disease was first encountered

    d. What the virus does to the body

 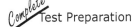

36. Viruses in the Ebola genus are recognizable

    a. Because of their hooked shape

    b. Because of their long filaments

    c. Due to their oblong heads

    d. Because of their unique color

37. One of the most common causes of death from the Ebola family of viruses is

    a. Hypovolemic shock due to blood vessel damage

    b. Bleeding of the brain that cannot be stopped

    c. A heart attack from blood loss and lack of fluids

    d. A high fever that cannot be lowered

38. The most deadly strain of the Ebola virus family is the

    a. The Reston strain

    b. The Ivory Coast strain

    c. The Zaire strain

    d. The Sudan strain

STRATEGY 11 - LOOK AT THE BIG PICTURE.

Details can be tricky when dealing with main idea and summary questions, but do not let the details distract you. Look at the big picture instead of the smaller parts to determine the right answer.

Directions: Read the passage below and answer the questions using this strategy.

As of late 2005, three fruit bat species have been identified as carrying the Ebola virus but not showing disease symptoms. They are now believed to be a natural host species, or reservoir, of the virus. Plants, arthropods, and birds have also been considered as reservoirs; however, bats are considered the most likely candidate. Bats were known to reside in the cotton factory where the first outbreaks in 1976 and 1979 occurred, and they have also been implicated in Marburg infections in 1975 and 1980. Of 24 plant species and 19 vertebrate species experimentally inoculated with Ebola virus, only bats became infected. The absence of clinical signs in these bats is characteristic of a reservoir species. In 2002-03, a survey of 1,030 animals from Gabon and the Republic of the Congo including 679 bats found Ebola virus RNA in 13 fruit bats (Hypsignathus monstrosus, Epomops franquetti and Myonycteris torquata). Bats are also known to be the reservoirs for a number of related viruses including Nipah virus, Hendra virus and Lyssaviruses. [59]

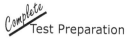

39. The species most suspected as a potential Ebola virus reservoir is

a. Birds

b. Insects

c. Plants

d. Bats

40. Most plant and animal species

a. Can carry the Ebola virus but not become infected

b. Can not carry and transmit the Ebola virus

c. Are responsible for new cases of Ebola viruses

d. Can be infected with one of the Ebola viruses

41. Bats are known for

a. Being carriers of many different viruses, including Ebola

b. Transmitting the Ebola virus through a scratch

c. Being susceptible to the virus and becoming infected

d. Transmitting the Ebola virus through infected droppings

STRATEGY 12 - BEST POSSIBLE ANSWER.

Try to determine the best possible answer according to the information given in the passage. Do not be distracted by answers that seem correct or are mostly correct.

Directions: Read the passage below and answer the questions using this strategy.

In the early stages, Ebola may not be highly contagious. Contact with someone in early stages may not even transmit the disease. As the illness progresses, bodily fluids represent an extreme biohazard. Due to lack of proper equipment and hygienic practices, large-scale epidemics occur mostly in poor, isolated areas without modern hospitals or well-educated medical staff. Many areas where the infectious reservoir exists have just these characteristics. In such environments, all that can be done is immediately cease all needle sharing or use without adequate sterilization procedures, to isolate patients, and to observe strict barrier nursing procedures with the use of a medical rated disposable face mask, gloves, goggles, and a gown at all times. This should be strictly enforced for all medical personnel and visitors. [59]

42. Ebola is highly contagious

a. Only when blood is present

b. Only in the first stages before hemorrhaging occurs

c. At all stages of the illness from incubation to recovery

d. Only in the later stages when the virus is very numerous

43. Exposure to the Ebola virus means

a. A death sentence for most patients

b. Isolation for the patient, and proper precautions for all medical personnel to contain the virus

c. The virus will spread rapidly and there is no treatment available

d. A full recovery usually, with very few symptoms

44. Ebola outbreaks commonly occur

a. Because sterilization and containment procedures are not followed or available

b. Due to infected animals in the area

c. Because of rat droppings in homes

d. Because of a contaminated water supply

45. Ebola is

a. More common in advanced nations where treatment makes the disease minor

b. More common in third world and developing countries

c. Fatal in more than ninety-five percent of the cases

d. Highly contagious during the incubation period

Answers to Sample Multiple Choice Strategy Questions

Strategy 1 - Keywords in the question tells what the question is asking

1. B
The question asks about the free range *method* of farming. Here method refers to *type* of farming. "Method" here is the keyword and can be marked or underlined.

2. D
The Question is, "Free-range farming is *practiced* ..." The keyword here is "practiced." Looking at the choices, which all start with "to," it is clear the answer will be about *why* free range ... Also notice that one of the choices is "All of the above," which in this case is the correct answer. However, when "All of the above" is an option, this is a potential Elimination strategy. All you have to do is find one option that is incorrect and you can use Strategy 5 - Elimination to eliminate two choices and increase your odds from one in four, to one in two.

3. A
The question is, "Free range farming husbandry ..." From the question, and the *lack* of keywords, together with the choices presented, the answer will be a definition free range farming husbandry.

4. C
The question is, "Free-range certification is *most important* to farmers because ... " The keywords here are "most important." Be careful to choose the best possible answer.

Strategy 2 - Negatives

These four questions all have negatives: does not mean, is never, do not, and is not. These questions exclude possibilities, so if you see any choices that are true, you can eliminate them right away.

5. D
The question asks what sexual dimorphism does *not* mean. Circle the word "not" and keep it firmly in mind. Next, what is sexual dimorphism. Reading the text quickly, sexual dimorphism is not defined explicitly but related to the female bears being smaller than the males. Probably there are other aspects, but this general definition is all that is needed to answer the question.

First, notice that "All of the above" is Choice D. In addition the question is a negative. So in order for Choice D to be correct, Choices A, B and C must be *incorrect*. This narrows down your options. If any of Choices A, B or C are correct, then you can eliminate that choice as well as Choice D.

Either all of the choices are *incorrect*, in which case, Choice D, "All of the above" is correct.

 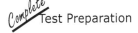

Choice A, male and females are the same size is incorrect.
Choice B, all grizzly bears look the same and are the same size, is incorrect.
Choice C, grizzly bears (plural so *all* grizzly bears) can be large and weigh more than half a ton. This is incorrect since while all grizzly bears are large, female bears weight less than half a ton.

All three choices are incorrect so Choice D is the correct answer, All of the above are incorrect.

6. A

First, circle or underline never to show this is a negative question. Now look at the options to find an option that is not true.

Choice A is true as male bears are 1,000 pounds. Place a mark beside this one. It may be tempting to select this option as your answer, but it is important to look at all choices before making a final decision.

Choice B is not true - size does not depend on the sex.
Choice C is not true - size does not depend on diet.
Choice D is not true - males often stand 8 feet.
So Choice A is correct.

7. A

First circle "do not" to mark this as a negative question.

Choice A is correct, Yukon River grizzly bears do not get as big as other grizzlies, so put a mark beside it for later consideration. Examine the other choices before making a final decision.

Choice B is not mentioned in the text, and can be eliminated.

Choice C is not mentioned in the text and can be eliminated.

Choice D is true, but this is a negative question so it is false.

Some of the above choices may be true from a common sense point of view, but if they aren't mentioned specifically in the passage, they can be eliminated.

Choice A is correct.

Strategies 3 - Read the stem completely.

Read the question, and then look for the answer in the text before reading the choices. Reading the choices first will confuse, just as it is meant to do! Do not fall into this trap!

8. B

The choices here are very confusing and are meant to be! Four variations on the Latin species name, Ursus Arctos are given, so the question is what version of this Latin name is correct, which gives a very straight-forward strategy to solving. Since the name is Latin, it is going to stand out in the text. Take the first option, "Arctas Ursinas," and

 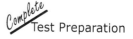

scan the text for something that looks like that. At the end of the second sentence is "Ursus Arctos," which is very close. Next confirm what this sentence refers to, which gives the correct answer, Choice B.

9. D
This question asks why Kodiak brown bears are a different subspecies, and the options are designed to confuse a careless, stressed test-taker. Scan the text for "Kodiak," which appears in the second to last sentence, and answers the question.

10. C
This question asks about the relationship between brown bears and grizzly bears. If you are not careful you will be confused by the choices.

11. A
Read the question, then read the text before trying to answer and avoid confusion.

Strategy 4 - Read every choice before deciding.

In Strategy 3, we learned to find the correct answer in the text before reading the choices. OK, now you have read the text and have the right answer. The next thing is Strategy 4 - Read *all* of the choices. Once you have read all of the choices, select the correct choice.

12. D
First, notice that "All of the above" is a choice. So if you find one option that is incorrect, you can eliminate that option and option D, "All of the above." Reading the question first, (Strategy #3) then looking in the text, and then reading all of the choices before answering, you can see that choices A, B and C are all correct, so choice D, All of the Above, is the correct choice.
If you had not read all the choices first, then you might be tempted to impulsively choose A, B, or C as the answer.

13. C
Looking at the choices, they are designed to confuse with different choices and combinations. Recognizing this, it is therefore important to be extra careful in making your choice. If you are stressed, in a hurry, or not paying attention, you will probably get this question wrong by making an impulsive choice and not reading through all the choices before making a selection.

Referring to the text, you will find the sentence, "… it was a hybrid, with the mother a polar bear and the father a grizzly," which answers the question.

14. D
Reading through all of the choices, B and C can be eliminated right away as they are not referred to in the text. They might appear as good answers but they are not from the passage.

Looking at A and D, the issue is if this has happened before, or has it happened only in zoos. Referring to the text, the last sentence tells us the answer, "It is the first documented case in the wild, though it was known that this hybrid was biologically possible

 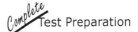

and other hybrids have been bred in zoos in the past."

15. B

Reading through the four choices, the question concerns, what does science know? Does it happen all the time? Completely understood? They do survive? Is it possible? Look in the text for how much is known. The last sentence, "It is the first documented case in the wild, though it was known that this hybrid was biologically possible" gives the answer.

Strategy 5 - Elimination.

For every question, no matter what type, eliminating obviously incorrect answers narrows the possible choices. Elimination is probably the most powerful strategy for answering multiple choice.

16. A

Using this strategy the choices can be narrowed down to A and D. I have never seen a peacock with red in their tail, so C can *probably* be eliminated, but check back. Most birds and many animals have a pattern where the male is colorful and the female less colorful. Choice B can be eliminated as it refers to "both sexes" having colorful tails. Choice D is a good candidate as the text refers to molting season, however, the text does not say how long this is, so there is some doubt. This makes A the best choice as it is referred to directly in the text.

17. B

Choice D can be eliminated right away, as it is rare for a male bird to sit on eggs.

Skimming the passage, choices A and C can be eliminated, as they are not mentioned directly in the text, leaving only D.

18. C

Choices A and D can be eliminated right away, since "cock" always refers to a male bird. Referring to the text, "The male peafowl, or peacock, has long been ..." making C the best choice.

19. D

Choices A and B can be eliminated either right away or with a quick check of the passage, since they are not mentioned. Choice C is suspicious since the grey feathers are under the tail feathers, so it is difficult to see how they could be visible when the tail feathers are lowered.

Strategy 6 - Opposites

If there are opposites, one of them is generally the correct answer. If it helps, make a table that lays out the different options and the correct option will become clear.

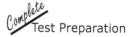

20. D
Notice that A and D are opposites. Referring to the text, "Smallpox is an infectious disease unique to humans ..." eliminates choice A.

21. C
Notice that all of the choices are opposites. 30 - 35% mortality, or survival rate, or 60%. Therefore, the task is to review the text, looking for 30% or 60%, survival or mortality, stay clear, and do not get confused. Sometimes making notes or a table can help to clarify.

The question is asking about percent, so it is easy and fast to skim the passage for a percent sign.

The first percent sign is in the second paragraph, 30 - 35%. Write this in the margin. Next, see what this percent refers to, which is the mortality rate. Write "mortality" next to 30 - 35%. Now, working backwards, see what the 30 - 35% mortality rate refers to. At the beginning of that sentence, is Variola Major. Now we have a clear understanding of what the passage is saying, which we have retrieved quickly and easily, and now hopefully we will not get confused by the different choices.

Choice A and B can be eliminated right away. Choice C looks correct. Check Choice D quickly, and confirm that it is incorrect. Choice C is the correct answer.

22. B
Choices A and B are opposites. Is Variola Minor more or less severe, with more or fewer pox, and more or less scarring? The other two choices, "no pox" and "no treatment" can be eliminated quickly. Either choice A or B are going to be wrong, which is confirmed by the text.

Make a quick table like this:

Major - more serious - scars, blindness
Minor - milder

The passage does not mention scarring from Variola minor, but we can infer that it is milder. Looking at the options, Choice A is clearly talking about Variola major, and we can infer that Choice B is talking about Variola minor and is the correct answer. We can confirm our inference from the text.

23. A
Choices A and B are not exactly opposite, but very close and designed to confuse if you do not read them properly. How many people die from the virus? Between 30 and 35%? Or between 35 and 60%? Scan the text with these numbers in mind.

This question is asking about a percent figures, so quickly scan the passage for a percent sign, which first appears in the second paragraph. Working back from there confirm that the percent figures is related to mortality, which it is.

 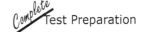

Strategy 7 - Look for Differences.

Look at two choices that appear to be correct and examine them carefully.

24. B
Choices A, B and C are very similar and designed to confuse and distract someone who does not look carefully at the text. What is astraphobia exactly? This is a definition question for an unusual word, astraphobia. Scan the text for "astraphobia." Choice B is correct.

25. C
Choices A, B and C are similar and designed to confuse, or tempt a stressed or careless test-taker into making a quick and incorrect choice. Checking the passage, in the first paragraph, lightning occurs in thunderstorms, volcanic eruptions and in dust storms, so choice C is correct.

26. C
All four answers are similar and designed to confuse. Seeing how similar the choices are, it is very important to be clear on the exact definition. This is a definition question, so scan the text quickly for the word "fulgurites." From the first paragraph, fulgurites are formed when lightning is ".. hot enough to fuse silica sand into glass channels ..." so the correct answer, and the option that answers the question the best, is choice C, "Made of silica turned into glass."

Strategy 8 - Context clues

Look at the sentences, and the context to determine the best option. In some cases, the answer to the question may be located right in the passage or question.

27. B
You do not have to know the exact meaning - just enough to answer the question. The phrase is used in the passage, "After the Moon, it is the brightest natural object in the night sky, reaching an apparent magnitude of −4.6" where Venus is compared to the brightness of the moon, so the apparent magnitude must have something to do with brightness, which is enough information to answer the question. Notice also, how the choices are opposites. Choice A and B are opposites as are choices C and D.

28. A
The exact meaning is not necessary, you only need only enough information to answer the question. The passage is, "Because Venus is an inferior planet from Earth, it never appears to venture far from the Sun: its elongation reaches a maximum of 47.8°." Elongation in this sentence is something connected with distance from the sun, but also something to do with Earth. Choices C and D can be eliminated right away. Choice A is the most likely correct because it mentions, "as seen from earth."

29. A
Terrestrial has many similar meanings, but choice A is the best. From the passage, "Venus is one of the four solar terrestrial planets, meaning that, like the Earth, it is a rocky body." Choice C can be eliminated right away. No mention is made of size or people, so

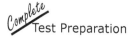

choices C and D are also incorrect.

Note that Choice B is a grammatical error and can be eliminated right away. The question is, "Terrestrial planets are," and Choice B is, "Have people on them."
This is a great strategy, looking for grammatical errors and eliminating, and what you might expect to see on a test that a professor has made themselves. However, most standardized tests are generated by computer, and proofed by many different people who have considerable expertise in correcting this type of easy question. Keep this in mind, but don't expect to see this type of thing on a standardized test.

30. A
All of the choices are similar and designed to confuse. Venus is the second closest planet to the sun so there must be one planet that is closer. Planets closer to the sun will rotate the sun faster, so the answer must be choice A.

Strategy 9 - Try out every option for word meaning questions.

For definition questions, try out all of the options - one option will fit better than the rest. As you go through the options, use Strategy 5 - Elimination to eliminate obviously incorrect choices as you go.

31. B
The answer is taken directly from the passage. Notice that choices A and B are opposites, so one of them will be incorrect. Look in the text carefully for the exact definition. If you are uncertain, make a table in the margin.

32. B
The choices are designed to confuse. The sentences talking about the jet stream and monsoons are next to each other. Trying each definition and comparing to the text, only choice B fits. If you are uncertain, make a table in the margin.

33. B
Trying each definition choice, Choice B is the only answer that makes sense referring to the text. The choices are designed to confuse, making it very important that you be extra careful to find the exact definition from the text.

34. A
The passage from the text is, "Because the Earth's axis is tilted relative to its orbital plane, sunlight is incident at different angles at different times of the year." Substituting all of the choices given into this sentence, slanted, choice 1, is the only sensible answer. Here is what substitutions look like:

    a. In June the Northern Hemisphere is *slanted* towards the sun...

    b. In June the Northern Hemisphere is *rotating* towards the sun...

    c. In June the Northern Hemisphere is *connected to* towards the sun...

    d. In June the Northern Hemisphere is *bent* towards the sun...

Choice A is the only one that makes sense.

Strategy 10 - You have to work for it! Check carefully for supporting details.

All of these answers can be found by carefully reading the text. The questions paraphrase the text found in the passage.

35. C
The passage has a lot of details so read carefully and stay clear.

36. B
The choices are designed to confuse. Check the text for the exact definition and do not be distracted by other choices.

37. A
Here is a quick tip. On choice A, the word Hypovolemic is used. This is an unusual word and specific medical vocabulary. None of the other choices uses any specific vocabulary like this, so it is very likely to be the right answer. You can quickly scan the text for this word to confirm. Scanning the text for an unusual word is easy and fast, and one of the most powerful techniques for this type of question.

38. C
Scan the text for Zaire.

Strategy 11 - Look at the big picture

Details can be tricky when dealing with main idea and summary questions, but do not let the details distract you. Look at the big picture instead of the smaller parts to determine the right answer.

39. D
The passage says in 2005 it was found there are 3 fruit bat species most suspected of carrying the virus. The details (3 species, fruit bats and 2005) do not matter. Only the fact that bats are suspected.

40. B
The relevant passage is, "Of 24 plant species and 19 vertebrate species experimentally inoculated with Ebola virus, only bats became infected." The inference is that these plant and animal species cannot be infected, (i.e. carry and transmit the disease) so Choice B is correct.

41. A
The relevant passage is, "Bats are also known to be the reservoirs for a number of related viruses including Nipah virus, Hendra virus and Lyssaviruses."

Strategy 12 - Make the best choice based on the information given.

42. D
Choices B and C are incorrect by the passage, "In the early stages, Ebola may not be

highly contagious." Choice A is not mentioned, leaving choice D.

43. B
The passage does not say anything about the information in choices A and D. Choice C is irrelevant to the question.

44. A
Choices B and C are not mentioned in the passage. Choice D is a good possibility, however, choice A covers choice D and is referred to in the passage.

45. B
Choice A is incorrect. Choices C and D are not mentioned.

How to Prepare for a Test

MOST STUDENTS HIDE THEIR HEADS AND PROCRASTINATE WHEN FACED WITH PREPARING FOR AN EXAMINATION, HOPING THAT SOMEHOW THEY WILL BE SPARED THE AGONY OF TAKING THAT TEST, ESPECIALLY IF IT IS A BIG ONE THAT THEIR FUTURES RELY ON. Avoiding the all-important test is what many students do best and unfortunately, they suffer the consequences because of their lack of preparation.

Test preparation requires strategy. It also requires a dedication to getting the job done. It is the perfect training ground for anyone planning a professional life. In addition to having a number of reliable strategies, the wise student also has a clear goal in mind and knows how to accomplish it. These tried and true concepts have worked well and will make your test preparation easier.

The Study Approach.

Take responsibility for your own test preparation.

It is a common- but big - mistake to link your studying to someone else's. Study partners are great, but only if they are reliable. It is your job to be prepared for the test, even if a study partner fails you. Do not allow others to distract you from your goals.

Prioritize the time available to study.

When do you learn best, early in the day or in the dark of night? Does your mind absorb and retain information most efficiently in small blocks of time, or do you require long stretches to get the most done? It is important to figure out the best blocks of time available to you when you can be the most productive. Try to consolidate activities to allow for longer periods of study time.

Find a quiet place where you will not be disturbed.

Do not try to squeeze in quality study time in any old location. Find someplace peaceful and with a minimum of distractions, such as the library, a park or even the laundry room. Good lighting is essential and you need to have comfortable seating and a desk surface large enough to hold your materials. It is probably not a great idea to study in your bedroom. You might be distracted by clothes on the floor, a book you have been planning to read, the telephone or something else. Besides, in the middle of studying, that bed will start to look very comfortable. Whatever you do, avoid using the bed as a place to study since you might fall asleep as a way of avoiding your work! That is the last thing you should be doing during study time.

The exception is flashcards. By far the most productive study time is sitting down and studying and studying only. However, with flashcards you can carry them with you and make use of odd moments, like standing in line or waiting for the bus. This isn't as productive, but it really helps and is definitely worth doing.

Determine what you need in order to study.

Gather together your books, your notes, your laptop and any other materials needed to focus on your study for this exam. Ensure you have everything you need so you don't waste time. Remember paper, pencils and erasers, sticky notes, bottled water and a snack. Keep your phone with you in case you need it to find out essential information, but keep it turned off so others can't distract you.

Have a positive attitude.

It is essential that you approach your studies for the test with an attitude that says you will pass it. And pass it with flying colors! This is one of the most important keys to successful study strategy. Believing that you are capable actually helps you to become capable.

THE STRATEGY OF STUDYING

Make materials easy to review and access.

Consolidate materials to help keep your study area clutter free. If you have a laptop and a means of getting on line, you do not need a dictionary and thesaurus as well since those things are easily accessible via the internet. Go through written notes and consolidate those, as well. Have everything you need, but do not weigh yourself down with duplicates.

Review class notes.

Stay on top of class notes and assignments by reviewing them frequently. Re-writing notes can be a terrific study trick, as it helps lock in information. Pay special attention to any comments that have been made by the teacher. If a study guide has been made available as part of the class materials, use it! It will be a valuable tool to use for studying.

Estimate how much time you will need.

If you are concerned about the amount of time you have available it is a good idea to set up a schedule so that you do not get bogged down on one section and end up without enough time left to study other things. Remember to schedule break time, and use that time for a little exercise or other stress reducing techniques.

 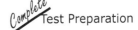

Test yourself to determine your weaknesses.

Look online for additional assessment and evaluation tools available for a particular subject. Once you have determined areas of concern, you will be able to focus on studying the information they contain and just brush up on the other areas of the exam.

Mental Prep – How to Psych Yourself Up for a Test

Because tests contribute mightily to your final class grade or to whether you are accepted into a program, it is understandable that taking tests can create a great deal of anxiety for many students. Even students who know they have learned all of the required material find their minds going blank as they stare at the words in the questions. One of the easiest ways to overcome that anxiety is to prepare mentally for the test. Mentally preparing for an exam is really not difficult. There are simple techniques that any student can learn to increase their chances of earning a great score on the day of the test.

Do not procrastinate.

Study the material for the test when it becomes available, and continue to review the material up until the test day. By waiting until the last minute and trying to cram for the test the night before, you actually increase the amount of anxiety you feel. This leads to an increase in negative self-talk. Telling yourself "I can't learn this. I am going to fail" is a pretty sure indication that you are right. At best, your performance on the test will not be as strong if you have procrastinated instead of studying.

Positive self-talk.

Positive self-talk serves both to drown out negative self-talk and to increase your confidence in your abilities. Whenever you begin feeling overwhelmed or anxious about the test, remind yourself that you have studied enough, you know the material and that you will pass the test. Use only positive words. Both negative and positive self-talk are really just your fantasy, so why not choose to be a winner?

Do not compare yourself to anyone else.

Do not compare yourself to other students, or your performance to theirs. Instead, focus on your own strengths and weaknesses and prepare accordingly. Regardless of how others perform, your performance is the only one that matters to your grade. Comparing yourself to others increases your anxiety and your level of negative self-talk before the test.

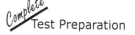

Visualize.

Make a mental image of yourself taking the test. You know the answers and feel relaxed. Visualize doing well on the test and having no problems with the material. Visualizations can increase your confidence and decrease the anxiety you might otherwise feel before the test. Instead of thinking of this as a test, see it as an opportunity to demonstrate what you have learned!

Avoid negativity.

Worry is contagious and viral - once it gets started it builds on itself. Cut it off before it gets to be a problem. Even if you are relaxed and confident, being around anxious, worried classmates might cause you to start feeling anxious. Before the test, tune out the fears of classmates. Feeling anxious and worried before an exam is normal, and every student experiences those feelings at some point. But you cannot allow these feelings to interfere with your ability to perform well. Practicing mental preparation techniques and remembering that the test is not the only measure of your academic performance will ease your anxiety and ensure that you perform at your best.

 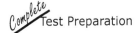

How to Take a Test

EVERYONE KNOWS THAT TAKING AN EXAM IS STRESSFUL, BUT IT DOES NOT HAVE TO BE THAT BAD! There are a few simple things that you can do to increase your score on any type of test. Take a look at these tips and consider how you can incorporate them into your study time.

How to Take a Test - The Basics.

Some tests are designed to assess your ability to quickly grab the necessary information; this type of exam makes speed a priority. Others are more concerned with your depth of knowledge, and how accurate it is. When you receive a test, look it over to determine whether the test is for speed or accuracy. If the test is for speed, like many standardized tests, your strategy is clear; answer as many questions as quickly as possible.

Watch out, though! There are a few tests that are designed to determine how fully and accurately you can answer the questions. Guessing on this type of test is a big mistake, because the teacher expects any student with an average grade to be able to complete the test in the time given. Racing through the test and making guesses that prove to be incorrect will cost you big time!

Every little bit helps.

If you are permitted calculators, or other materials, make sure you bring them, even if you do not think you will need them. Use everything at your disposal to increase your score.

Make time your friend.

Budget your time from the moment your pencil hits the page until you are finished with the exam, and stick to it! Virtually all standardized tests have a time limit for each section. The amount of time you are permitted for each portion of the test will almost certainly be included in the instructions or printed at the top of the page. If for some reason it is not immediately visible, rather than wasting your time hunting for it you can use the points or percentage of the score as a proxy to make an educated guess regarding the time limit.

Use the allotted time for each section and then move on to the next section whether you have completed the first section or not. Stick with the instructions and you will be able to answer the majority of the questions in each section.

With speed tests you may not be able to complete the entire test. Rest assured that you are not really expected to! The goal of this type of examination is to determine how quickly you can reach into your brain and access a particular piece of information, which is one way of determining how well you know it. If you know a test you are taking is a speed test, you will know the strategies to use for the best results.

Read the directions carefully.

Spend a few minutes reading the directions carefully before starting each section. Studies show students who read the instructions get higher marks! If you just glance at them, you may misunderstand and could blow the whole thing. Very small changes in the wording of the instructions or the punctuation can change the meaning completely. Do not make assumptions. Just because the directions are written one way in one section does not mean they will be exactly the same in all sections. Focus your attention and read what the instructions actually say, not what you think they are saying.

When reading the directions, underline the important parts. For example, if you are directed to circle the best answer, underline "circle" and "best". This flags the key concepts and will keep you focused.

If the exam is given with an answer booklet, copy the instructions to the top of the first page in the booklet. For complicated instructions, divide the directions into smaller steps and number each part.

Easy does it.

One smart way to tackle a test is to locate the easy questions and answer those first. This is a time-tested strategy that never fails, because it saves you a lot of unnecessary fretting. First, read the question and decide if you can answer it in less than a minute. If so, complete the question and go on to the next one. If not, skip it for now and continue on to the next question. By the time you have completed the first pass through this section of the exam, you will have answered a good number of questions. Not only does it boost your confidence, relieve anxiety and kick your memory up a notch, you will know exactly how many questions remain and can allot the rest of your time accordingly. Think of doing the easy questions first as a warm-up!

If you run out of time before you manage to tackle all the difficult questions, do not let it throw you. All that means is you have used your time in the most efficient way possible by answering as many questions correctly as you could. Missing a few points by not answering a question whose answer you do not know just means you spent that time answering one whose answer you did.

A word to the wise: Skipping questions for which you are drawing a complete blank is one thing, but we are not suggesting you skip every question you come across that you are not 100 % certain of. A good rule of thumb is to try to answer at least eight of every 10 questions the first time through.

 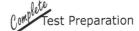

Do not watch your watch.

At best, taking an important exam is an uncomfortable situation. If you are like most people, you might be tempted to subconsciously distract yourself from the task at hand. One of the most common ways to do so is by becoming obsessed with your watch or the wall clock. Do not watch your watch! Take it off and place it on the top corner of your desk, far enough away that you will not be tempted to look at it every two minutes. Better still, turn the watch face away from you. That way, every time you try to sneak a peek, you will be reminded to refocus your attention to the task at hand. Give yourself permission to check your watch or the wall clock after you complete each section. If you know yourself to be a bit of a slow-poke in other aspects of life, you can check your watch a bit more often. Even so, focus on answering the questions, not on how many minutes have elapsed since you last looked at it.

Divide and conquer.

What should you do when you come across a question that is so complicated you may not even be certain what is being asked? As we have suggested, the first time through the section you are best off skipping the question. But at some point, you will need to return to it and get it under control. The best way to handle questions that leave you feeling so anxious you can hardly think is by breaking them into manageable pieces. Solving smaller bits is always easier. For complicated questions, divide them into bite-sized pieces and solve these smaller sets separately. Once you understand what the reduced sections are really saying, it will be much easier to put them together and get a handle on the bigger question.

Reason your way through the toughest questions.

If you find that a question is so dense you can't figure out how to break it into smaller pieces, there are a few strategies that might help. First, read the question again and look for hints. Can you re-word the question in one or more different ways? This may give you clues. Look for words that can function as either verbs or nouns, and try to figure out from the sentence structure which it is in this case. Remember that many nouns in English have a number of different meanings. While some of those meanings might be related, in some cases they are completely distinct. If reading the sentence one way does not make sense, consider a different definition or meaning for a key word.

The truth is, it is not always necessary to understand a question to arrive at a correct answer! A trick that successful students understand is using Strategy 5, Elimination. In many cases, at least one answer is clearly wrong and can be crossed off of the list of possible correct answers. Next, look at the remaining answers and eliminate any that are only partially true. You may still have to flat-out guess from time to time, but using the process of elimination will help you make your way to the correct answer more often than not - even when you don't know what the question means!

 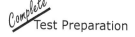

Do not leave early.

Use all the time allotted to you, even if you can't wait to get out of the testing room. Instead, once you have finished, spend the remaining time reviewing your answers. Go back to those questions that were most difficult for you and review your response. Another good way to use this time is to return to multiple choice questions in which you filled in a bubble. Do a spot check, reviewing every fifth or sixth question to make sure your answer coincides with the bubble you filled in. This is a great way to catch yourself if you made a mistake, skipped a bubble and therefore put all your answers in the wrong bubbles!

Become a super sleuth and look for careless errors. Look for questions that have double negatives or other odd phrasing; they might be an attempt to throw you off. Careless errors on your part might be the result of skimming a question and missing a key word. Words such as "always", "never", "sometimes" , "rarely" and the like can give a strong indication of the answer the question is really seeking. Don't throw away points by being careless!

Just as you budgeted time at the beginning of the test to allow for easy and more difficult questions, be sure to budget sufficient time to review your answers. On essay questions and math questions where you are required to show your work, check your writing to make sure it is legible.

Math questions can be especially tricky. The best way to double check math questions is by figuring the answer using a different method, if possible.

Here is another terrific tip. It is likely that no matter how hard you try, you will have a handful of questions you just are not sure of. Keep them in mind as you read through the rest of the test. If you can't answer a question, looking back over the test to find a different question that addresses the same topic might give you clues.

We know that taking the test has been stressful and you can hardly wait to escape. Just keep in mind that leaving before you double-check as much as possible can be a quick trip to disaster. Taking a few extra minutes can make the difference between getting a bad grade and a great one. Besides, there will be lots of time to relax and celebrate after the test is turned in.

In the Test Room – What you MUST do!

If you are like the rest of the world, there is almost nothing you would rather avoid than taking a test. Unfortunately, that is not an option if you want to pass. Rather than suffer, consider a few attitude adjustments that might turn the experience from a horrible one to...well, an interesting one! Take a look at these tips. Simply changing how you perceive the experience can change the experience itself.

Get in the mood.

After weeks of studying, the big day has finally arrived. The worst thing you can do to yourself is arrive at the test site feeling frustrated, worried, and anxious. Keep a check on your emotional state. If your emotions are shaky before a test it can determine how well you do on the test. It is extremely important that you pump yourself up, believe in yourself, and use that confidence to get in the mood!

Don't fight reality.

Oftentimes, students resent tests, and with good reason. After all, many people do not test well, and they know the grade they end up with does not accurately reflect their true knowledge. It is easy to feel resentful because tests classify students and create categories that just don't seem fair. Face it: Students who are great at rote memorization and not that good at actually analyzing material often score higher than those who might be more creative thinkers and balk at simply memorizing cold, hard facts. It may not be fair, but there it is anyway. Conformity is an asset on tests, and creativity is often a liability. There is no point in wasting time or energy being upset about this reality. Your first step is to accept the reality and get used to it. You will get higher marks when you realize tests do count and that you must give them your best effort. Think about your future and the career that is easier to achieve if you have consistently earned high grades. Avoid negative energy and focus on anything that lifts your enthusiasm and increases your motivation.

Get there early enough to relax.

If you are wound up, tense, scared, anxious, or feeling rushed, it will cost you. Get to the exam room early and relax before you go in. This way, when the exam starts, you are comfortable and ready to apply yourself. Of course, you do not want to arrive so early that you are the only one there. That will not help you relax; it will only give you too much time to sit there, worry and get wound up all over again.

If you can, visit the room where you will be taking your exam a few days ahead of time. Having a visual image of the room can be surprisingly calming, because it takes away one of the big 'unknowns'. Not only that, but once you have visited, you know how to get there and will not be worried about getting lost. Furthermore, driving to the test site once lets you know how much time you need to allow for the trip. That means three potential stressors have been eliminated all at once.

Get it down on paper.

One of the advantages of arriving early is that it allows you time to recreate notes. If you spend a lot of time worrying about whether you will be able to remember information like names, dates, places, and mathematical formulas, there is a solution for that. Unless the exam you are taking allows you to use your books and notes, (and very few do) you will have to rely on memory. Arriving early gives to time to tap into your memory and jot down key pieces of information you know will be asked. Just make certain you are allowed to make notes once you are in the testing site; not all locations will permit it. Once you get your test, on a small piece of paper write down everything you are afraid you will forget. It will take a minute or two but by dumping your worries onto the page you have effectively eliminated a certain amount of anxiety and driven off the panic you feel.

Get comfortable in your chair.

Here is a clever technique that releases physical stress and helps you get comfortable, even relaxed in your body. You will tense and hold each of your muscles for just a few seconds. The trick is, you must tense them hard for the technique to work. You might want to practice this technique a few times at home; you do not want an unfamiliar technique to add to your stress just before a test, after all! Once you are at the test site, this exercise can always be done in the rest room or another quiet location.

Start with the muscles in your face then work down your body. Tense, squeeze and hold the muscles for a moment or two. Notice the feel of every muscle as you go down your body. Scowl to tense your forehead, pull in your chin to tense your neck. Squeeze your shoulders down to tense your back. Pull in your stomach all the way back to your ribs, make your lower back tight then stretch your fingers. Tense your leg muscles and calves then stretch your feet and your toes. You should be as stiff as a board throughout your entire body.

Now relax your muscles in reverse starting with your toes. Notice how all the muscles feel as you relax them one by one. Once you have released a muscle or set of muscles, allow them to remain relaxed as you proceed up your body. Focus on how you are feeling as all the tension leaves. Start breathing deeply when you get to your chest muscles. By the time you have found your chair, you will be so relaxed it will feel like bliss!

Fight distraction.

A lucky few are able to focus deeply when taking an important examination, but most people are easily distracted, probably because they would rather be anyplace else! There are a number of things you can do to protect yourself from distraction.

Stay away from windows. If you select a seat near a window you may end up gazing out at the landscape instead of paying attention to the work at hand. Furthermore, any sign of human activity, from a single individual walking by to a couple having an argument or exchanging a kiss will draw your attention away from your important work. What goes on outside should not be allowed to distract you.

Choose a seat away from the aisle so you do not become distracted by people who leave early. People who leave the exam room early are often the ones who fail. Do not compare your time to theirs.

Of course you love your friends; that's why they are your friends! In the test room, however, they should become complete strangers inside your mind. Forget they are there.

The first step is to physically distance yourself from friends or classmates. That way, you will not be tempted to glance at them to see how they are doing, and there will be no chance of eye contact that could either distract you or even lead to an accusation of cheating. Furthermore, if they are feeling stressed because they did not spend the focused time studying that you did, their anxiety is less likely to permeate your hard-earned calm.

Of course, you will want to choose a seat where there is sufficient light. Nothing is worse than trying to take an important examination under flickering lights or dim bulbs.

Ask the instructor or exam proctor to close the door if there is a lot of noise outside. If the instructor or proctor is unable to do so, block out the noise as best you can. Do not let anything disturb you.

Make sure you have enough pencils, pens and whatever else you will need. Many entrance exams do not permit you to bring personal items such as candy bars into the testing room. If this is the case with the exam you are sitting for, be sure to eat a nutritionally balanced breakfast. Eat protein, complex carbohydrates and a little fat to keep you feeling full and to supercharge your energy. Nothing is worse than a sudden drop in blood sugar during an exam.

Do not allow yourself to become distracted by being too cold or hot. Regardless of the weather outside, carry a sweater, scarf or jacket in case the air conditioning at the test site is set too high, or the heat set too low. By the same token, dress in layers so that you are prepared for a range of temperatures.

Bring a watch so that you can keep track of time management. The danger here is many students become obsessed with how many minutes have passed since the last question. Instead of wearing the watch, remove it and place it in the far upper corner of the desk with the face turned away. That way, you cannot become distracted by repeatedly glancing at the time, but it is available if you need to know it.

Drinking a gallon of coffee or gulping a few energy drinks might seem like a great idea, but it is, in fact, a very bad one. Caffeine, pep pills or other artificial sources of energy are more likely to leave you feeling rushed and ragged. Your brain might be clicking along, all right, but chances are good it is not clicking along on the right track! Furthermore, drinking lots of coffee or energy drinks will mean frequent trips to the rest room. This will cut into the time you should be spending answering questions and is a distraction in itself, since each time you need to leave the room you lose focus. Pep pills will only make it harder for you to think straight when solving complicated problems on the exam.

At the same time, if anxiety is your problem try to find ways around using tranquilizers during test-taking time. Even medically prescribed anti-anxiety medication can make you less alert and even decrease your motivation. Being motivated is what you need to get you through an exam. If your anxiety is so bad that it threatens to interfere with your ability to take an exam, speak to your doctor and ask for documentation. Many testing sites will allow non-distracting test rooms, extended testing time and other accommodations as long as a doctor's note that explains the situation is made available.

 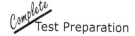

Keep Breathing.

It might not make a lot of sense, but when people become anxious, tense, or scared, their breathing becomes shallow and, in some cases, they stop breathing all together! Pay attention to your emotions, and when you are feeling worried, focus on your breathing. Take a moment to remind yourself to breathe deeply and regularly. Drawing in steady, deep breaths energizes the body. When you continue to breathe deeply you will notice you exhale all the tension.

It is a smart idea to rehearse breathing at home. With continued practice of this relaxation technique, you will begin to know the muscles that tense up under pressure. Call these your "signal muscles." These are the ones that will speak to you first, begging you to relax. Take the time to listen to those muscles and do as they ask. With just a little breathing practice, you will get into the habit of checking yourself regularly and when you realize you are tense, relaxation will become second nature.

Avoid Anxiety Prior to a Test

Manage your time effectively.

This is a key to your success! You need blocks of uninterrupted time to study all the pertinent material. Creating and maintaining a schedule will help keep you on track, and will remind family members and friends that you are not available. Under no circumstances should you change your blocks of study time to accommodate someone else, or cancel a study session in order to do something more fun. Do not interfere with your study time for any reason!

Relax.

Use whatever works best for you to relieve stress. Some folks like a good, calming stretch with yoga, others find expressing themselves through journaling to be useful. Some hit the floor for a series of crunches or planks, and still others take a slow stroll around the garden. Integrate a little relaxation time into your schedule, and treat that time, too, as sacred.

Eat healthy.

Instead of reaching for the chips and chocolate, fresh fruits and vegetables are not only yummy but offer nutritional benefits that help to relieve stress. Some foods accelerate stress instead of reducing it and should be avoided. Foods that add to higher anxiety include artificial sweeteners, candy and other sugary foods, carbonated sodas, chips, chocolate, eggs, fried foods, junk foods, processed foods, red meat, and other foods containing preservatives or heavy spices. Instead, eat a bowl of berries and some yogurt!

 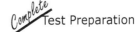

Get plenty of ZZZZZZZs.

Do not cram or try to do an all-nighter. If you created a study schedule at the beginning, and if you have stuck with that schedule, have confidence! Staying up too late trying to cram in last-minute bits of information is going to leave you exhausted the next day. Besides, whatever new information you cram in will only displace all the important ideas you've spent weeks learning. Remember: You need to be alert and fully functional the day of the exam

Eat a healthy meal before the exam.

Whatever you do - do not go into the test room hungry! Eat a meal that is rich in protein and complex carbohydrates before the test. Avoid sugary foods; they will pump you up initially, but you might crash hard part way through the exam. While you do not want to consume a lot of unhealthy fat, you do need a little of the healthy stuff such as flaxseed or olive oil on a salad. Avoid fried foods; they tend to make you sleepy.

Have confidence in yourself!

Everyone experiences some anxiety when taking a test, but exhibiting a positive attitude banishes anxiety and fills you with the knowledge you really do know what you need to know. This is your opportunity to show how well prepared you are. Go for it!

Be sure to take everything you need.

Depending on the exam, you may be allowed to have a pen or pencil, calculator, dictionary or scratch paper with you. Have these gathered together along with your entrance paperwork and identification so that you are sure you have everything that is needed.

Do not chitchat with friends.

Let your friends know ahead of time that it is not anything personal, but you are going to ignore them in the test room! You need to find a seat away from doors and windows, one that has good lighting, and get comfortable. If other students are worried their anxiety could be detrimental to you; of course, you do not have to tell your friends that. If you are afraid they will be offended, tell them you are protecting them from your anxiety!

Common Test-Taking Mistakes

Taking a test is not much fun at best. When you take a test and make a stupid mistake that negatively affects your grade, it is natural to be very upset, especially when it is something that could have been easily avoided. So what are some of the common mistakes that are made on tests?

Do not fail to put your name on the test.

How could you possibly forget to put your name on a test? You would be amazed at how often that happens. Very often, tests without names are thrown out immediately, resulting in a failing grade.

Not following directions.

Directions are carefully worded. If you skim directions, it is very easy to miss key words or misinterpret what is being said. Nothing is worse than failing an examination simply because you could not be bothered with reading the instructions!

Marking The Wrong Multiple Choice Answer.

It is important to work at a steady pace, but that does not mean bolting through the questions. Be sure the answer you are marking is the one you mean to. If the bubble you need to fill in or the answer you need to circle is 'C', do not allow yourself to get distracted and select 'B' instead.

Answering A Question Twice.

Some multiple choice test questions have two very similar answers. If you are in too much of a hurry, you might select them both. Remember that only one answer is correct, so if you choose more than one, you have automatically failed that question.

Mishandling A Difficult Question.

We recommend skipping difficult questions and returning to them later, but beware! First of all, be certain that you do return to the question. Circling the entire passage or placing a large question mark beside it will help you spot it when you are reviewing your test. Secondly, if you are not careful to actually skip the question, you can mess yourself up badly. Imagine that a question is too difficult and you decide to save it for later. You read the next question, which you know the answer to, and you fill in that answer. You continue on to the end of the test then return to the difficult question only to discover you didn't actually skip it! Instead, you inserted the answer to the following question in the spot reserved for the harder one, thus throwing off the remainder of your test!

 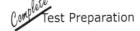

Incorrectly Transferring An Answer From Scratch Paper.

This can happen easily if you are trying to hurry! Double check any answer you have figured out on scratch paper, and make sure what you have written on the test itself is an exact match!

Don't Ignoring The Clock, And Don't Marry It, Either.

In a timed examination many students lose track of the time and end up without sufficient time to complete the test. Remember to pace yourself! At the same time, though, do not allow yourself to become obsessed with how much time has elapsed, either.

Thinking Too Much.

Oftentimes, your first thought is your best thought. If you worry yourself into insecurity, your self-doubts can trick you into choosing an incorrect answer when your first impulse was the right one!

Be Prepared.

Running out of ink and not having an extra pen or pencil is not an excuse for failing an exam! Have everything you need, and have extras. Bring tissue, an extra erasure, several sharpened pencils, batteries for electronic devices, and anything else you might need.

Conclusion

CONGRATULATIONS! You have made it this far because you have applied yourself diligently to practicing for the exam and no doubt improved your potential score considerably! Getting into a good school is a huge step in a journey that might be challenging at times but will be many times more rewarding and fulfilling. That is why being prepared is so important.

Study then Practice and then Succeed!

Good Luck!

Thanks!

If you enjoyed this book and would like to order additional copies for yourself or for friends, please check with your local bookstore, favourite online bookseller or visit www.test-preparation.ca and place your order directly with the publisher.

Feedback to the publisher may be sent by email to feedback@test-preparation.ca

Customizing and White Label Service

Have your logo and school name on the front cover in a special edition produced for your school or institution. Visit http://test-preparation.ca/customization.html or please contact us for details at sales@test-preparation.ca

Endnotes

Text where noted below is used under the Creative Commons Attribution-ShareAlike 3.0 License

http://en.wikipedia.org/wiki/Wikipedia:Text_of_Creative_Commons_Attribution-Share-Alike_3.0_Unported_License

[1] Immune System. In *Wikipedia*. Retrieved November 12, 2010 from, en.wikipedia.org/wiki/Immune_system.

[2] White Blood Cell. In Wikipedia. Retrieved November 12, 2010 from en.wikipedia.org/wiki/White_blood_cell.

[3] Convection. In *Wikipedia*. Retrieved November 12, 2010 from en.wikipedia.org/wiki/Convection.

[4] Herr, N. (2008). The Sourcebook for Teaching Science: Strategies, Activities, and Instructional Resources. San Francisco, CA: John Wiley & Sons, Inc.

[5] Brimblecombe, S., Gallannaugh, D., & Thompson, C. (1998). QPB Science Encyclopedia: An A to Z Guide to Everything You Need to Know About Science. New York, NY: Helicon Publishing Group Ltd.

[6] Biology. In Wikipedia. Retrieved May 10, 2012 from http://en.wikipedia.org/wiki/Biology.

[7] Chemistry. In Wikipedia. Retrieved May 10, 2012 from http://en.wikipedia.org/wiki/Chemistry.

[8] Human Hoeostatsis. In *Wikipedia*. Retrieved November 12, 2010 from http://en.wikipedia.org/wiki/Human_homeostasis.

[9] Infectious Disease. In *Wikipedia*. Retrieved November 12, 2010 from en.wikipedia.org/wiki/Infectious_disease.

[10] Virus. In *Wikipedia*. Retrieved November 12, 2010 from en.wikipedia.org/wiki/Virus.

[11] Thunderstorm. In *Wikipedia*. Retrieved November 12, 2010 from en.wikipedia.org/wiki/Thunderstorm.

[12] Meteorology. In *Wikipedia*. Retrieved November 12, 2010 from en.wikipedia.org/wiki/Outline_of_meteorology.

[13] Butterfly. In *Wikipedia*. Retrieved November 12, 2010 from en.wikipedia.org/wiki/Butterfly.

[14] U.S. Navy Seal. In *Wikipedia*. Retrieved November 12, 2010 from en.wikipedia.org/wiki/United_States_Navy_SEALs.

[15] Gardening. In *Wikipedia*. Retrieved January 2, 2012 from en.wikipedia.org/wiki/Gardening.

[16] Coral Reef. In *Wikipedia*. Retrieved January 2, 2012 from http://en.wikipedia.org/wiki/Coral_reef

[17] Wiktionary. http://www.wiktionary.org/

[18] The Four Fundamental Forces. (n.d.) Oracle Education Foundation. Retrieved from http://library.thinkquest.org/27930/forces.htm

[19] Heat Transfer. (n.d.) HyperPhysics Online. Retrieved from hyperphysics.phy-astr.gsu.edu/hbase/thermo/heatra.html

[20] What Causes DNA Mutations? (n.d.) Learn.Genetics http://learn.genetics.utah.edu/archive/sloozeworm/mutationbg.html

[21] Extracting Energy from Glucose. (n.d.). Muscle Physiology. http://muscle.ucsd.edu/musintro/glucose.shtml

[22] Body Systems/Tissue. (n.d.). virtualmedicalcentre.com http://www.virtualmedical-centre.com/anatomy.asp

[23] Parker, S.P., Biderman, A., Well, J., Richman, B., & Albers, P.A. (eds.) (1994). Dictionary of Bioscience (5th ed.). New York: McGraw-Hill.

[24] What is the Musculoskeletal System? (n.d).Wisegeek.com http://www.wisegeek.com/what-is-the-musculoskeletal-system.htm

[25] Law of Definite Proportions. (n.d.) In In Encyclopædia Britannica online. Retrieved from http://www.britannica.com/EBchecked/topic/155796/law-of-definite-proportions

[26] Cell Membrane. In *Wikipedia*. Retrieved November 12, 2010 from http://en.wikipedia.org/wiki/Cell_membrane.

[27] Mitosis. In *Wikipedia*. Retrieved November 12, 2010 from http://en.wikipedia.org/wiki/Mitosis.

[28] Prophase. In *Wikipedia*. Retrieved November 12, 2010 from http://en.wikipedia.org/wiki/Prophase.

[29] Metaphase. In *Wikipedia*. Retrieved November 12, 2010 from http://en.wikipedia.org/wiki/Metaphase.

[30] Anaphase. In *Wikipedia*. Retrieved November 12, 2010 from http://en.wikipedia.org/wiki/Anaphase.

[31] Telophase. In *Wikipedia*. Retrieved November 12, 2010 from http://en.wikipedia.org/wiki/Telophase.

[32] Epithelial Tissue. In *Wikipedia*. Retrieved November 12, 2010 from http://en.wikipedia.org/wiki/Epithelial_tissue.

[33] Respiratory System. In *Wikipedia*. Retrieved November 12, 2010 from en.wikipedia.org/wiki/Respiratory_system.

[34] Mythology. In *Wikipedia*. Retrieved November 12, 2010 from en.wikipedia.org/wiki/Mythology.

[35] Tree. In *Wikipedia*. Retrieved November 12, 2010 from en.wikipedia.org/wiki/Tree.

[36] Insect. In *Wikipedia*. Retrieved November 12, 2010 from en.wikipedia.org/wiki/Insect.

[37] Circulatory System. In *Wikipedia*. Retrieved November 12, 2010 from en.wikipedia.org/wiki/Circulatory_system

[38] Blood. In Wikipedia. Retrieved November 12,2010 from http://en.wikipedia.org/wiki/Blood.

[39] The Skeletal System. (n.d.). virtualmedicalcentre.com http://www.virtualmedicalcentre.com/anatomy.asp

[40] Membrane. Retrieved from http://faculty.clintoncc.suny.edu/faculty/michael.gregory/files/bio%20101/bio%20101%20lectures/membranes/membrane.htm

[41] DNA. In *Wikipedia*. Retrieved November 12, 2010 from http://en.wikipedia.org/wiki/DNA.

[42] Tight Junction. In *Wikipedia*. Retrieved November 12, 2010 from http://en.wikipedia.org/wiki/Tight_junction.

[43] Cell Membrane. In *Wikipedia*. Retrieved November 12, 2010 from http://en.wikipedia.org/wiki/Cell_membrane.

[44] Balanced Equations. (n.d.) In General Chemistry Online! Retrieved from http://antoine.frostburg.edu/chem/senese/101/glossary/b.shtml

[45] Covalent Bonds. (n.d.) In Plos Biology. Retrieved from staff.jccc.net/pdecell/chemistry/bonds.html

[46] Boyle's law. (n.d.) In General Chemistry Online! Retrieved from http://antoine.frostburg.edu/chem/senese/101/glossary/b.shtml

[47] Brownian motion. (n.d.) In General Chemistry Online! Retrieved from http://antoine.

frostburg.edu/chem/senese/101/glossary/b.shtml

[48] Wavelength. (n.d.) In General Chemistry Online! Retrieved from http://antoine.frostburg.edu/chem/senese/101/glossary/b.shtml

[49] Wavefunction. (n.d.) In General Chemistry Online! Retrieved from http://antoine.frostburg.edu/chem/senese/101/glossary/b.shtml

[50] Periodic Table. In *Wikipedia*. Retrieved November 12, 2010 from http://en.wikipedia.org/wiki/Periodic_table.

[51] Law of Constant Composition. In *Wikipedia*. Retrieved November 12, 2010 from http://en.wikipedia.org/wiki/Law_of_constant_composition.

[52] Main Group Element. In *Wikipedia*. Retrieved November 12, 2010 from http://en.wikipedia.org/wiki/Main_group_element.

[53] Boyles Law. In *Wikipedia*. Retrieved November 12, 2010 from http://en.wikipedia.org/wiki/Boyle%27s_Law.

[54] Gas Laws. In *Wikipedia*. Retrieved November 12, 2010 from http://en.wikipedia.org/wiki/Gas_laws.

[55] What is Free Range Chicken In *Answers.com*. Retrieved Feb 14, 2009, from http://wiki.answers.com/Q/What_is_free-range_chicken.

[56] Grizzly Bear. In *Wikipedia*. Retrieved Feb 14, 2009, from http://en.wikipedia.org/wiki/Grizzly_Bear.

[57] Grizzly Polar Bear Hybrid. In *Wikipedia*. Retrieved Feb 14, 2009, from http://en.wikipedia.org/wiki/Grizzly%E2%80%93polar_bear_hybrid.

[58] Peafowl. In *Wikipedia*. Retrieved Feb 14, 2009, from en.wikipedia.org/wiki/Peafowl.

[59] Smallpox. In *Wikipedia*. Retrieved Feb 14, 2009, from http://en.wikipedia.org/wiki/Smallpox.

[60] Venus. In *Wikipedia*. Retrieved Feb 14, 2009, from http://en.wikipedia.org/wiki/Venus.

[61] Weather. In *Wikipedia*. Retrieved Feb 14, 2009, from http://en.wikipedia.org/wiki/Weather.

Images

1 http://en.wikipedia.org/wiki/Digestive_system
2 http://en.wikipedia.org/wiki/File:Endocrine_reproductive_system_en.svg
3 http://en.wikipedia.org/wiki/File:Skin.jpg
4 http://en.wikipedia.org/wiki/Female_reproductive_system_%28human%29
5 http://en.wikipedia.org/wiki/Male_reproductive_system_%28human%29
6 http://en.wikipedia.org/wiki/Respiratory_system
7 http://en.wikipedia.org/wiki/Skeletal_system
8 http://en.wikipedia.org/wiki/Hinge_joint
9 http://upload.wikimedia.org/wikipedia/en/0/0b/NSdiagram.png
10 http://en.wikipedia.org/wiki/Spinal_cord
11 http://en.wikipedia.org/wiki/Neuron
12 http://en.wikipedia.org/wiki/Kidney
13 http://en.wikipedia.org/wiki/Urinary_system
14 http://en.wikipedia.org/wiki/Molecule

Made in the USA
Lexington, KY
08 January 2013